CANCER ETIOLOGY, DIAGNOSIS AND TREATMENTS

GASTRIC CANCER

FROM STAGING TO SURGICAL TREATMENT. PROCEDURES, COMPLICATIONS AND ONCOLOGICAL RESULTS

Cancer Etiology, Diagnosis and Treatments

Additional books in this series can be found on Nova's website
under the Series tab.

Additional E-books in this series can be found on Nova's website
under the E-book tab.

CANCER ETIOLOGY, DIAGNOSIS AND TREATMENTS

GASTRIC CANCER

FROM STAGING TO SURGICAL TREATMENT. PROCEDURES, COMPLICATIONS AND ONCOLOGICAL RESULTS

ANNIBALE D'ANNIBALE
VITO PENDE
AND
IGOR MONSELLATO
EDITORS

Nova Science Publishers, Inc.
New York

For permission to use material from this book please contact us:
Telephone 631-231-7269; Fax 631-231-8175
Web Site: http://www.novapublishers.com

Library of Congress Cataloging-in-Publication Data

ISBN: 978-1-62081-294-5

Library of Congress Control Number: 2012936703

Published by Nova Science Publishers, Inc. † New York

Contents

Preface

Gastrectomy for gastric cancer is a complex procedure also for skilled surgeons. Radical gastrectomy with lymphadenectomy represents the sole curative treatment for gastric cancer. In the last decade, nevertheless, many advances have been made in terms of staging, neoadjuvant and adjuvant therapies, thanks to the discover of new drugs with reduced toxicity, the standardization of lymphadenectomy according to Japanese Society for Gastric Cancer guidelines *and the gradual application in gastric cancer of minimally invasive techniques and robotics, which have already been experienced in colorectal diseases*.

This book is structured in eleven chapters, written by leading experts in the field of gastric cancer and includes the most interesting topics: surgical anatomy, clinical staging, analysis of prognostic factors in early and advanced stages, sentinel node biopsy results, surgical standard, laparoscopic and robotic techniques of gastrectomy with D2 lymphadenectomy, perioperative and postoperative complications, neoadjuvant and adjuvant therapies and preoperative, perioperative and postoperative nutrition.

The authors hope therefore, that the book is useful both for surgeons in training and experienced surgeons for its completeness and actuality of the treated topics.

In: Gastric Cancer
Editors: A. D'Annibale, V. Pende and I. Monsellato
ISBN: 978-1-62081-294-5

Chapter I

Surgical Anatomy of the Stomach

Francesco Ruotolo[1], Monica De Angelis[2], Giovanni Alfano[2], Igor Monsellato[2]* and Annibale D'Annibale[2]
[1]Research Professor at San Giovanni Addolorata Hospital, Rome, Italy
[2]Minimally-Invasive and Robotic Surgery Unit,
San Giovanni Addolorata Hospital, Rome, Italy

Embryological Signs

Development of the Posterior Mesogastrium – Gastric Rotation – Development of the Hepato-Enteric Cavity

At an early-stage of embryonic development, the stomach, distal portion of the anterior primitive intestine, appears as a fusiform dilatation, laterally flattened. It remains in the sagittal position, connected to the dorsal abdominal wall by a peritoneal fold, *dorsal mesogastrium,* whose thickness contains the celiac trunk (CT) and the buds of pancreas and spleen (figure 1). During the progressive embryonic development, the stomach is gaining its form: it has two surfaces one turned to the right and the other to the left, and two borders, one dorsal (greater curvature) and one ventral (lesser curvature).

The stomach rotates through 90° so that its primitive left surface becomes anterior, and its right surface becomes posterior. The dorsal border (greater curvature) moves forward and left while the anterior border (lesser curvature) moves back and right: that is why in the abdomen the left vagus nerve is anterior while the right is posterior (remember the mnemonic LARP: left anterior, right posterior).

The clockwise rotation of the stomach around the longitudinal axis is associated with the invagination of the dorsal mesogastrium which becomes deeper behind the stomach and in front of the pancreas. It forms the omental bursa or retrocavity of the epiploon and the greater omentum (figures 2-3).

* Email address: imonsellato@libero.it

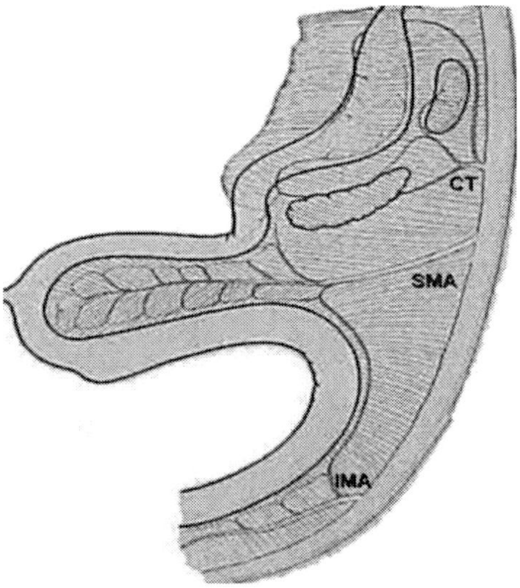

Figure 1. Sagittal position of the primitive intestine and dorsal mesentery embryonic peritoneal vessels.

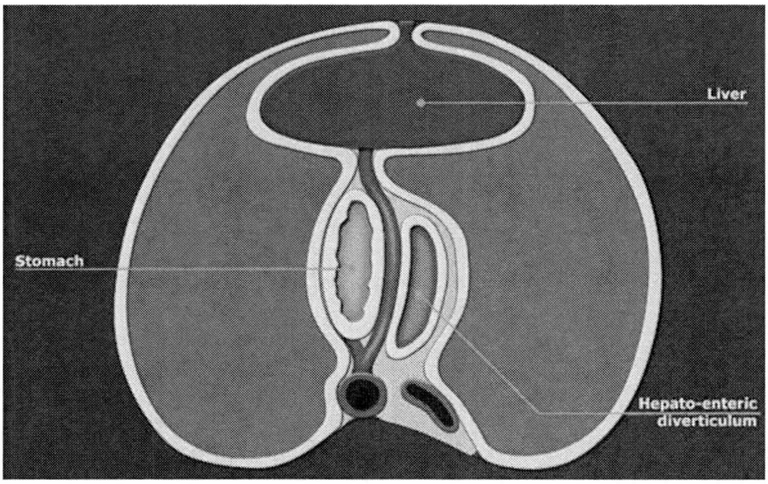

Figure 2. Sagittal position of embrionic stomach.

Phases of Attachment: Fasciae – Cleavage Planes

Active processes of peritoneal attachment reduce the size of the omental retrocavity and determine the final location and shape of the stomach and of its attached organs. The final mesogastrium attaches to the posterior parietal coelomic peritoneum to form the mesogastric fascia, continuation upwards of the left mesocolic fascia of Toldt and cleavage plane along which the dissection of the spleno-pancreatic block is made. The attachment is made larger at the postero-upper gastric surface generating the gastro-phrenic ligament and the fixed area of the gastric fundus. The posterior parietal attachment of the left gastric and common hepatic arteries, raising the peritoneum, results in the formation of the gastro-pancreatic ligament or Huschke's fold and of the duodeno-pancreatic ligament, while the attachment of the supramesocolic fascia of the posterior omental lamina to colon and transverse mesocolon leads to the *colo-epiploic attachment* (figures 4-6).

At the right-side of the median sagittal plane, the two omental laminae join the supra-mesocolic upper two-third of the anterior surface of the pancreatic head and of the second duodenal portion forming the *supramesocolic omental fascia*, while the transverse mesocolon, below the right side of its root, makes contact with the pre-duodenal peritoneum forming the *preduodenopancreatic submesocolic fascia of Fredet* (figure 7-8).

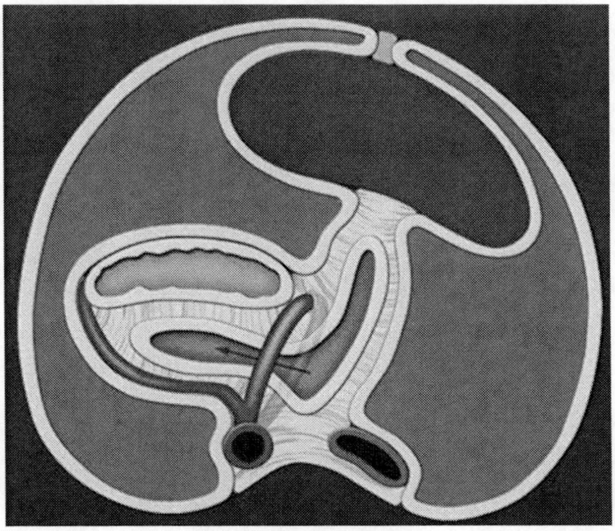

Figure 3. Development of hepato-enteric cavity and gastric rotation.

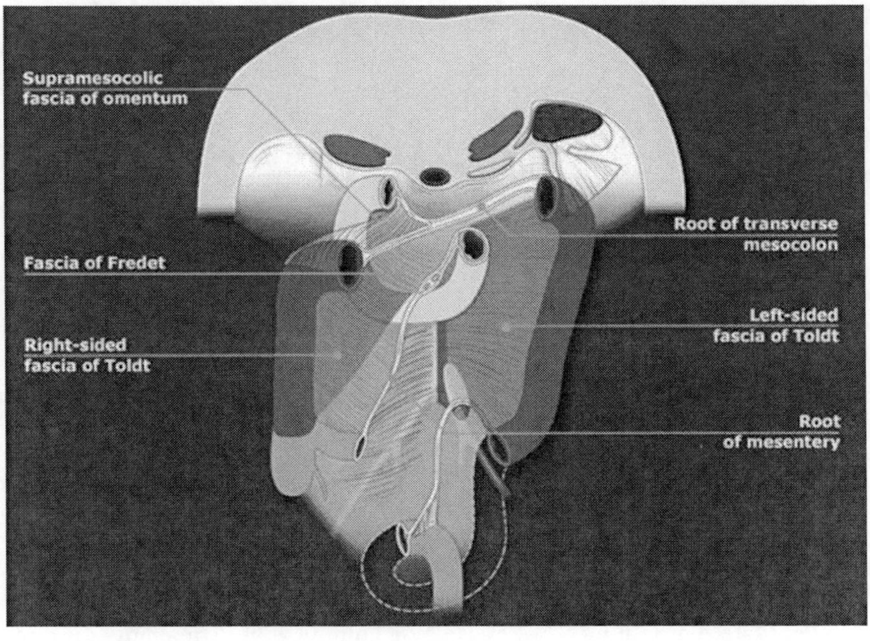

Figure 4. Fusion of the fasciae –anterior view.

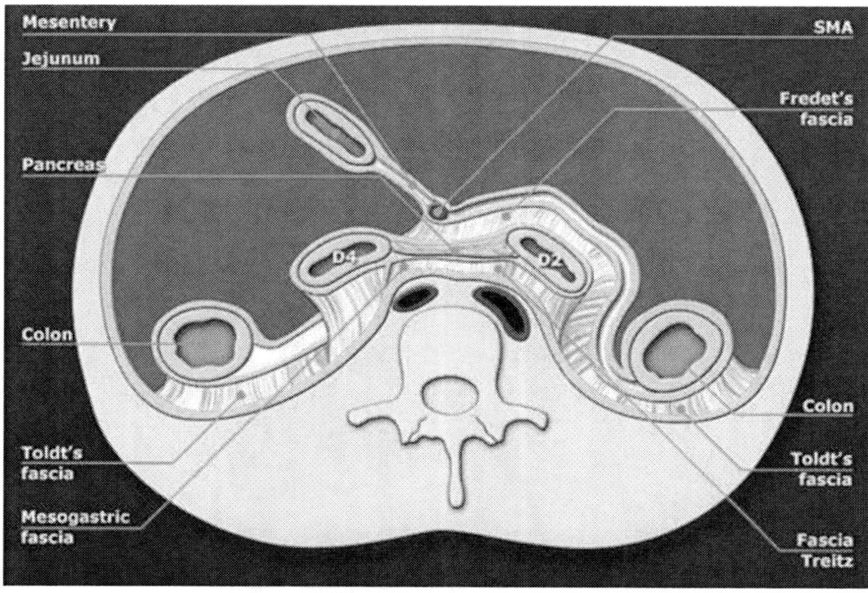

Figure 5. Fusion of the fasciae – transverse section.

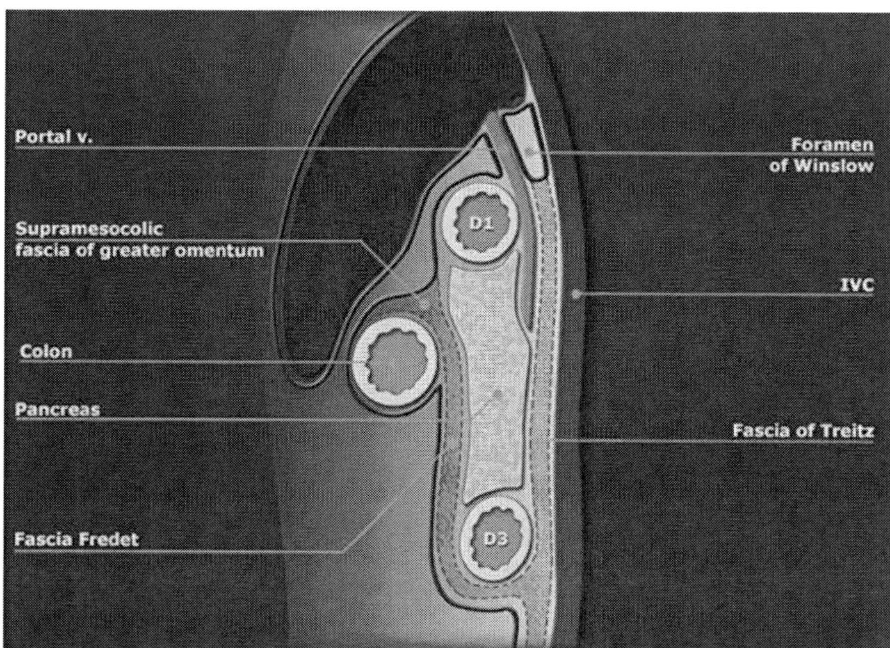

Figure 6. Peripancreatic fasciae – sagittal section.

These fasciae, laterally to the duodenum, are combined to the ***posterior*** *duodenopancreatic fascia of Treitz* resulting from the fusion process involving the posterior mesoduodenum with the posterior parietal peritoneum. In the plane of this fascia, which continues lower, with the right mesocolic fascia of Toldt, Kocher's maneuver is done.

In the submesocolic area, the fusion between the anterior and posterior laminae of the greater omentum, gives it the appearance of single lamina or omental apron (figure 9).

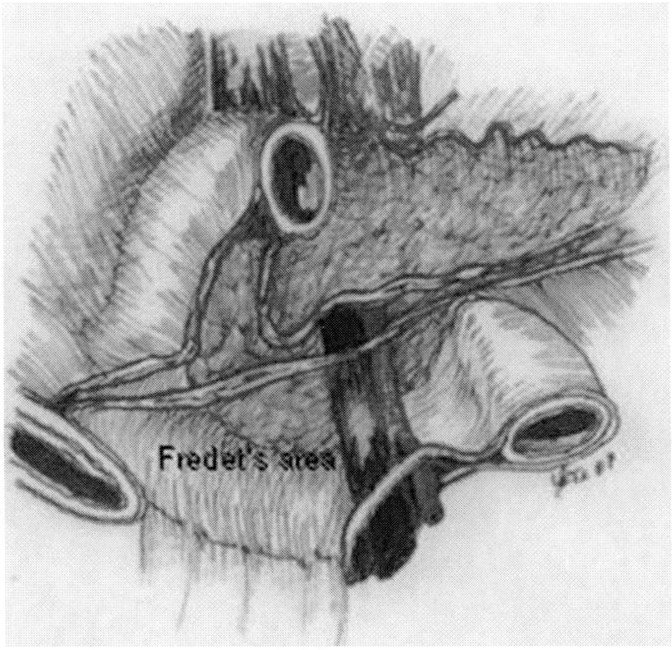

Figure 7. Inframesocolic preduodenopancreatic area of Fredet (a).

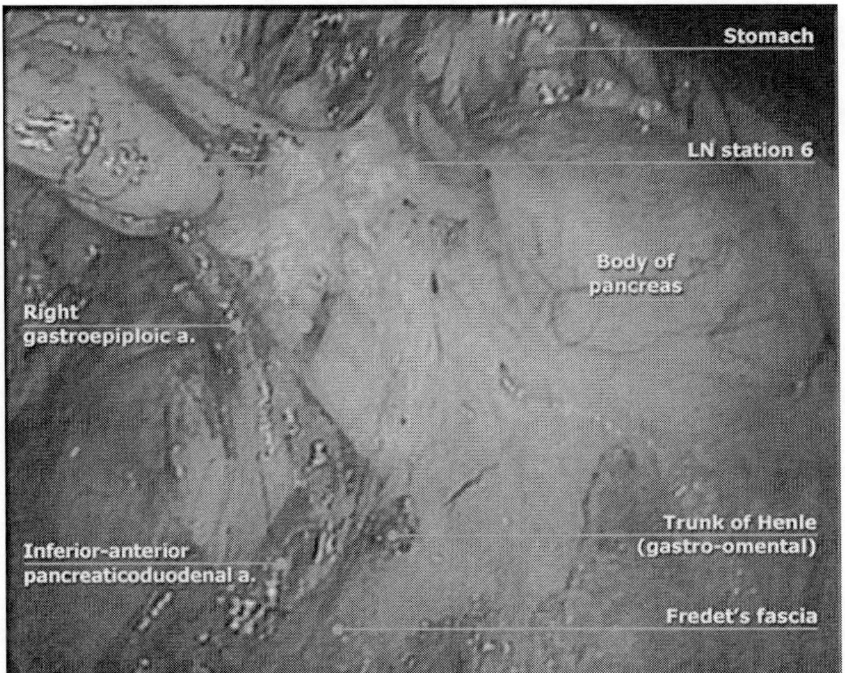

Figure 8. Inframesocolic preduodenopancreatic area of Fredet (b).

Notes of Descriptive and Topographic Anatomy

The stomach, placed in the supramesocolic area, fills the left hypochondrium and most of the epigastrium, locating below the liver and the diaphragm and above the transverse colon and relative mesocolon. The stomach is divided into three main parts: fundus, body and pylorus. The fundus has a hemispherical form and is located to the left of the cardia. A horizontal plane passing just above the cardia artificially markets its limit towards the body. The body has a nearly vertical direction and continues in the pylorus with a right or obtuse angle.

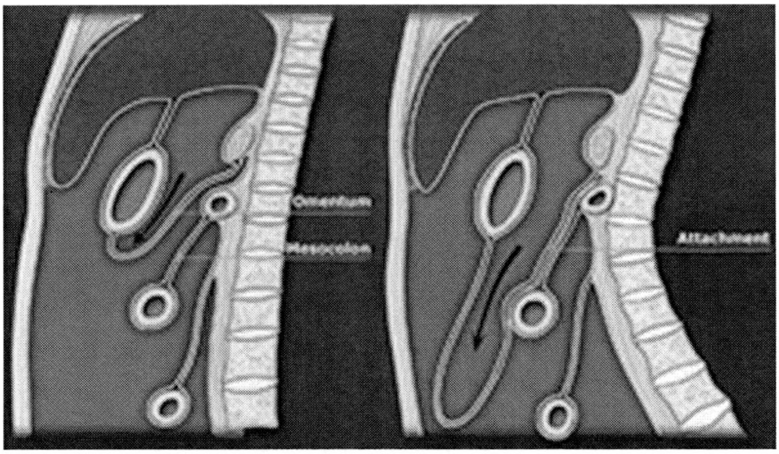

Figure 9. Omento-mesocolic attachment.

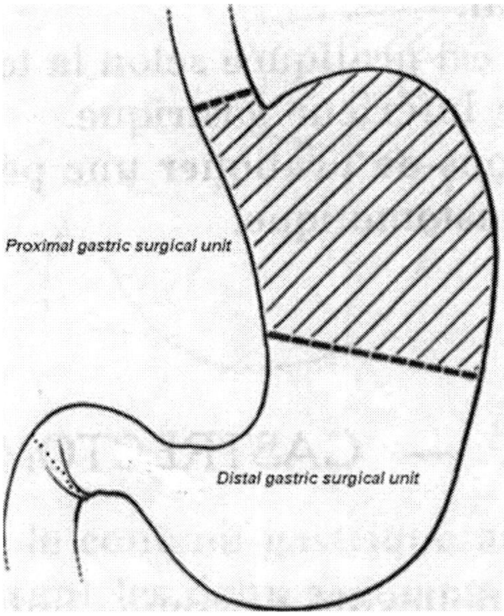

Figure 10. Proximal and distal gastric unit.

The pylorus is the lower, horizontal part of the stomach and includes two portions: pyloric antrum and pyloric canal. From the surgeon's viewpoint, the stomach is part of two almost separated systems, each with its special pathology and surgical approach. The first, called the *proximal gastric unit* (figure 10), contains the proximal stomach, distal esophagus, and esophageal hiatus of the diaphragm.

The most important relation of the proximal gastric unit is with the left gastric artery, which should be ligated at its origin to include the lymph nodes associated with it and the celiac axis. The second is the *distal gastric unit* (figure 10), and includes the gastric antrum and pylorus, together with the first part of the duodenum.

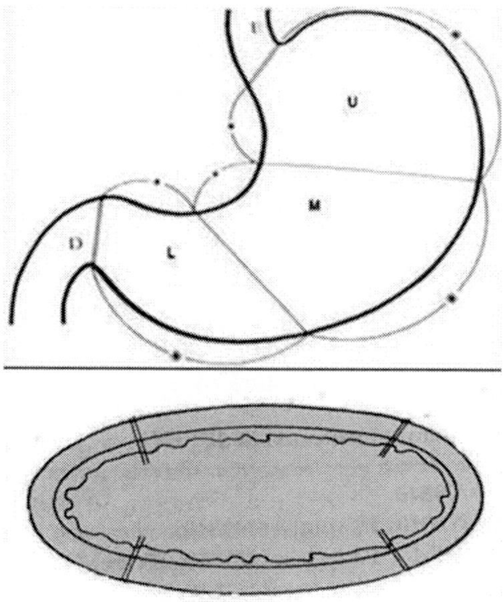

Figure 11. Gastric subdivisions.

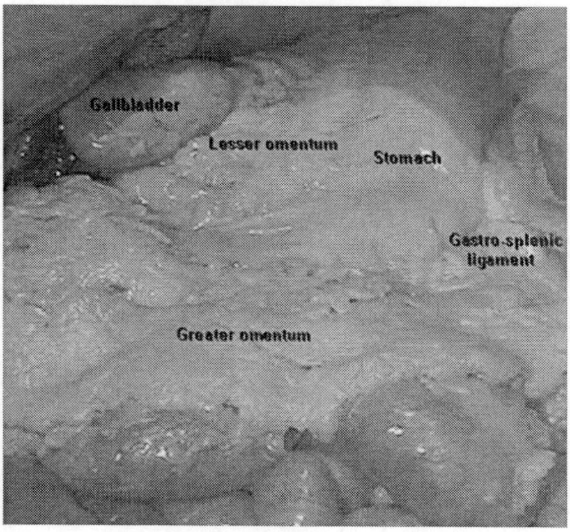

Figure 12. Peritoneal reflections – omental ligaments.

The boundary of the antrum on the lesser curvature usually lies at the incisura angularis, inconstant and often absent in operating room. The surgeon can use the *crow's foot* of the anterior descending vagal trunk as a landmark. In surgical oncology, the division of lesser and greater curvature into three equidistant zones, united by straight lines, divides the stomach into three parts: Upper (U), Middle (M), Lower (L) (figure 11). Subdividing, then, the gastric circumference into four equal parts, for each of these three portions four further sites are distinguished: greater curvature (Great), lesser curvature (Less), anterior wall (Ant) and posterior wall (Post).

The stomach is kept in place by its continuity with esophagus and duodenum, by the celiac trunk and especially by the coronarostomacic artery, which connects the lesser curvature to the aorta, and by peritoneal folds which connect lesser curvature, fundus and greater curvature to the liver, spleen, diaphragm and transverse colon (figure 12). Posteriorly, the peritoneal serosa stops toward the upper body, so that the posterior surface of the esophagus and a portion of gastric fundus have no peritoneal covering (bare area).

On the other points of the circumferential line of the viscera, i.e. at the lesser curvature, greater curvature and upper-external part of the fundus, both anterior and posterior peritoneal layers join together to form membranes, derivates of the dorsal mesentery, securing the stomach to the near viscera: gastro-hepatic epiploon (ligament) (*omentum minus*), gastro-splenic epiploon (ligament) (*omentum medium*) (figure 13) and gastro-colic epiploon (ligament) (*omentum maius*).The gastro-hepatic epiploon is that part of the small epiploon which extends from the lesser gastric curvature to the lower surface of the liver inserting in the fissure of the venous duct of Arantius. It is characterized by a *pars flaccida* and a *pars condensa*. The gastro-splenic epiploon joins the great tuberosity of the stomach to the medial surface of the spleen and between its two layers the short vessels and the left gastroepiploic artery run. It continues, above the spleen, with the *gastro-phrenic ligament*, that extends from the great tuberosity of the stomach to the diaphragmatic cupola.

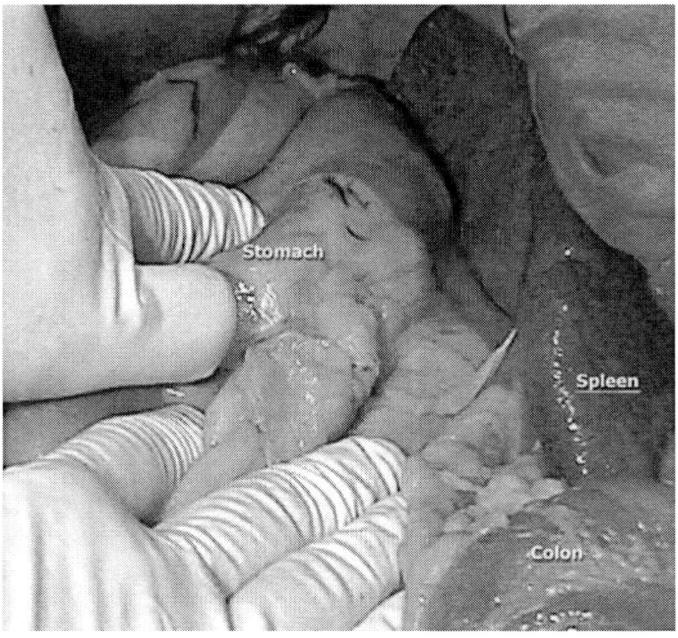

Figure 13. Gastro-splenic ligament.

The gastro-colic epiploon moves away from the greater gastric curvature, joins the mesocolon- transverse colon, descending behind the anterior abdominal wall in front of the intestinal coil. In its early development the greater omentum appears as a pouch, which is formed by two walls, anterior and posterior, each of them consists of two peritoneal layers attached to each other.

Later, the four layers join together creating the descending (or posterior or direct) omental lamina and the ascending (or anterior or reflected) omental lamina. During gastric surgery, an inappropriate traction on the *spleno-omental criminal fold* (figure 14) can injure the spleen resulting in an avulsion of its capsule. The omental bursa or retrocavity of the epiploon is a large diverticulum of the peritoneal cavity, greatly flattened in antero-posterior, which extends in width from the epiploic foramen of Winslow to the hilum of the spleen (*splenic recess*), and in height from the superior border of Spigelian lobe to the plane of the transverse mesocolon and the most declivous part of the greater omentum. This arrangement, typical of the embryonic period, changes in the adult following the fusion of the two laminae of the greater omentum; thus the retrocavity doesn't extend beyond the transverse colon.

In the omental bursa there are two parts: the vestibulum and the proper omental bursa (figure 15-16).

The vestibulum follows Winslow's foramen and corresponds to that portion which is placed behind the gastro-hepatic epiploon. The proper omental bursa, that corresponds forward to the posterior gastric surface, behind to the anterior pancreatic surface, to the left adrenal gland and to the upper part of the ipsilateral kidney, down to the mesocolon and transverse colon, to which the peritoneum of the omental bursa is already intimately joined at an early stage of its development. The vestibulum and the proper retrocavity are connected through the *foramen of omental bursa* which is limited at the top, behind and medially by the gastropancreatic fold of Huschke (figure 17). It is extended from the superior part of the lesser curvature to the *omental tuber* on the upper pancreatic surface, and resulting from the raising of the parietal peritoneum by coronarostomacic vessels.

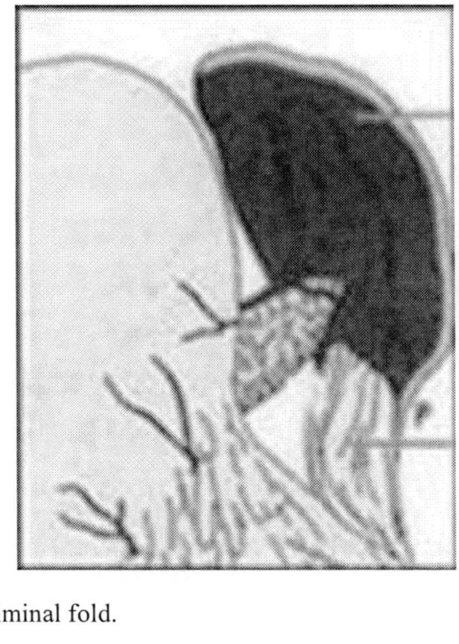

Figure 14. Spleno-omental criminal fold.

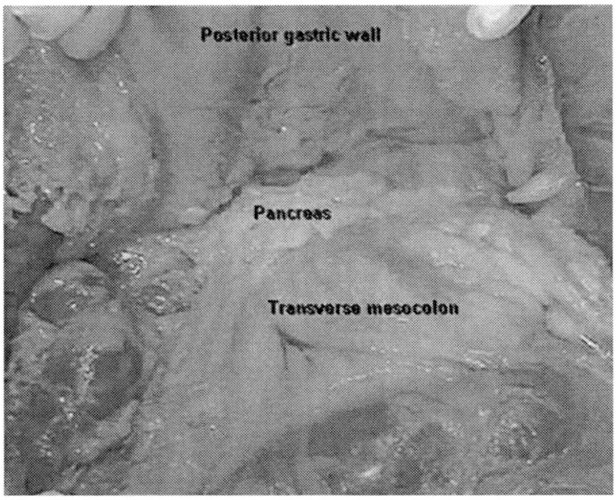

Figure 15. Omental bursa - inside view.

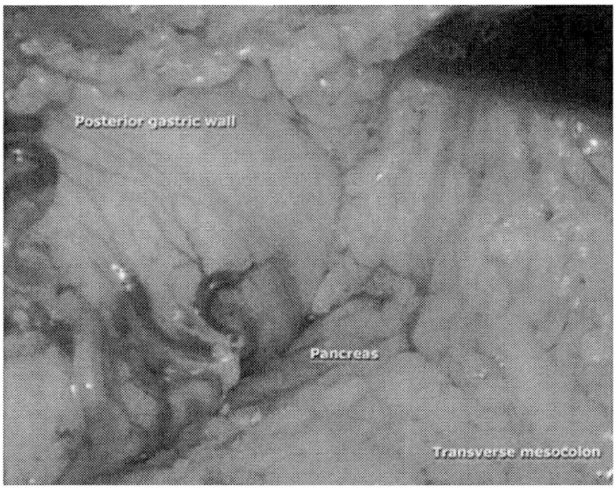

Figure 16. Omental bursa - inside view.

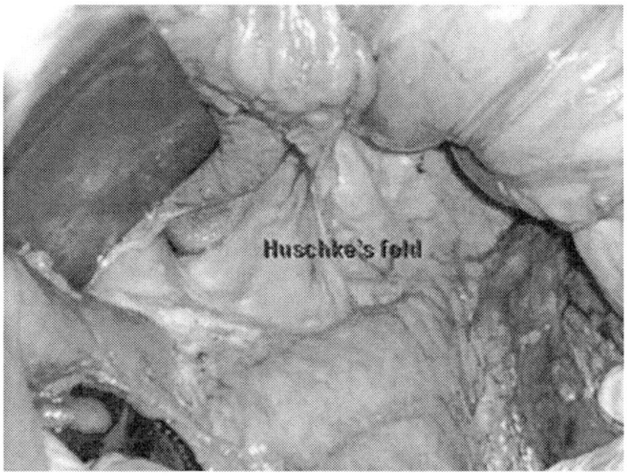

Figure 17. Gastro-pancreatic ligament of Huschke.

Vascularization of the Stomach

Principal blood supplies derive directly or indirectly from the celiac trunk (CT) of Haller which appears in the fifth week of embryonic development at the level of the seventh cervical segment; its final position is at the lower third of the first lumbar vertebra (figure 18-19).The three constitutive arteries often arise *ad modum tridentis*, but in most cases the left gastric artery is the first that originates from the superior surface of the CT which, after 2-3 mm, divides into hepatic and splenic artery (figure 19). Not only the stomach is served by many arteries, but its wall also contains a rich anastomotic network of vessels extrinsically and intrinsically.

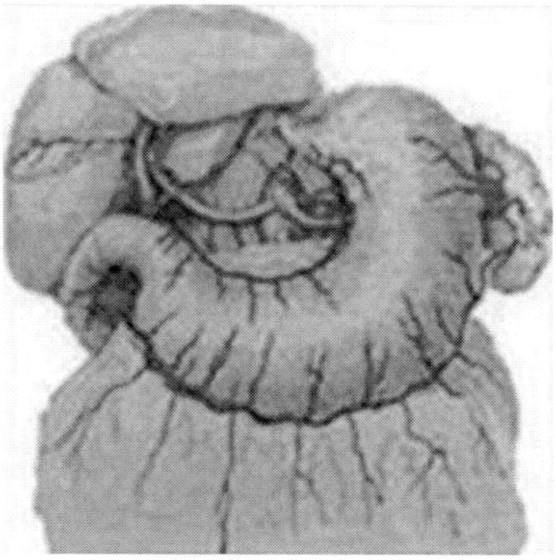

Figure 18. Arterial blood supply of the stomach.

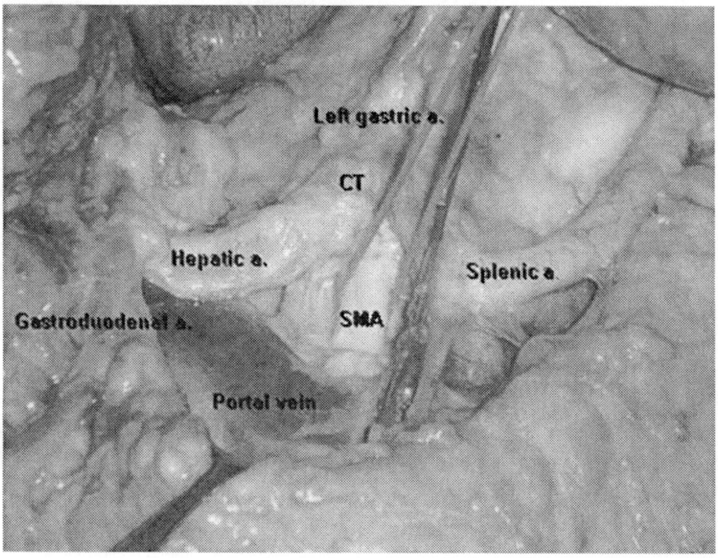

Figure 19. Celiac trunk (CT) and superior mesenteric artery.

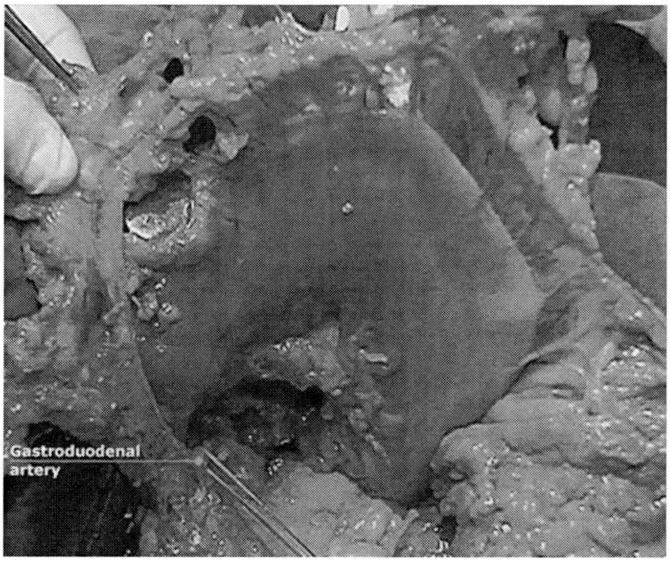

Figure 20. Gastroepipolic arch of Winslow (stomach has been lifted up).

The left gastric or coronarostomacic artery usually arises from the CT (85-90%) and takes its place in the gastro-pancreatic fold of Huschke. At first it directs up and left supplying the cardio-esophageal extremity and the right side of the great tuberosity; then it suddenly folds and descends along the lesser curvature between the two layers of the lesser omentum dividing into two branches, anterior and posterior.

The anterior branch is distributed to the gastric anterior wall with numerous small ramifications and it forms a *vascular "crow's foot"* of Payne similar to the anterior gastric nerve of Latarjet, while the posterior branch follows the lesser curvature and anastomoses with the right gastric artery, supplying most of the gastric posterior wall. The left gastric artery can provide accessory inferior diaphragmatic arteries which supply the gastric fundus and in 30% of cases, a left aberrant hepatic artery (Hyrtl's artery). The right gastric or pyloric artery usually originates from the proper hepatic artery, sometimes from the common hepatic or gastroduodenal artery and supply the first part of the duodenum and the posterior and anterior walls of the pyloric canal and anastomoses with the posterior branch of the left gastric artery.

The right gastroepiploic artery arises from the gastroduodenal artery, branch of the hepatic artery, at the inferior border of the first duodenal portion. After supplying the lower half of the pyloric canal, it runs along the greater curvature of the stomach through the layers of the greater omentum, to the middle part of it, where it anastomoses in 90% of cases with the left gastro-omental artery, branch of the splenic artery, forming the arch of Winslow (figure 20). The anastomosis is defined "strong" if it is with full-channel (in about 75% of cases) and "weak" if it is through intramural gastric anastomotic plexuses.

The ascending branches starting from this arch, anastomose with the descending branches coming from the arch of the lesser curvature, while the descending or epiploic branches (and in particular the right epiploic artery) join the corresponding branches of the left gastro-omental artery (and in particular to the voluminous left epiploic branch) to form the subcolic intraepiploic arch of Haller and Barkow. For omental viability during distal gastrectomy, the right gastroepiploic artery should be preserved by one of the following methods: ligating its gastric branches or ligating the right gastroepiploic distal and close to the origin of right epiploic. The left gastroepiploic artery arises from the splenic artery at the level of the posterior wall of the great tuberosity of the stomach. It runs in the thickness of the gastro-splenic ligament, then crosses the greater curvature from left to right in the thickness of the anterior lamina of the greater omentum to Van Goethem's point (figure 21), where usually anastomoses with the right gastro-omental artery, after providing ascending or gastric branches and descending or epiploic branches.

In 66% of cases it arises from the splenic artery by a common stem with the inferior polar splenic branch, the splenogastric omental trunk.

The short gastric vessels, whose number varies from two to ten, derive from the terminal branches of the division of the splenic artery. They are directed, included in the thickness of the gastro-splenic ligament, to the great tuberosity and there they branch anastomosing with the gastric branches of the previous artery and with the cardiac branches of the left gastric artery, completing the arterial circulation of the stomach.

With subtotal gastrectomy, the gastric remnant remains viable with circulation from the left gastroepiploic artery and the short gastric vessels, because the left gastric artery is ligated. The posterior gastric artery, if present, participates in the survival of the remnant.

All the arterial system represents the great gastric circle that, starting from the cardia, initially follows the lesser curvature, then descends behind the pylorus, surrounds the greater curvature and rises along the great tuberosity to the cardia, its starting point.

The secondary arterial supplies originate from numerous arteries: supraduodenal, superior pancreaticoduodenal, retroduodenal, dorsal pancreatic and transverse pancreatic, aberrant left gastric, left inferior phrenic, posterior gastric and oesophageal.

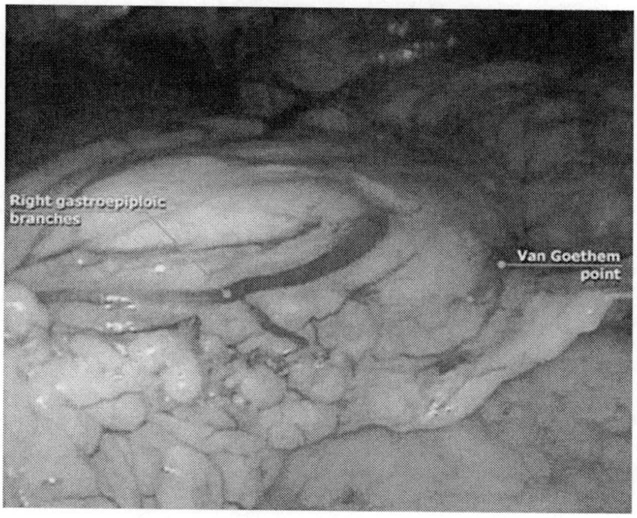

Figure 21. Van Goethem's point.

Particularly interesting are:

- *the left inferior phrenic artery*, which arises from the aorta in 90% of cases or from the celiac trunk. Before reaching the diaphragm, it provides recurrent branches for the cardiotuberosity region and for the terminal portion of the esophagus. In 15% of cases, there are not intramural anastomoses between the gastric branches of the phrenic artery and the short vessels, so the left posterior half wall of gastric fundus is vascularized by the short vessels and eventually by the posterior gastric artery. The opinion that this artery, alone, can ensure the vitality of the gastric fundus is not shared by all (figure 22);

- *the posterior gastric artery* (ramus esofago-gastricus ascendens posterior of the Japanese Research Society for Gastric Cancer), which is inconstant (intraoperatively has been detected in 66-84% of cases) and arises from the trunk of the splenic artery usually about 5 cm from its origin. It goes up and left to reach the posterior gastric surface, 2-3 cm below and left of the cardia, dividing into small branches designed to the gastric walls and also to the spleen to which it provides a superior polar branch (gastrosplenic artery of Trubel). The awareness of the existence and location of the posterior gastric artery is the fundamental basis of its preservation in order to avoid unexpected bleeding and necrosis of the fundus or of the gastric stump in case of subtotal distal gastrectomy for cancer (figure 22);
- *the median esophageal arteries,* which arise from the bronchial arteries, intercostal arteries and from the trunk of the aorta and the inferior esophageal arteries which arise in part from the inferior phrenic arteries and in part from the left gastric artery. Despite the frequent presence of significant anastomoses between these esophageal vessels, it's impossible to say with certainty, that they are able to provide by themselves the vascularization of the gastric fundus.

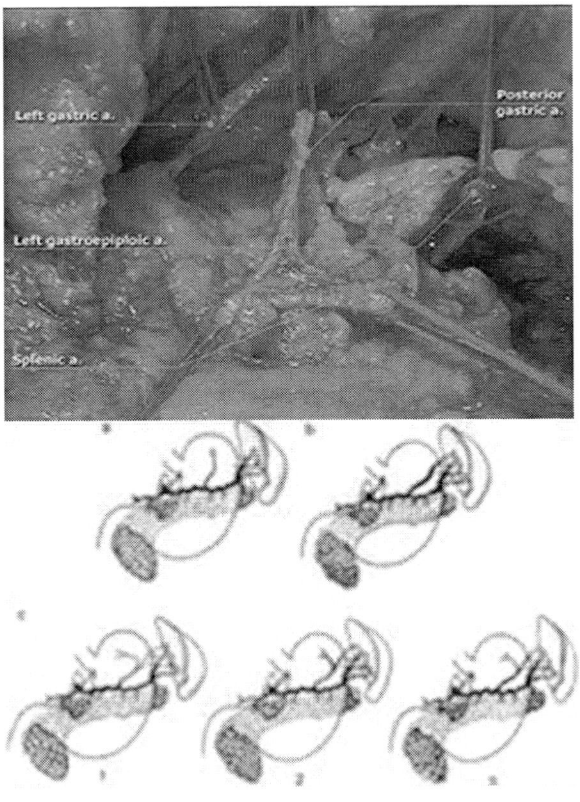

Figure 22. Splenic artery and posterior gastric artery.

In gastric cancer surgery, the knowledge of the anomalies of the CT and of the SMA according to Tandler allows to avoid ischemic damages, especially during the lymph node dissection. In particular, the anomalies of the hepatic arterial perfusion should be recognized to prevent necrosis of the liver deriving from the ligation of abnormal vessels.

In 80% of cases, the common hepatic artery arises from the celiac artery. It becomes proper hepatic artery after the origin of the gastroduodenal artery and then it divides into 2 or 3 terminal branches (right, left and median), while in 3-7% of cases it can originate from the SMA (figure 23).

From the last one often derives (up to 25% of cases) an aberrant right hepatic artery, whose existence should be suspected and then searched in presence of the proper hepatic artery reduced in size. It ascends to the liver on the deep or posterior aspect of the hepatoduodenal ligament.The incidence (up to 30% of cases) of an aberrant left hepatic artery (Hyrtl's artery) (figures 24-25) arising from the coronarostomacic artery is high.

This artery in the embryo divides into two main branches: a transversal one (artery of the gastric body) and the other ascending to the left hepatic lobe which is, in most cases, designed to obliteration. The hepatic branch, which runs through the layers of the lesser omentum and goes up to the left-sided end of the transverse furrow of Haller, where it anastomoses with the left branch of the hepatic artery, is sometimes so large to provide a substantial share of blood to the left liver. In these cases, it is advisable to tie the left gastric artery distally to the origin of the left aberrant hepatic artery, thus making a complete lymphectomy along the preserved tract of the gastric artery (figure 26).

A right aberrant hepatic artery and a left aberrant hepatic artery with the size-reduced proper hepatic artery are present in less than 10% of cases. Another anomaly of the left gastric artery is the left gastro-hepatic artery of Haller consisting of a single vessel that supplies the left hepatic lobe, of which it represents, in half of the cases, the only blood supply, and from whose ascending portion branches depart for the lesser gastric curvature.

In case of lymphectomy it is not possible to tie the gastro-hepatic artery at the origin, but it's necessary to respect the common trunk just tying the gastric branches only. The perfusion of the gastric fundus is usually provided by three sources: left gastric artery, splenic artery (through the posterior gastric artery and the short vessels) and left inferior phrenic artery. The esophageal vessels are involved in the vascularization of the juxta-cardial region for a share which is probably insignificant. To avoid the ischemic necrosis of the stump after subtotal gastrectomy (STG), it is necessary to preserve at least one of these sources.

The problem is extremely important in the treatment of the gastric cancer because in distal gastric resections for benign disease it is not necessary to stop the branches that arise from the splenic artery, while the left gastric artery is dissected, not at the origin but close to the lesser curvature. The venous gastric circulation is tributary of the portal system, which communicates through many roots with the venous networks of the venae cavae system. At the cardia, the roots of the left gastric vein anastomose with the esophageal veins, which open into the intercostal and azygos ones. Other anastomoses have been described between veins of the gastric fundus and left renal vein and between gastric short veins and phrenic veins.

Of surgical interest is the gastrocolic trunk of Henle (figure 27), which arises from the *variable confluence* of the right gastroepiploic, anterior-inferior pancreatic-duodenal, middle colic and right superior colic veins and leads into the superior mesenteric vein (SMV) at the inferior pancreatic border in the area of the submesocolic pre-duodenal pancreatic fascia of Fredet.

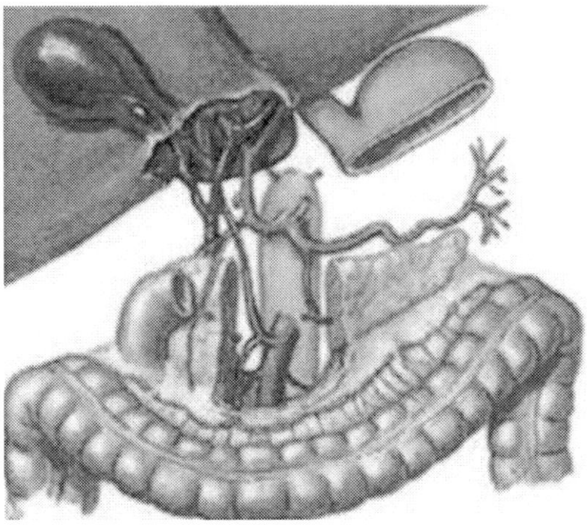

Figure 23. Right aberrant hepatic artery arising from the SMA.

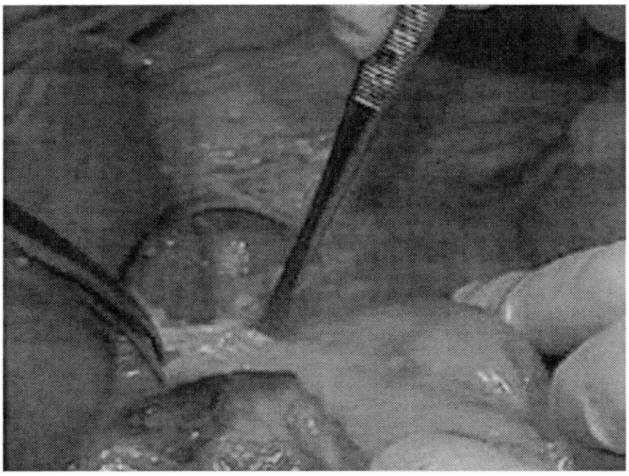

Figure 24. Hyrtl's artery.

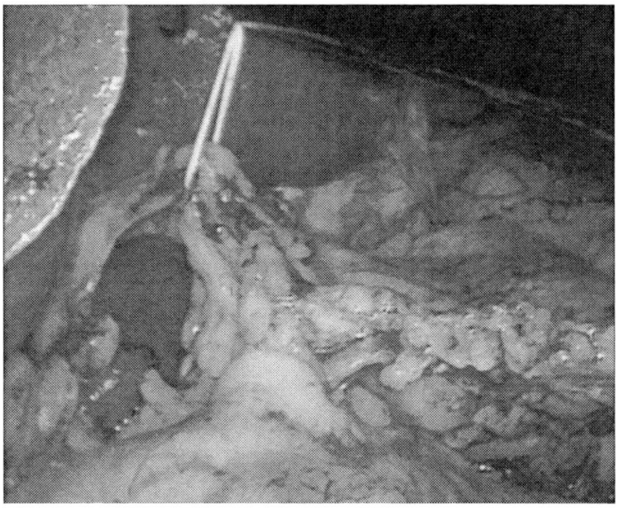

Figure 25. Hyrtl's artery and Huschke's fold.

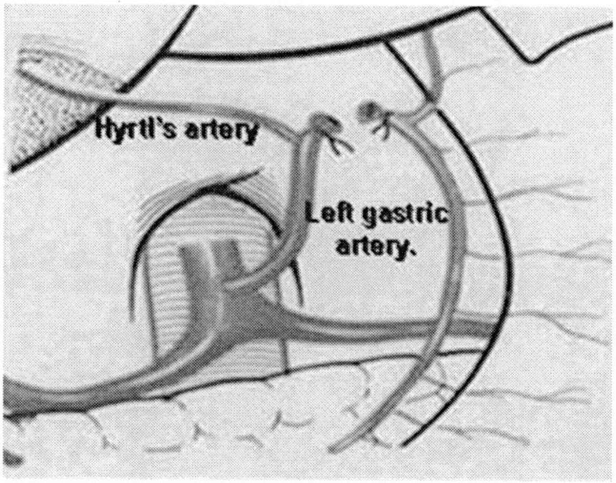

Figure 26. Section of left gastric artery distal to emergence of Hyrtl's artery.

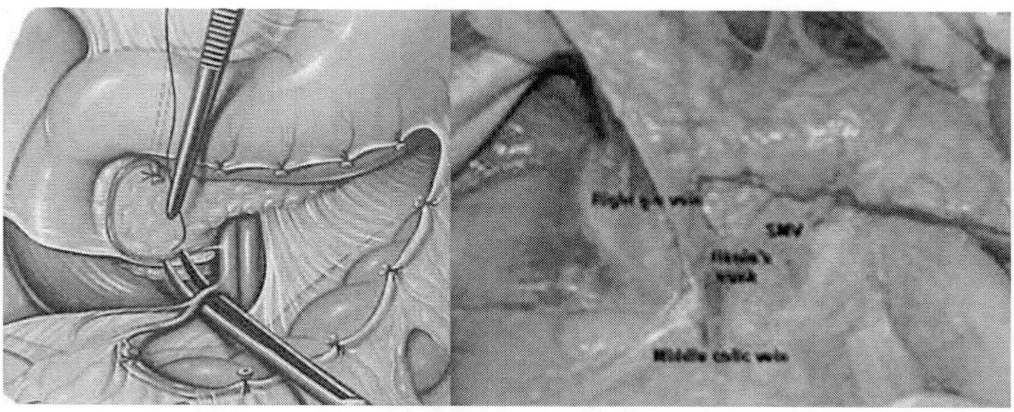

Figure 27. Gastrocolic venous trunk of Henle.

The anatomy of the region at the inferior border of the head and neck of the pancreas is one of the most challenging aspects for two reasons: the fusion between the greater omentum and the transverse mesocolon at this level, and the complex anatomy of the vulnerable venous tributaries of the superior mesenteric vein. During the lymphatic dissection of the sub pyloric station, of the middle colic and the SMV, the colic root of the trunk must be preserved.

Innervation of the Stomach

The hindbrain parasympathetic, contained in the vagus nerves, makes the anterior and posterior gastric plexuses for the corresponding gastric surfaces (figure 28).

The anterior vagal trunk gives rise at level of the cardia to some hepatic branches, it runs along the lesser curvature and reaches the pyloric antrum to which it gives Letarjet's nerve (or anterior antral motor branch). The posterior vagal trunk divides into two branches: the biggest moves to the celiac plexus, while from the smallest, along the lesser curvature, branches for the posterior gastric wall are originated.

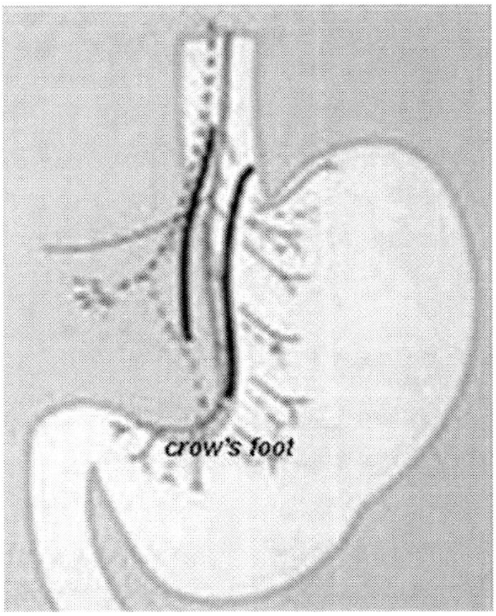

Figure 28. Vagal trunks - crow's foot of the nerve of Latarjet.

The thoracolumbar sympathetic gives raise to periarterial plexuses, in particular the superior gastric plexus, which accompanies the left gastric artery and the inferior gastric plexus, which accompanies the gastroepiploic arteries.

The meta-sympathetic has two plexuses in the gastric walls, Auerbach's myoenteric and Meissner's submucosal plexus; they operate independently from the nerves coming from the outside.

Lymphatic Drainage of the Stomach - Anatomosurgical Bases of the Gastric Cancer Lymphadenectomy

The rational assumption of the therapeutic role of extended lymphadenectomy in the gastric cancer is based on the principle of Moynihan (1908) *["The surgery of the malignant disease is not the surgery of the organs, it is the anatomy of the lymphatic system"]* and, then, on the removal of a lymph node level superior to the one in which metastatic cells are present (D> N).The topographic description of the lymphatic gastric system according to Cuneo and Delamare (figure 29), Rouvière, Coller and Maruyama (figure 30) is based on the satellitosis of lymphatic vessels respect to arterial branches and on the substantial regularity of lymphatic flows: all roads lead to Rome, and, in other words, to celiac axis lymph nodes.

The lymphatics arising from the mucous and muscular coats reach the subserosa network, from which three lymphatic chains, which are satellites of arteries, depart:

- *chain of the left gastric artery*, in which the upper half of the lesser curvature drains,
- *chain of the splenic artery*, in which the left side of body and fundus drains;
- *chain of the hepatic artery*, in which the antrum and the lower half of the greater curvature drains.

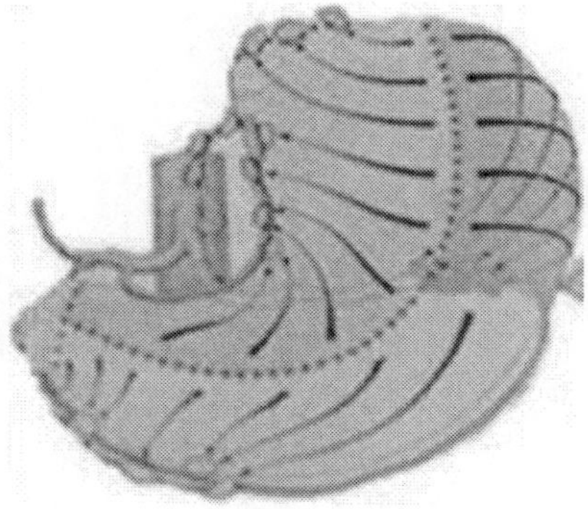

Figure 29. Lymphatic drainge according according to Cuneo E Delamare.

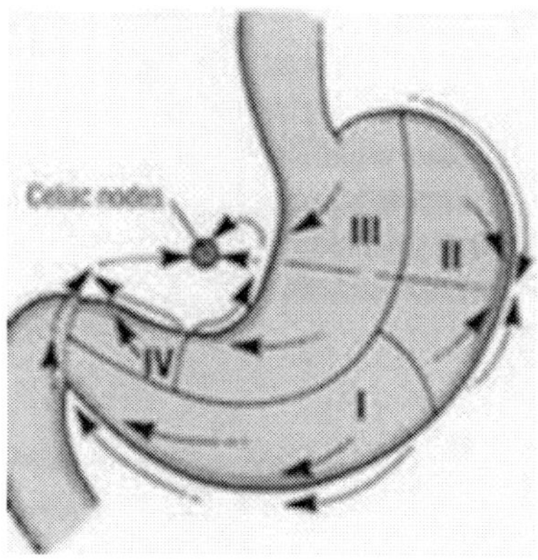

Figure 30. Four drainage zones of the gastric lymphatics according to Coller.

The researches on lymph node involvement in gastric cancers provide a systematization of lymphatic drainage, identifying 16 lymph node stations, defining their level of invasion according to the site of the primary tumor and distinguishing them in locoregional and metastatic (figure 31). The first correspond to the stations located along the lesser and greater curvature, along the left gastric, common hepatic, splenic and celiac and hepato-duodenal arteries; the second to retropancreatic, mesenteric and para-aortic stations.

Depending on the extension of the lymphatic dissection, three types of lymphectomy, of progressively increasing engagement and whose execution requires a perfect knowledge of the anatomy of the abdominal vessels which are the real landmarks of lymphatic dissection, can be described (figure 32).

According to the JRSGC classification, the lymphatic stations which are subjected to dissection are:

- *n. 1* – right paracardial lymph nodes located along the cardioesophageal branch of the left gastric artery close to the esophagogastric junction. They are removed during the dissection of the *pars condensa* of the lesser omentum (figure 33);

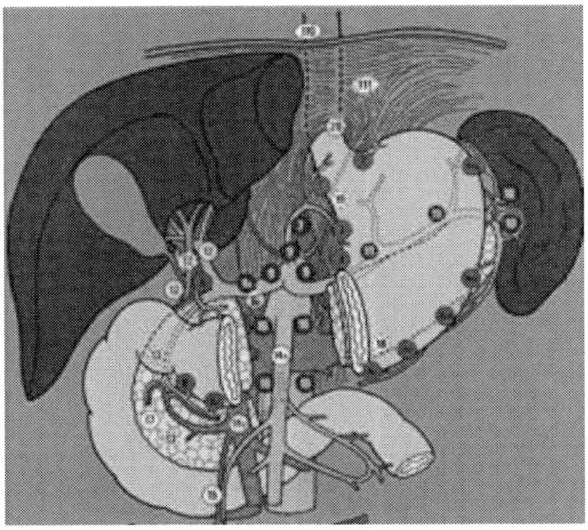

Figure 31. Gastric lymphatics according to JRSG.

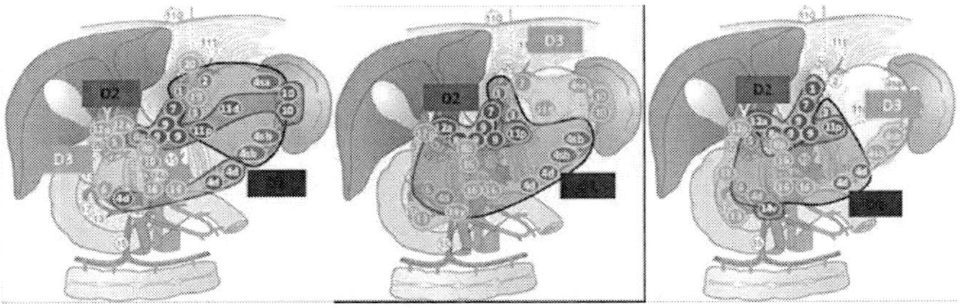

Figure 32. Lymphadenectomy UpperThird Lymphadenectomy MiddleThird Lymphadenectomy LowerThird.

- *n. 3 and 5* - group 3 is placed near the lesser curvature, along the left gastric artery, while the satellite lymph nodes of the pyloric artery represent station 5 which is located in the superior part of the pylorus. The lymph nodes of station 3 are removed during the dissection of the gastro-hepatic ligament, the ones of station 5 during the section of the duodenum distal to the pylorus and after the section of the right gastric artery at its origin from the proper hepatic artery (figure 34);
- *n. 4* - the lymph nodes of the greater curvature, satellites of Winslow's vascular arch, are divided into 4sa (at the level of the short vessels), 4sb (along the left gastroepiploic artery) and 4d (along the right gastroepiploic artery) and they are removed by the dissection of gastro-splenic epiploon and of greater omentum, respectively (figure 35);
- *n. 6* - subpyloric lymph nodes are satellites of the first tract of the gastro-omental right artery. The research of Henle's gastro-colic trunk leads to the ligation of the gastroepiploic right vein, followed by the dissection of the homonymous artery at the origin of the gastroduodenal artery (figure 36);
- The preferential involvement of the inferior para-aortic lymph nodes (n. 16 b1) in tumors of the middle and distal stomach would confirm the existence of a way that, from infrapyloric lymph nodes, leads to that station, through the root of the SMA;

- *n. 7, 8 and 9 - group 7* corresponds to the satellite lymph nodes of the left gastric artery, from its origin from the CT to the terminal portion of its arch along the gastro-pancreatic fold of Huschke, whose dissection allows the excision. The lymph nodes of *group 8* (divided into 8a: anterior and 8p: posterior) follow the common hepatic artery until the emergence of the gastroduodenal artery. The dissection begins at this level in the duodenopancreatic ligament and continues toward the CT, where is located *station 9*, which is removed resecting the connective tissue placed around the celiac artery and the diaphragmatic pillars. The gastric mobilization resulting from the duodenum and epiploon dissection facilitates the excision of these groups (figure 37-39);

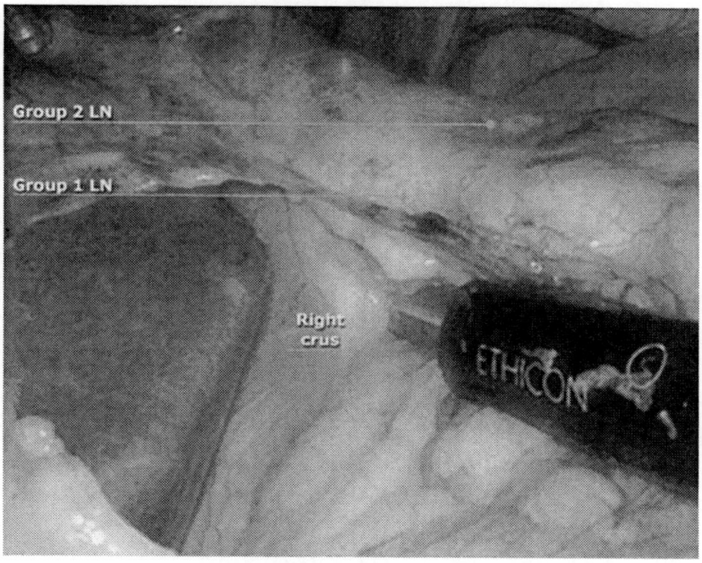

Figure 33. Right and left pericardial LN - groups 1-2.

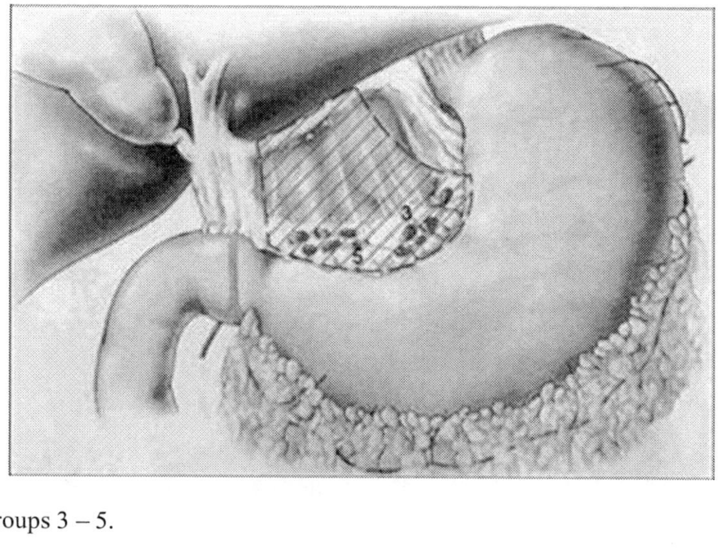

Figure 34. LN groups 3 – 5.

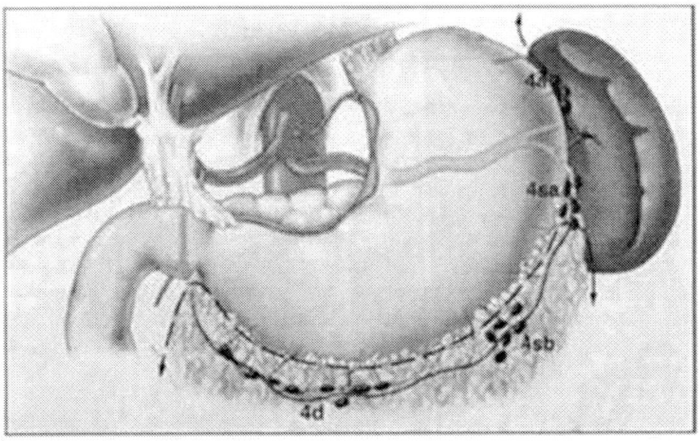

Figure 35. LN group 4 4sa – 4sb – 4d.

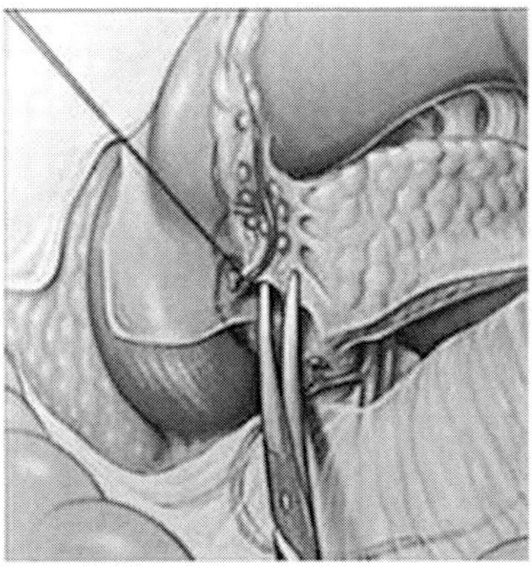

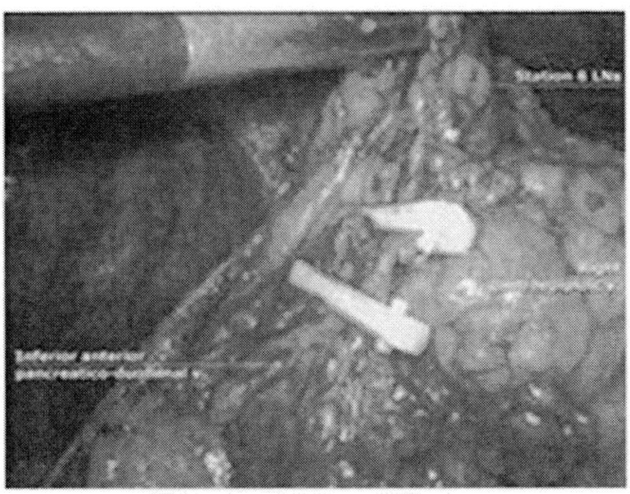

Figure 36. Dissection of Henle's trunk and right gastroepiploic vessels - sub-pyloric LN station.

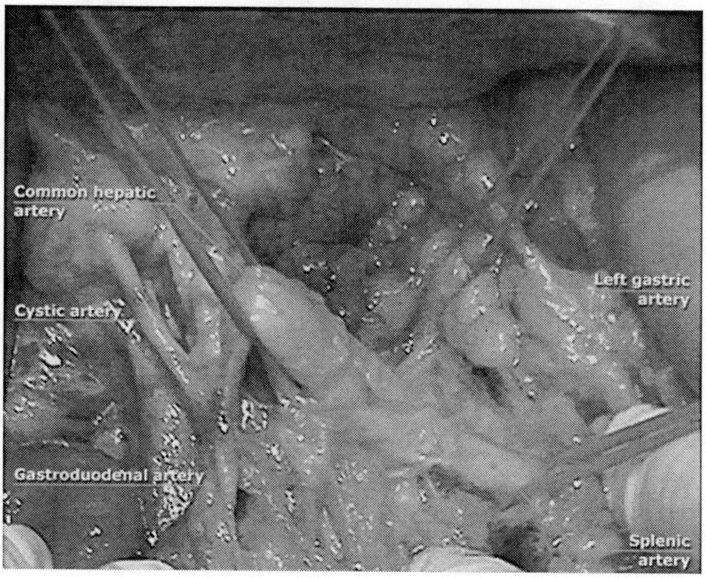

Figure 37. Celiac artery dissection of lesser omentum.

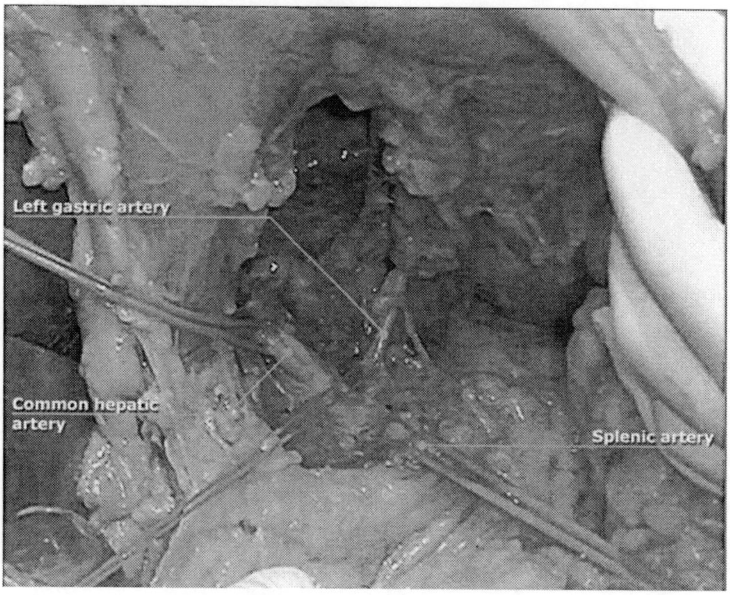

Figure 38. Celiac trunk seen within omental bursa.

- *n. 2* - left paracardial lymph nodes are satellites of the cardiotuberosity branches of the left inferior phrenic artery and it is necessary to mobilize the cardia, to expose the retroperitoneum of the posterior mesogastrium, for their removal. There is also a preferential lymphatic way that from the paracardial lymph nodes, is directed to the retroperitoneal lymphatic stations and to superior para-aortic lymph nodes (16a), following the branches of the inferior phrenic artery designed to the adrenal area and, backward, to the posterior gastric artery (figure 40);

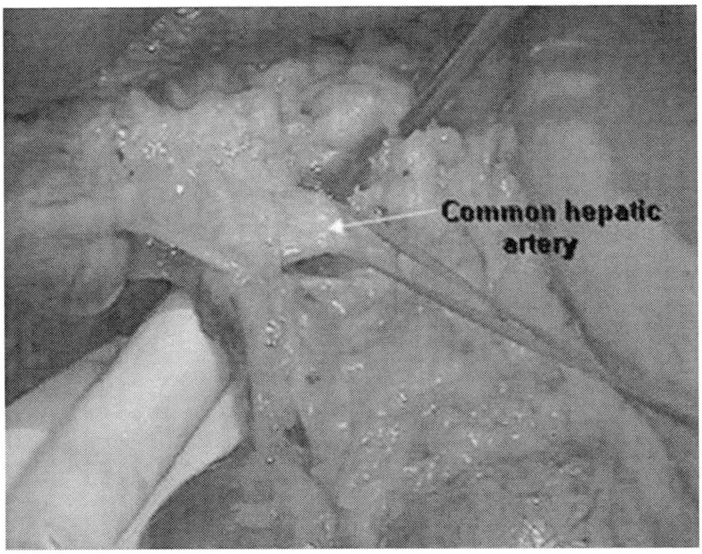

Figure 39. LN group 8.

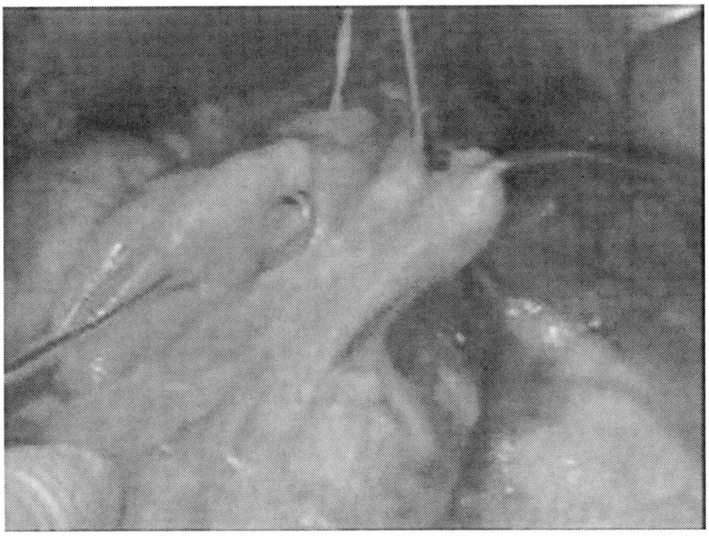

Figure 40. Left pericardial LN - group 2.

- *n. 10 and 11* - the dissection of the splenic hilum lymph node (10) usually requires the splenectomy, while the excision of the chain of the splenic artery (11p: proximal lymph nodes and 11d: distal lymph nodes respect to the origin of the posterior gastric artery) can be performed either by distal splenopancreatectomy, either with *pancreas-preserving* technique, or by Jinnai's maneuver that, through the mobilization of the spleno-pancreatic block, allows the emptying of the lymph nodes placed along the splenic artery and at the hilum with preservation of the spleen. A left splenopancreatectomy is indicated only in cases of macroscopic infiltration of the pancreas (suspected T4), otherwise it is better to perform a splenectomy with *pancreas-preserving technique*. The assumptions of this technique are the following:

after adequate mobilization of the distal splenopancreatic block, the block formed by the spleen, by the tract of the splenic artery distal to the origin of the pancreatic magna artery (great pancreatic artery) and by the 10 and 11 lymphatic stations, is removed. The splenic artery is ligated and divided after the origin of the pancreatic magna artery to preserve the vascularization of the pancreatic body-tail and the splenic vein is sectioned at the pancreatic tail as for a classical splenectomy (figure 41-42).

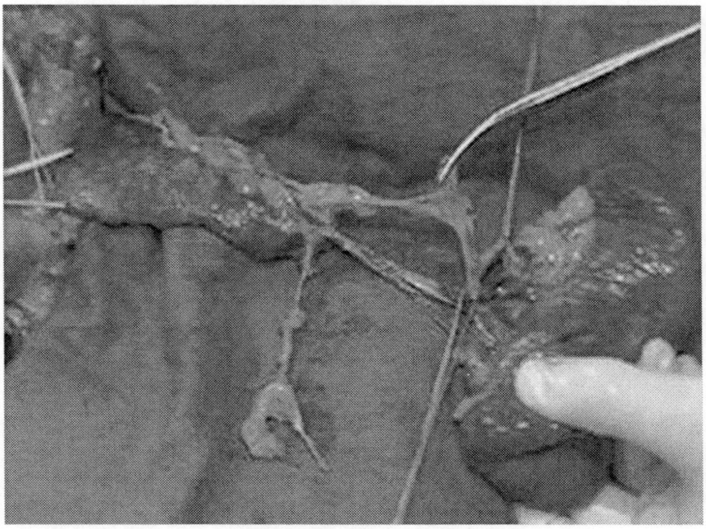

Figure 41. Dissection of LN splenic stations – groups 11 (11p - 11d) and 10 (a).

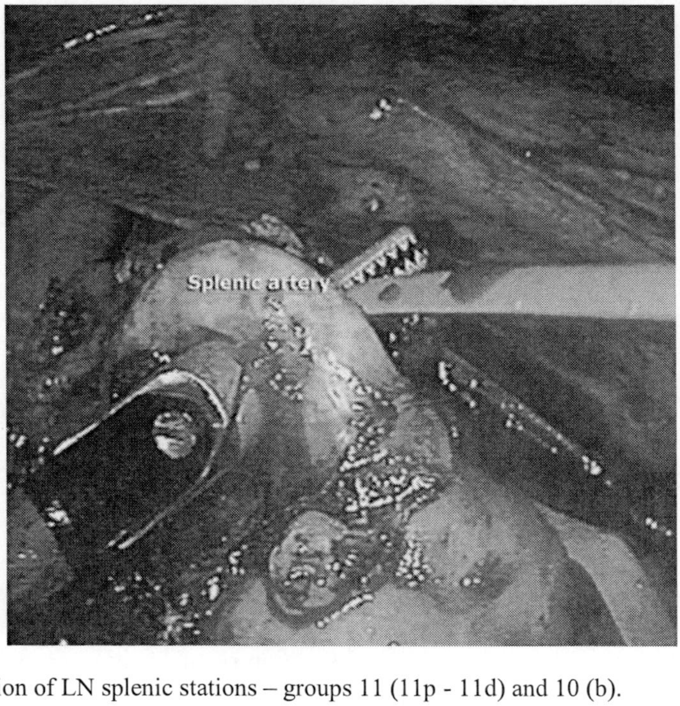

Figure 42. Dissection of LN splenic stations – groups 11 (11p - 11d) and 10 (b).

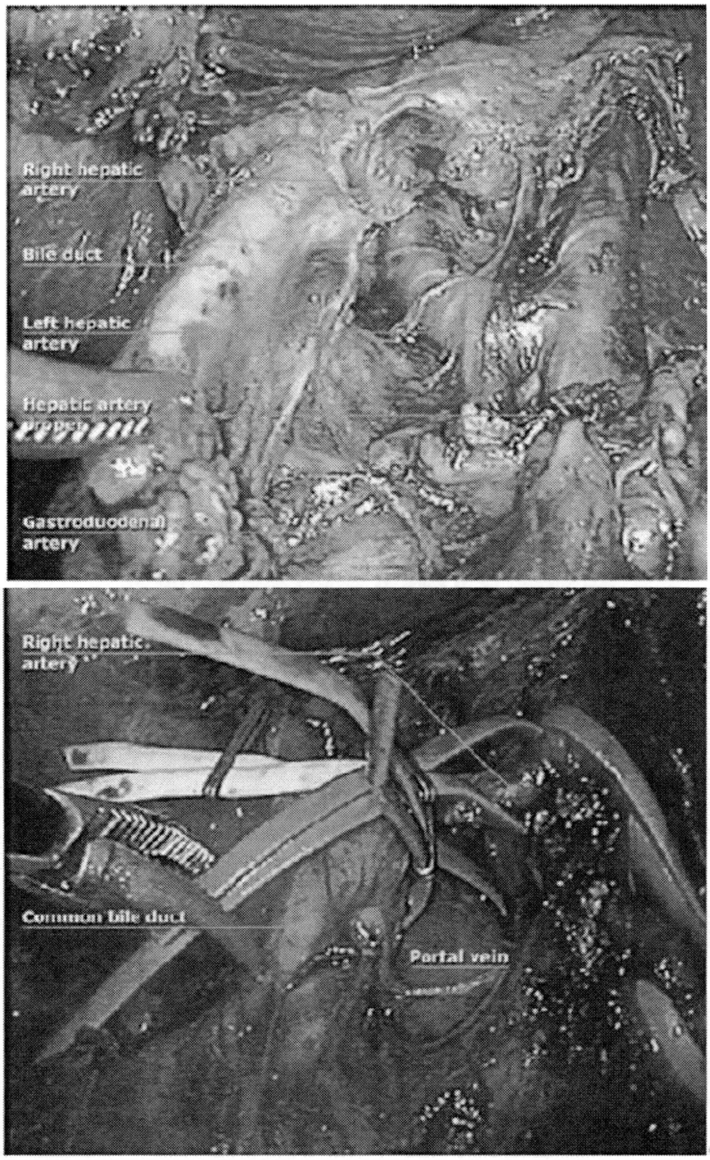

(a)

(b)

Figure 43. Dissection of LN stations of the hepatoduodenal ligament.

- *n. 12* - the lymphatic dissection of the hepatoduodenal ligament (12a: lymph nodes of the hepatic artery, 12b: choledocic lymph nodes, 12p: portal or foraminal lymph nodes, 12c: Mascagni cystic lymph node) results in skeletonization of the hepatic pedicle from the hilum to the retropancreatic area. The possible presence of an aberrant right hepatic artery or of an anterior portal vein requires special care (figure 43).
- *n. 13* - the mobilization of the duodeno-pancreatic block in the plane of Treitz's fascia (Kocher maneuver or process of Wiart and Vautrin) exposes the posterior surface of the pancreatic head, where at the level of the posterior pancreatic-duodenal arteries this station is located. The dissection of this station requires caution due to the risk of pancreatic fistula (figure 44);

- *n. 14 and 15* - the dissection of the lymph nodes located at the mesenteric root along the SMV (14v) and the SMA (14a) occurs in the submesocolic pre-duodeno-pancreatic fascia of Fredet which can be accessed by mobilizing the right colic angle and the proximal tract of the transverse colon. The dissection of the satellite lymph nodes of the middle colic vessels (15) requires the removal of the upper layer of the transverse mesocolon and must be continued along the middle colic vein until the trunk of Henle, which leads to the SMV (figure 45);
- *n. 16* - para-aortic lymph nodes are divided into 4 levels in the craniocaudal direction:

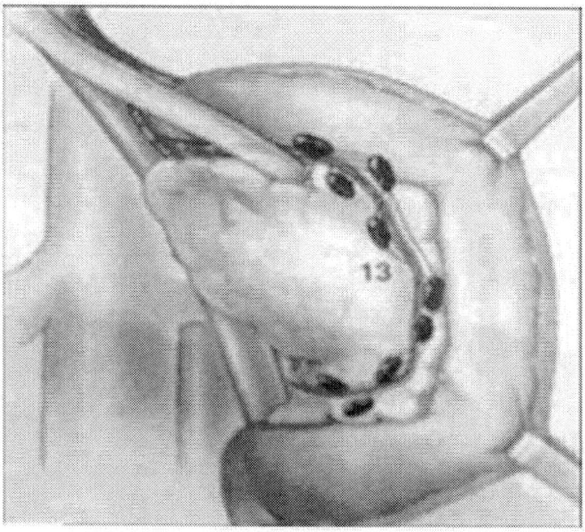

Figure 44. Dissection of LN retrocephalopancreatic station - group 13.

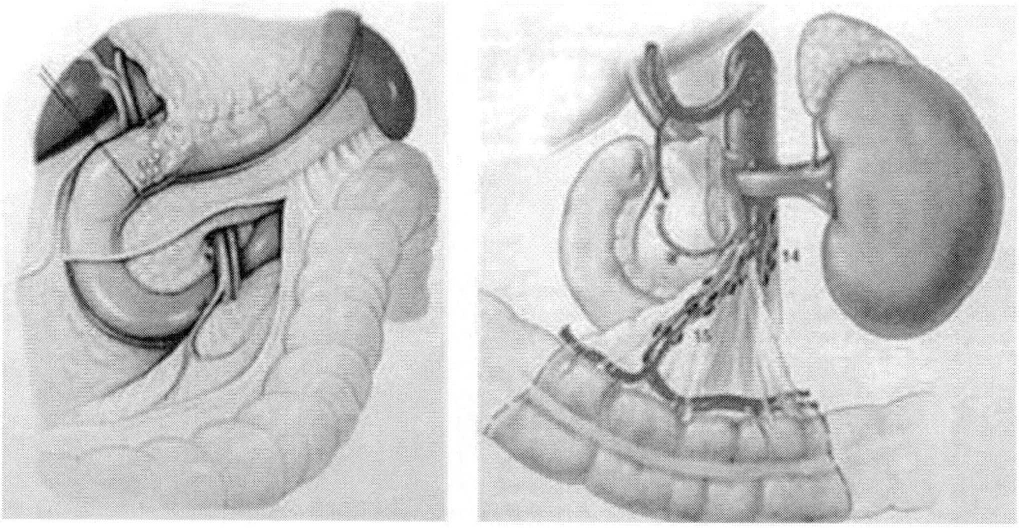

Figure 45. Dissection of Fredet's area – LN groups 14 (14 v-14 a)-15.

- a1: from the inferior border of the esophageal hiatus to the origin of the CT;
- a2: from the origin of the CT to the lower margin of the left renal vein;
- b1: from the lower margin of the left renal vein to the origin of the IMA;
- b2: from the IMA origin to the aortic bifurcation.

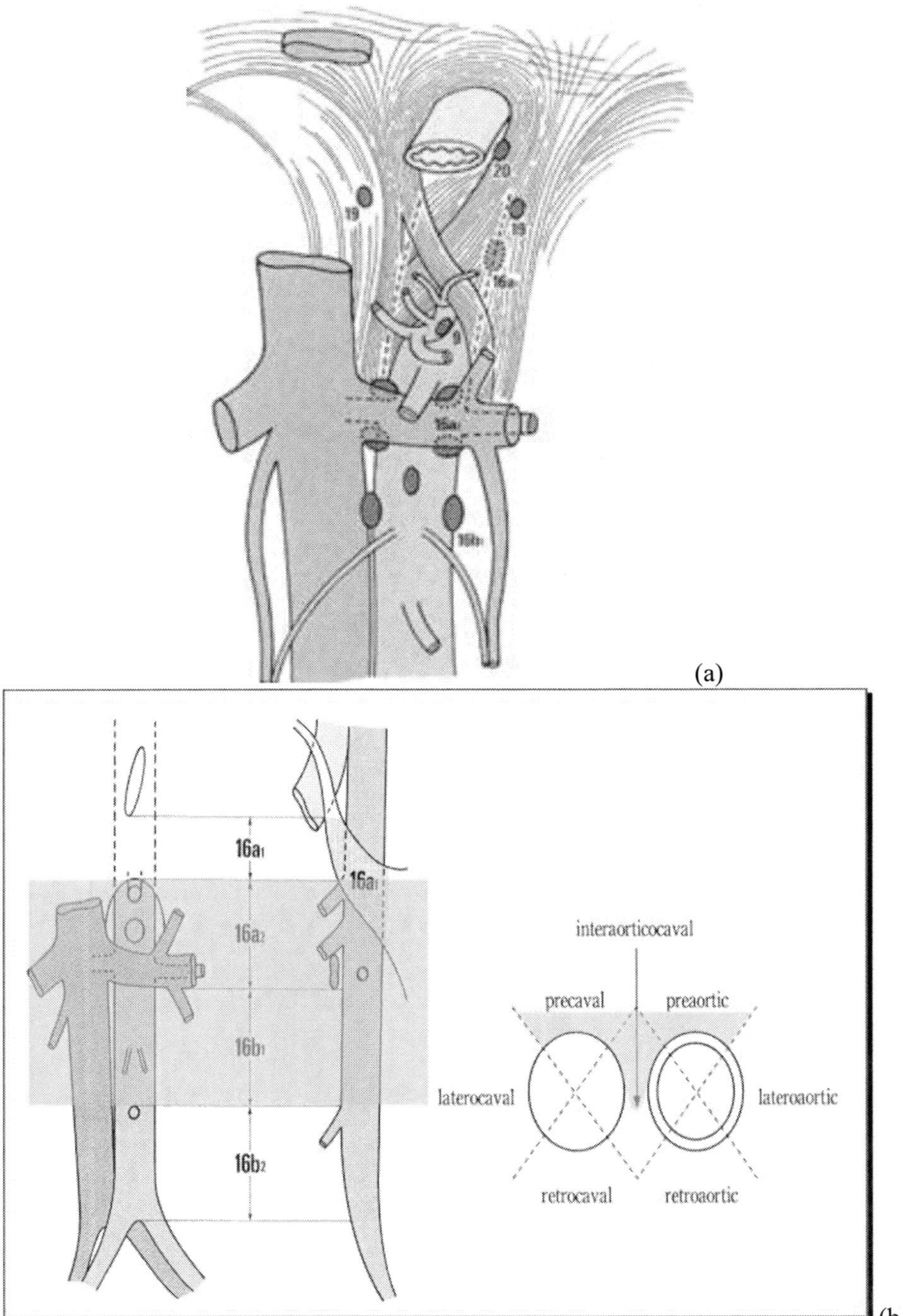

Figure 46. Dissection of LN paraortic stations – groups 16a1, 16 a2, 16b1, 16b2.

As regards to the inferior vena cava and the aorta, paraaortic lymph nodes are divided into 7 sectors: interaortocaval, laterocaval, retrocaval, precaval, lateroaortic, retroaortic and preaortic lymph nodes. During a D3 lymphectomy, the interaortocaval and lateroaortic lymph nodes between the esophageal hiatus and IMA must be removed.

In particular, the dissection of lymph nodes 16a1 (interaortocaval and lateroaortic) requires the complete mobilization of the left kidney (Mattox's maneuver) and the removal of the ipsilateral adrenal gland, with complete skeletonization of the left diaphragmatic pillar.

During the dissection of lymphatic station 16a2, after Jinnai's maneuver, great caution is necessary during the dissection of the left renal vein, as the great lumbar lymphatic trunks afferent to the cistern of Pecquet run after it and for the frequent presence of the freno-azygos-lumbar vein trunk of Lejars that ends up on its posterior wall, and for the proximity of the left lumbar sympathetic chain (figure 46).

The classification of the JRSGC also includes the following nodal stations:

- *n. 17* - lymph nodes placed on the anterior surface of the pancreatic head
- *n. 18* - lymph nodes along the inferior margin of the pancreas
- *n. 19* – infra-diaphragmatic lymph nodes (along the course of the left inferior phrenic artery)
- *n. 20* - lymph nodes of esophageal hiatus of the diaphragm
- *n. 110* - distal thoracic paraesophageal lymph nodes
- *n. 111* – supra-diaphragmatic lymph nodes
- *n. 112* - posterior mediastinal lymph nodes

In the treatment of gastric cancer in stage II (T1N2 - T2N1 - T3N0) D2-D3 lymph node dissection associated with total gastrectomy (TG) or subtotal gastrectomy (STG) showed a satisfactory local control of the disease and an acceptable survival.

If a super-extended lymphadenectomy should be necessary, the dissection of stations 16 a1, a2 and b1 requires many procedures, such as the posterior mesogastric mobilization and the maneuvers of Jinnai, Mattox, Cattell and Kocher which allow a wide access to the retroperitoneal space and, in particular, to the para-aortic lymphatic stations.

Surgical Maneuvers

The surgical manoeuvres described above are based on precise embryologic and anatomical grounds, allowing the dissection to proceed along specific ontogenetic planes with full respect of all organs and tissues.

Gastric Derotation – Mesogastrectomy

The total mesogastric detachment is obtained associating the derotation of mesogastric area to the mobilization of the duodeno-cephalo-pancreatic block. In this way, the embryonic layout is reproduced: the greater curvature is situated in the upper-posterior side together with greater omentum, spleen and pancreatic body-tail. The lesser curvature with the duodenum and the pancreatic head are located forward and down.

The derotation of the mesogastric area begins with colo-epiploic and epiploic-mesocolon dissection and, advancing in the sub-retro-supra-pancreatic plane of mesogastric fascia, comes to the fixed area of the gastric fundus (embryonic access to the retrocavity of the epiploon and to the mesogastric retroperitoneum).

Then the splenic posterior peritoneal attachment is dissected and the spleno-phrenic and gastro-phrenic ligaments are divided proceeding to the mobilization of the spleno-pancreatic block in the plane of the mesogastric fascia. The dissection is pushed medially to the plane of the pancreatic isthmus, where the mesogastric fascia and the posterior mesogastric area end (Figure 47).

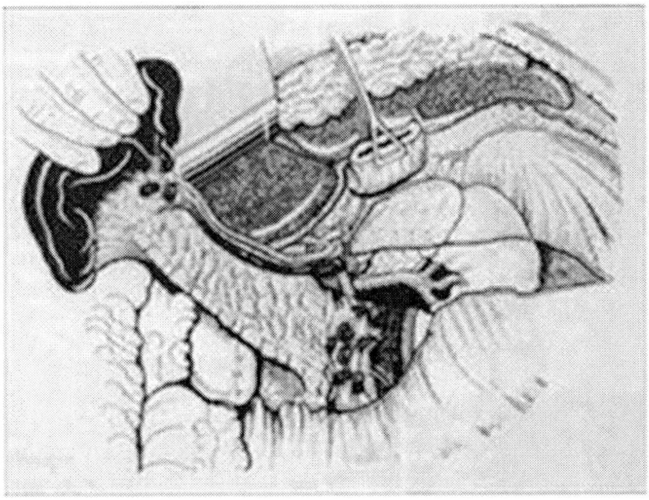

Figure 47. Dissection of the posterior mesogastrium – mesogastrectomy.

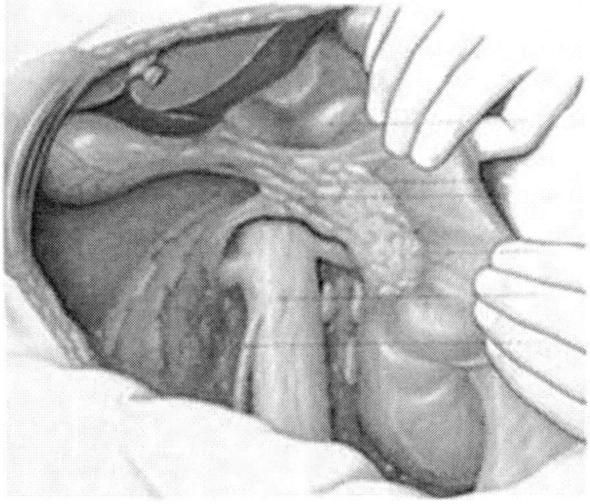

Figure 48. Kocher's maneuver.

Duodeno-Pancreatic Detachment: Kocher's Maneuver

This maneuver, described by Lane and Kocher, mobilizes the head of the pancreas and the duodenal loop from the underlying plane of the inferior vena cava (IVC). In this way the plane between retroduodenopancreatic fascia of Treitz and Gerota's fascia is exposed. Kocher's manoeuvre can be extended to the midline to fully expose the IVC, the renal veins, the aorta and the SMA (supramesocolic access acc. to Borelly).

The duodenal loop and pancreatic head turned over medially and to the left show their posterior surface allowing full access to the retropancreatic and choledocal LN, in the so called Quénu quadrilateral (Wiart and Vautrin maneuver (Figure 48).

Spleno-Pancreatic Mobilization According to Jinnai

The mobilization of the splenopancreatic complex includes initially the opening of the lesser sac by the separation of the greater omentum from transverse colon and mesocolon; the splenic flexure is mobilized by dividing the phrenocolic ligament (*sustentaculum lienis*) and the splenocolic ligament (Tillaux's ligament); the greater curvature is mobilized by dividing the gastro-splenic ligament. The posterior peritoneum is divided along the inferior margin of body and tail of the pancreas, corresponding to the insertion of the root of the transverse mesocolon to the inferior margin of the pancreas.

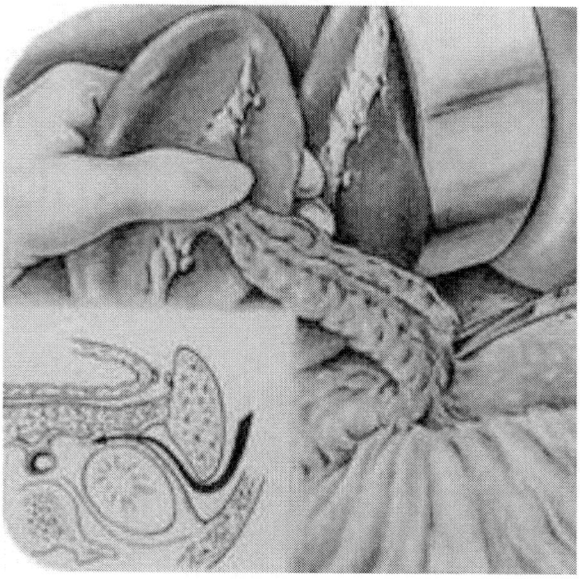

Figure 49. Jinnai's maneuver.

This section starts at the left border of SMV and continues leftwards along the inferior margin of the pancreas and the posterior margin of the spleen, from lower to upper pole. The dissection proceeds by dividing the posterior leaflet of the splenopancreatic ligament and separating the splenopancreatic complex along the plane between the mesogastric fascia investing the pancreatic vessels and the posterior abdominal wall. The mobilization continues medially to the confluence of the splenic vein and SMV. The splenopancreatic complex is exteriorized allowing to the dissection of the splenic artery and the splenic hilar LN with conservation of the spleen. Jinnai's manoeuvre and splenic LN dissection are too difficult to be done laparoscopically. Maruyama's technique *(pancreas preserving)* is to be preferred: the middle and distal parts of the splenic artery, with its dense network of peri-pancreatic lymphatics are removed with the spleen, resulting in an oncologically satisfactory lymphadenectomy (Figure 49).

Access to the Omental Bursa and to Mesogastric Retroperitoneum

The detachment of the greater omentum from the transverse colon and mesocolon represents our first choice and is fully respectful of the embryonic planes. It is therefore possible, advancing in the plane of the mesogastric fascia first below, then behind and above the pancreas, to obtain the full detachment of the territory derived from the posterior mesogastrium (Figure 50).

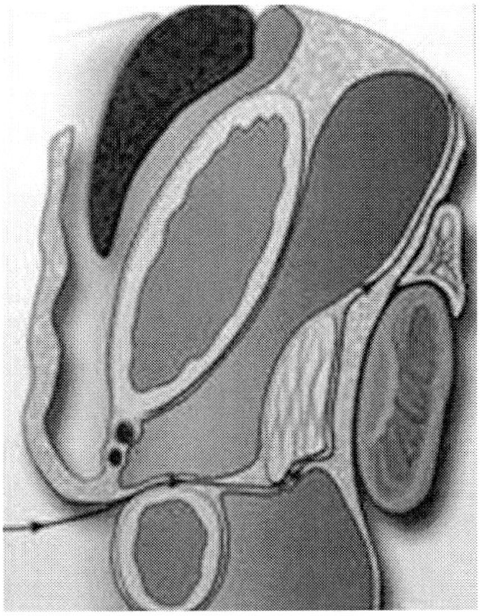

Figure 50. Access to omental bursa following dissection along megastric fascia.

Derotation of the Middle Bowel or Umbilical Loop

Two very similar techniques described by Cattell-Braasch and by Valdoni obtain the same result of de-rotating the territory of the common mesentery, also called midgut or umbilical loop.

The maneuver includes the following steps:

- Mobilization of the ascending colon along the plane between Toldt's and Gerota's fasciae. In this way the right ureter and gonadal vessels are separated from the mesocolic plane;

- section of the secondary root of the mesentery, separated from the posterior abdominal wall up to the third part of the duodenum, just below the superior mesenteric vessels;
- mobilization of the hepatic flexure and the right half of transverse colon along the plane of the preduodenopancreatic inframesocolic fascia of Fredet and supramesocolic omental fascia; the anterior surface of the pancreatic head and the second part of duodenum are exposed;
- duodenopancreatic mobilization (Kocher's or Wiart's maneuvers);
- separation of the greater omentum from the transverse colon and mesocolon: the dissection is continued by dividing the posterior lamina of the greater omentum to enter the lesser sac or by advancing in the plane of the supramesocolic fascia of the posterior omental lamina;
- mobilization of the duodenojejunal junction: the muscle of Treitz is divided, the fourth part of the duodenum is freed, being careful not to damage the IMV and the vascular arch of Treitz;
- derotation according to Valdoni: the entire intestine, corresponding to the primitive umbilical loop, is completely freed from its attachments to the posterior parietal peritoneum, and remains hanging on its vascular pedicle, reproducing the condition called *mesenterium commune.* To obtain this result, the small bowel loops are rotated and brought to the right passing underneath the SMA. In so doing the second, third and fourth part of duodenum and the first jejunal loop will sit in a para-medial sagittal line to the right of the superior mesenteric vessels. The remaining small bowel loops will go to the right, while the right and transverse colon will move to the left. As a consequence the SMA will move to the right of the SMV (Figure 51).

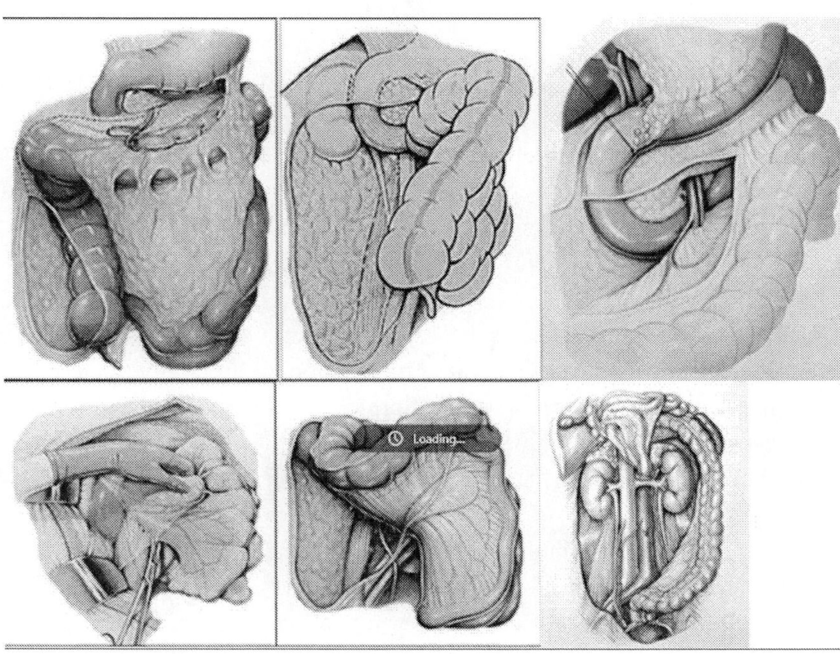

Figure 51. Access to the aortocaval plane according to Cattell-Valdoni maneuver.

Mattox's Maneuver

This was developed to expose the suprarenal aorta but can be used to dissect the lymphatic station 16a.

All abdominal viscera including the left kidney are mobilized and moved to the right resulting in excellent exposure of the aorta, CA, SMA and renal arteries. A similar access was described by Benjamin-Jackson to expose extraperitoneally the CA and SMA (Figure 52).

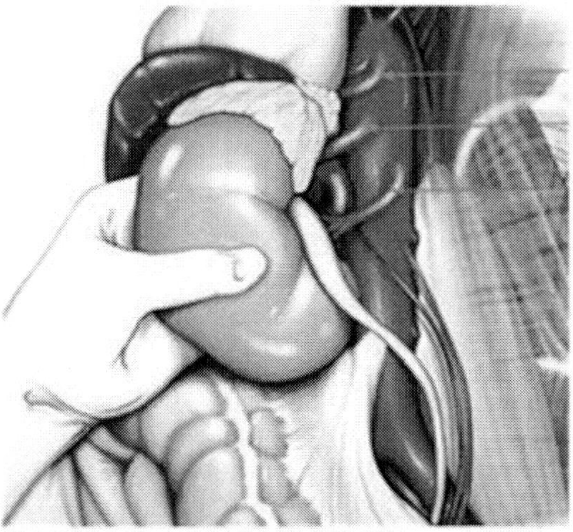

Figure 52. Mattox maneuver.

References

Bouchet A. Structure et vascularisation du grand épiploon, *Arch. Anat. Strasbourg.*, 1962, 45: 1-31.

Chiarugi L. Istituzioni di Anatomia dell'uomo. Vol. III, Soc. Ed. Libraria, Milano, 1944.

Corcione F, Miranda L, Ruotolo F. Chirurgia laparoscopica. Dall'anatomia alla tecnica chirurgica standardizzata. Idelson-Gnocchi, Napoli, 2008.

Cordiano C, De Manzoni G, Guglielmi A. Il trattamento del carcinoma gastrico. 98° Congr. SIC, Roma, 1996.

Cunéo B, Delamare G: Les lymphatiques de l'estomac. Journ. de l'Anat. et de la Phys., 1900.

D'annibale A, Pende V, Pernazza G et al. Full robotic gastrectomy with extended (D2) lymphadenectomy for gastric cancer: Surgical technique and preliminary results. *Journal of Surgical Research*, 2011; 166, 113-120.

Fredet P: Le péritoine in Traité d'Anatomie humaine de Poirier et Charpy. T. 4, 3 facs, Paris Masson Ed., 1905.

Guadagni S et al. Arterial vasculature of the stomach and oncologic gastrectomies. *Surg. Radiol. Anat.*, 1995; 17: 269-276.

Gullino D. Chirurgia del peritoneo e del sottoperitoneo. Trattato di Tecnica Chirurgica, vol. VIII, UTET, Torino, 1988.

Huschke E. Traité de splanchnologie. Enciclopedia anatomica. Paris, 1848.

Jinnai D, Ono M, Sakakibara N. *The necessity of the extended radical gastrectomy for gastric cancer*. Geke, 1961; 23: 1099-1107.

JRSGC. Japanese classification of gastric cancer. 1st english edition. Tokyo: Kanehara and Co, 1995.

Kosaka T et al. Lymphatic routes of the stomach demostrated by gastric carcinoma with solitary lymphonode metastasis. *Surg. Today*, 1999; 29: 695-700.

Leriche R, Villemin F. Recherches anatomiques sur les artères de l'estomac, *Biblio anat.,* 1907, 16: 111-125.

Levasseur Jc, Couinaud C. Etude de la distribution des artères gastriques. Incidences chirurgicales. *J. Chir.*, 1968, 95: 57-58 et 161-176.

Maruyama K et al. Lymph node metastases of gastric cancer. General pattern in 1931 patiens. *Ann Surg.,* 1989; 210:596-602.

Mattox KL. Management of upper abdominal vascular trauma. *Am. J. Surg*., 1974, 128: 823

Merkel FR. Trattato di Anatomia Topografica. Vol. II, UTET, Torino, 1903.

Rouvière H. Les lymphatiques de l'homme. Masson, Paris, 1932

Ruotolo F, Hüscher CGS et al. Anatomia chirurgica in Chirurgia laparoscopica dello stomaco, SVP, Padova, 2003.

Skandalakis JE. Surgical Anatomy. *The Embryologic and Anatomic Basis of Modern Surgery. V*ol. II, PMP, 2004.

Siewert JR et al. Problems of proximal third gastric carcinoma. *World J. Surg*., 1995; 19: 523-531.

Tandler J. Über die Varietaten der Arteria Coeliaca und derm Etwickelung. *Anat. Hefte*, 1904 ; 25: 472.

Testut L, Jacob O. Anatomia Topografica. Vol.II, UTET, Torino, 1922

Toldt C. Darmgekröse und Netze im gesetzmässigen und gesetzwidrigen Zustand: Wien, 1889.

Treitz W. Ueber einen neuen Muskel am Duodenum des Menschen, uber elastische Sehnen und einige andere anatomiche Verhaltuisse. Prager Vierteljahrscrift, XXXVII, Prague, 113-144, 1853.

Valdoni P. Chirurgia addominale. Tecniche operatorie. Vallardi Ed, Milano 1974.

Whalter AF. De arteriis caeliacis. Lipsia, 1729.

In: Gastric Cancer
Editors: A. D'Annibale, V. Pende and I. Monsellato
ISBN: 978-1-62081-294-5

Chapter II

Gastric Cancer Staging

Matthew Dixon[1], Wiley Chung[2] and Natalie Coburn[2]
[1]Department of Surgery, Maimonides Medical Center, Brooklyn, NY, US
[2]Department of Surgery, University of Toronto, Toronto, Ontario, Canada

Abstract

Worldwide, gastric adenocarcinoma is one of the most commonly found malignancies, and one of the most common causes of cancer-related death. Resection is the fundamental curative option for these patients while adjuvant therapies have also improved survival. Accurate staging forms the basis for which treatments are based. An understanding of the staging systems commonly used is important for physicians involved in the treatment of gastric cancer, and are reviewed. In addition, several staging modalities are routinely prescribed in an attempt to accurately stage the patient with gastric cancer. Each of these staging modalities has their own benefits and drawbacks with varying degrees of accuracy, sensitivity and specificity. The following staging modalities will be reviewed in detail: computed tomography, magnetic resonance imaging, abdominal ultrasound, ^{18}Fluorodeoxyglucose-positron emission tomography, esophagogastroduodenoscopy, endoscopic ultrasound, staging laparoscopy, and peritoneal cytology. The ultimate goal is correlation between staging modalities and pathology findings such that accurate staging is performed with delivery of the most appropriate stage-specific treatment.

Introduction

Surgical and endoscopic resections are the only curative treatments for gastric adenocarcinoma. In recent years, the addition of adjuvant therapies has demonstrated an improvement in overall survival [1-4], but this has increased the complexity of clinical decision-making. Management decisions for the treatment of gastric cancer by a multidisciplinary team are stage-specific and thus rely heavily on accurate staging. Inappropriate staging and pre-operative planning could potentially lead to under-staging, resulting in positive resection margins, or an unnecessary laparotomy for patients with incurable disease. It is also possible for patients to be over-staged, leading to the unfortunate circumstance of a potentially curative patient being incorrectly recommended for palliation rather than surgical resection.

Staging Systems

Two staging systems for gastric cancer have been proposed: the Tumor-Node-Metastasis (TNM) staging system outlined by the Union International Contre le Cancer (UICC) / American Joint Committee on Cancer (AJCC) [5] and the Japanese classification of gastric cancer as defined by the Japanese Gastric Cancer Association (JGCA) [6]. The two systems are similar, as they both describe the depth of the primary tumor invasion, the extent of lymph node (LN) involvement, and the presence or absence of distant metastasis.

UICC/AJCC T Stage

The T component of the TNM staging system corresponds to the depth of tumor invasion within the corresponding organ. The deeper the tumor invades into the wall of the organ, the higher the T stage it is assigned. In the updated 7th edition of the AJCC staging manual, the T categories for gastric cancer have been modified to be consistent with those corresponding to cancers of the esophagus and small and large intestine.

A stage of T0 is assigned when there is no evidence of a primary tumor. Tis, represents carcinoma in situ, where the pathology demonstrates malignant cells which have not yet violated the basement membrane of the mucosa. Any tumor greater than Tis has violated the basement membrane and is considered to be a malignant lesion. T1a lesions are confined to the mucosa, while T1b lesions have invaded through the mucosa into the submucosa. It can be important to differentiate between T1a and T1b lesions, as some T1a lesions may be amenable to endoscopic resection. If T1a lesions contain well to moderately differentiated adenocarcinoma or papillary carcinoma, is <2 cm in diameter and non-ulcerated, or ≤1 cm and flat and depressed, and with no venous or lymphatic involvement, these lesions are amendable to endoscopic resection as opposed to gastrectomy. Expanded criteria include ulcerated lesions ≤3 cm in addition to T1b lesions only if the cancer invades the upper 1/3 of the submucosa [7]. From a series of 1549 cases of surgically resected patients, the median 5-year survival of patients with T1a and T1b lesions are 90.2% and 86.7%, respectively [8] (Figure 1). When a cancer invades through the submucosa and into the muscularis propria, it is classified as a T2 lesion. The median 5-year survival of patients with these lesions is 75.2%. T3 lesions invade the subserosa, but do not invade the serosa or any of the structures adjacent to the stomach.

The median 5-year survival of these patients is 54.9%. T4 lesions, the highest classification assigned, are split into two subcategories. T4a lesions invade through the serosa and are exposed to the peritoneal cavity. T4b lesions are cancers that not only invade through the serosa, but invade adjacent structures as well. The 5-year survival of patients with T4a and T4b lesions are 31.1% and 17.5%, respectively (Figure 1).

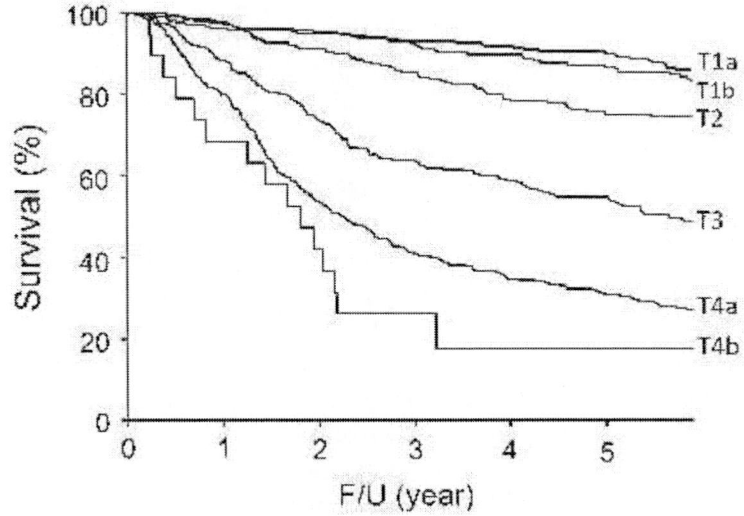

Figure 1. Kaplan-Meier cure of 5-year survival of patients with gastric cancer by T-stage. (From Fang WL, Huang KH, et al. *World J Surg*. 2011;35(12):2723-9).

Table 1. T staging of gastric cancer

T Stage	Description
TX	The primary tumor is not feasible
T0	No evidence of a primary tumor
Tis	Carcinoma in situ
T1	Tumor invasion of the lamina propria, muscularis mucosa, or submucosa
	T1a: Tumor invasion of the lamina propria or muscularis mucosa
	T1b: Tumor invasion of the submucosa
T2	Tumor invasion of the muscularis propria
T3	Tumor penetration of the subserosal connective tissue without evidence of visceral peritoneum or adjacent structures
T4	Tumor invasion of serosa or adjacent structures
	T4a: Tumor invasion of serosa
	T4b: Tumor invasion of adjacent structures

Knowledge of a tumor being classified as T4b can be crucial in pre-operative planning, as these lesions may require a multivisceral resection. For example, if a tumor is found to be invading the tail of the pancreas or colon, then en-bloc resection will be necessary for curative intent [9].

Similarly, if a tumor is found to be invading the head of the pancreas, then gastrectomy with en bloc pancreaticoduodenectomy could be considered for curative intent in selected patients [10].

Survival in these advanced cases is also influenced by burden of LN involvement, with most authors suggesting that a multi-visceral approach should be undertaken when five or fewer LN are involved with cancer [9-14]. In these cases of advanced disease, a neoadjuvant approach may be considered.

UICC/AJCC N Stage

The N component of the TNM staging system corresponds to the degree to which LN harbor gastric cancer. Nodal status is one of the most important prognostic indicators in many cancers, including gastric cancer.

The UICC/AJCC have evolved their classification system for N staging in gastric cancer. Prior to 1997, nodal staging was based upon the distance of involved LN to the primary cancer. In order to improve the ability to reliably compare nodal stage between series and institutions, to align the staging of gastric cancer to that of other gastrointestinal malignancies, and to minimize the impact of surgical dissection, in the fifth edition, the AJCC/UICC recommended that N stage be based upon the number of LN involved. They recommended a minimum of 15 LN to be assessed with N1 = 1–6 positive LN; N2 = 7–15 positive LN; and N3 = more than 15 positive LN. The cut-points were derived from retrospective databases [15]. Subsequent examinations [16, 17] have demonstrated the superior predictive ability of LN staging based on number of nodes involved rather than location of nodal involvement [18]. Part of the superior predictive ability has been attributed to the category N3 (>15 LN positive), a group with extremely poor prognosis. In the 7th edition, the UICC/AJCC revised the nodal classification system such that N1 = 1–2 positive LN; N2 = 3-6 positive LN; N3a = 7-15 positive LN; and N3b = 16 or more positive LN [19].

As such, the UICC/AJCC now recommends that a minimum of 16 LN be assessed for accurate nodal staging [20]. Unfortunately, if an inadequate number of LN are assessed, significant stage migration can occur [21, 22]. An appropriately performed resection should yield enough LN for adequate staging, as an average of 15 LN can be harvested from a D1 lymphadenectomy, 27 nodes from a D2 lymphadenectomy, and 43 nodes from a D3 lymphadenectomy [22].

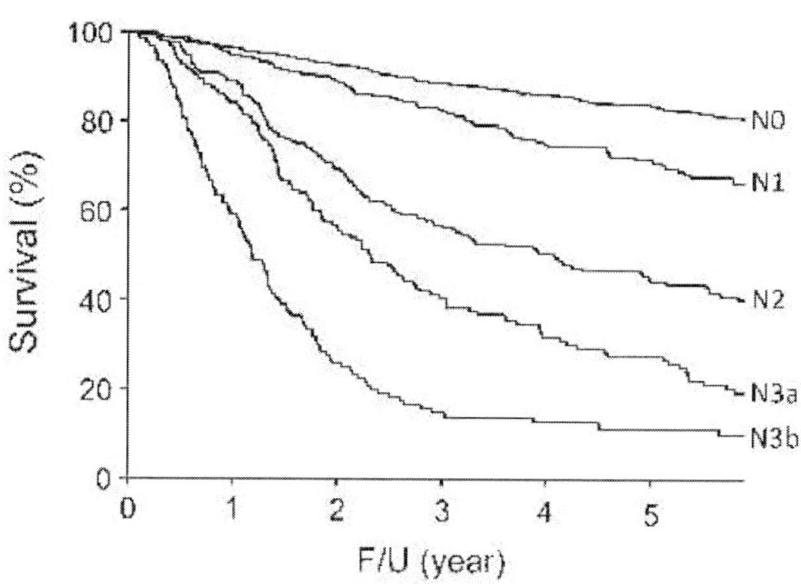

Figure 2. Kaplan-Meier cure of 5-year survival of patients with gastric cancer by N-stage. (From Fang WL, Huang KH, et al. *World J Surg*. 2011;35(12):2723-9).

There is a strong correlation between T and N stages. In patients with disease that is limited to the mucosa (i.e. T1a lesions), there is an approximate 3-5% risk of LN involvement. This risk increases to 11-25% in cases where disease is limited to the submucosa (i.e. T1b lesions). More advanced cancers have a substantial increase in risk of LN involvement, with T2 tumors having a risk of 50%, while T3 tumors have a risk of involvement of 83% [23, 25]. This can be attributed, in part, to the complex lymphatic system of the stomach, which freely communicates with other equally complex intermuscular and subserosal lymphatic networks [26, 27]. 5-year survival rates based on N-stage have also been defined. N0 disease has a 5-year survival of 83.5%; 57.8% for N1; 27.4% for N2, and 11.4% for N3 disease (Figure 2) [5, 8].

UICC/AJCC M Stage

The M component of the TNM staging system corresponds to the presence of any distant metastases, and is denoted as M1. M stage is highly predictive of patient survival. While the 5-year survival of patients with metastatic disease is 7%, those without evidence of metastatic disease have an estimated 5-year survival of up to 78% [28]. Unfortunately, over 30% of patients will have evidence of metastatic disease at presentation [29]. Common manifestations of distant metastases include the presence of liver metastases, ascites, carcinomatosis (diffuse peritoneal metastases), Blummer shelf (palpable mass on rectal examination secondary to drop metastases into the pelvis), Virchow node (palpable supraclavicular LN), or Sister Mary Joseph node (palpable periumbilical mass) [30, 31].

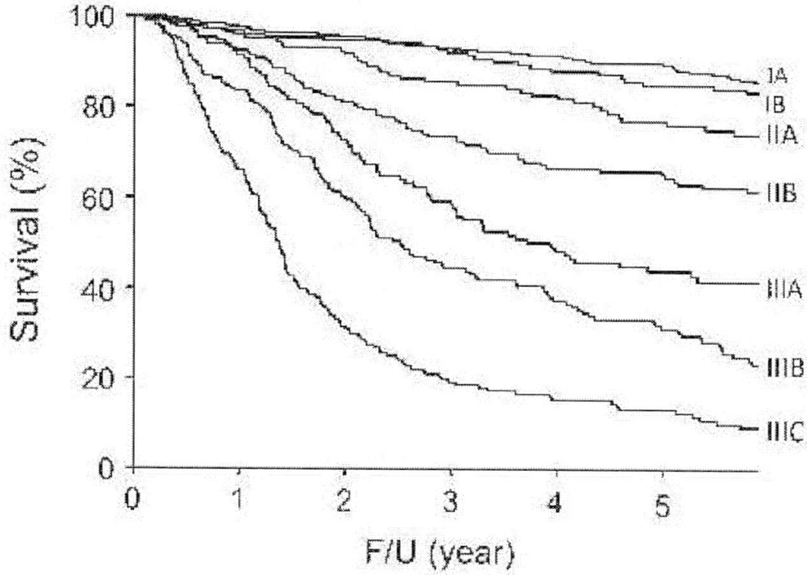

Figure 3. Kaplan-Meier cure of 5-year survival of patients with gastric cancer by Stage. (From Fang WL, Huang KH, et al. *World J Surg*. 2011;35(12):2723-9).

Confirmation of M stage in gastric cancer is a necessary and important component of the staging process. The presence of distant metastases has important implications on treatment.

While patients without evidence of metastatic disease should undergo curative-intent resection and possibly adjuvant therapy, patients with M1 disease should be referred for systemic chemotherapy, clinical trial enrollment, best supportive care or palliative treatments if symptomatic [32].

All of the possible combinations of T, N, and M status have been organized into different stages of disease; stage I disease represents the earliest malignant disease, while stage IV represents metastatic spread. Updates to the 7th edition of the UICC/AJCC staging system include the splitting of stage II disease into stage IIA and stage IIB, and the addition of stage IIIC. Additionally, all TNM stages now considered to be stage IIB were previously classified as stage IIIA, with the exception of T1N3M0, which was previously considered to be stage IV disease.

In the previous edition of the UICC/AJCC staging manual, N3 disease was considered to represent stage IV disease, regardless of T or M stage. This is no longer the case, as now only patients with metastases are considered to have stage IV disease [5]. Figure 3 shows the 5-year survival of patients by each stage with the exception of stage IV.

Japanese Gastric Cancer Association Staging Classification

The JGCA updated their staging classification system in 2011 with the release of the 3rd edition [6], which is very similar to the 7th edition of the UICC/AJCC.

However, the JGCA classification system offers more detailed descriptions of the cancer than the TNM staging system. The primary tumor is described in the JGCA by six characteristics: (1) size and number of lesions, (2) tumor location, (3) macroscopic types, (4) histological classification, (5) depth of tumor invasion, and (6) cancer stromal volume, infiltrative pattern, and capillary invasion.

For the size and number of lesions, the tumor is described in its two greatest dimensions. If there are multiple lesions, then the largest of the lesions is classified.

In describing the tumor's location, the stomach is anatomically divided into three areas: the upper (U), middle (M) and lower (L) portions. Gastric cancers are then described by the area of the stomach involved by tumor. In cases where the tumor involves more than one portion of the stomach, those portions are described in descending order of the degree of involvement, with the portion containing most of the tumor described first.

Table 2. N staging of gastric cancer

N stage	Description
NX	Regional lymph nodes cannot be assessed
N0	No evidence of lymph node metastases
N1	Metastases in ≤2 regional lymph nodes
N2	Metastases in 3-6 regional lymph nodes
N3	Metastases in ≥7 regional lymph nodes
	N3a : Metastases in 7-15 regional lymph nodes
	N3b : Metastases in 16 or more regional lymph nodes

Table 3. M staging of gastric cancer

M stage	Description
M0	No evidence of metastases
M1	Evidence of distant metastases

Table 4. TNM staging system of gastric cancer

Stage	T stage	N stage	M stage
Stage 0	Tis	N0	M0
Stage IA	T1	N0	M0
Stage IB	T2	N0	M0
	T1	N1	M0
Stage IIA	T3	N0	M0
	T2	N1	M0
	T1	N2	M0
Stage IIB	T4a	N0	M0
	T3	N1	M0
	T2	N2	M0
	T1	N3	M0
Stage IIIA	T4a	N1	M0
	T3	N2	M0
	T2	N3	M0
Stage IIIB	T4b	N0	M0
	T4b	N1	M0
	T4a	N2	M0
	T3	N3	M0
Stage IIIC	T4b	N2	M0
	T4b	N3	M0
	T4a	N3	M0
Stage IV	Any T	Any N	M1

Table 5. Macroscopic types of gastric cancer

Type	Description
Type 0 (superficial)	Typical of T1 tumor
Type 1 (mass)	Polypoid tumor with sharp demarcation from surrounding mucosa
Type 2 (ulcerative)	Ulcerated tumor with raised margins; surrounded by thickened gastric wall; clear margins
Type 3 (infiltrative ulcerative)	Ulcerated tumor with raised margins; surrounded by thickened gastric wall; unclear margins
Type 4 (diffuse infiltrative)	Marked ulceration or raised margins; gastric wall is thickened and indurated; unclear margin
Type 5 (unclassifiable)	Tumor cannot be classified

For example, if a tumor on the lesser curvature involves the upper and middle portions of the stomach, and most of the tumor is in the middle portion of the stomach, then it is described as MU. The macroscopic type describes the tumor by its appearance, and whether it has an infiltrative or an ulcerative pattern of growth, or a combination of both (Table 5).

Table 6. Tumor infiltrative (INF) pattern into surrounding tissues

Type	Description
INFa	Expanding growth with distinct border from surrounding tissue
INFb	Intermediate pattern between INFa and INFc
INFc	Infiltrative growth with no distinct border with surrounding tissue

Table 7. Lymphatic invasion pattern by gastric tumors

Type	Description
ly0	No lymphatic invasion
ly1	Minimal lymphatic invasion
ly2	Moderate lymphatic invasion
ly3	Marked lymphatic invasion

Table 8. Venous invasion pattern by gastric tumors

Type	Description
v0	No venous invasion
v1	Minimal venous invasion
v2	Moderate venous invasion
v3	Marked venous invasion

For the histological classification system, if there is more than one subtype, the different components are recorded in descending order of the amount of surface area occupied. Additionally, tumors are described by stromal volume, infiltrative pattern and capillary invasion. Stromal volume, which must be recorded for tumors whose depth of invasion are deeper than T1b, are classified by being medullary type (containing scanty stroma), scirrhous type (containing abundant stroma), or intermediate.

Tables 6, 7 and 8 summarize the classification scheme for infiltrative pattern, lymphatic invasion and venous invasion, respectively.

With recent changes, the depth of tumor invasion follows the T staging from the 7th edition of the UICC/AJCC, as outlined in Table 1. The 2nd edition of JGCA described tumor depth of invasion from T1 to T4 without any sub-classification [17]. Thus, differences between the 2nd and 3rd JGCA classifications system include expansion of T1 lesions into T1a and T1b lesions, as well as expansion of T4 lesions into T4a and T4b.

The evolution of the JGCA classification system from the 2nd to the 3rd edition has seen an abandonment of the classification of LN metastases based on anatomic location, and adoption of classification of LN metastases based on the number of involved nodes [6,17]. The 2nd edition of the JCGA system classified LN involvement with respect to anatomic location of the primary tumor. N1 disease was classified as metastases to group 1 nodes, which refer to perigastric nodes. N2 disease was classified as metastases to group 2 nodes, which refer to the nodes along the celiac axis and its branches. Finally, N3 disease was classified as involvement of group 3 nodes, which refer to retropancreatic or para-aortic nodes. Description of N stage by the JGCA currently follows the 7th edition of the UICC/AJCC staging manual (Table 2). Description of M stage by the JGCA classification system also follows the 7th edition of the UICC/AJCC staging manual, as outlined in Table 3. They further sub-classify metastases based on three locations: peritoneal metastases, positive peritoneal cytology, and hepatic metastases. Finally, definition of disease stage is the same as the 7th edition of the UICC/AJCC staging manual (Table 4).

Radiology

Radiological studies have an important role in the staging of gastric cancer. The refinement of technologies allows the examination of gastric cancer with greater resolution, permitting determination of stage with better accuracy.

CT Scan

The computed tomography (CT) scan (Figure 4) is the standard non-invasive imaging modality used in the pre-operative staging of the gastric cancer patient. Although limited in accuracy of determination of T stage [33], it is a powerful tool for examining LN involvement, ascites, pelvic involvement, liver metastases and peritoneal dissemination. Drawbacks of CT include exposure to ionizing radiation and iodine-based intravenous contrast agents, which can potentially result in contrast-induced nephropathy or anaphylaxis [36].

Importantly, there are considerable differences among CT scanners. Traditional single detection CT scanners are limited by large section thickness, low image resolution, and slow scanning, which lead to respiratory motion artifacts. Additionally, traditional CT scanners are unable to provide multi-planar reformations [35, 36], which can be especially useful when planning operative approach. MDCT has improved the speed at which images are acquired (which minimizes or eliminates respiratory motion artifact) [36], and allows for more accurate timing of contrast boluses during arterial, venous or parenchymal phases [37]. MDCT also has improved the spatial resolution and quality of the multi-planar reformation images, allowing the radiologist to choose the optimal imaging plane in which to accurately evaluate tumor depth of invasion of the gastric wall and perigastric fat plane infiltration [35]. Distention of the gastric wall with water or other low attenuation agents and intravenous contrast injection are required for optimal imaging [37]. MDCT has an overall accuracy of T stage determination of 80%. With multi-planar reformation images, this increases to 82% [33]. Determination of N stage with CT, while important, also suffers from low accuracy. The ability of many imaging modalities to detect potentially metastatic nodes is determined primarily by the size of the nodes [38]. It should be noted that not all tumor positive LN are enlarged [39].

Similarly, not all enlarged LN contain metastases [40], making accuracy of N staging suboptimal with any modality that evaluates primarily based upon size or shape criteria, including CT, ultrasound, or MRI.

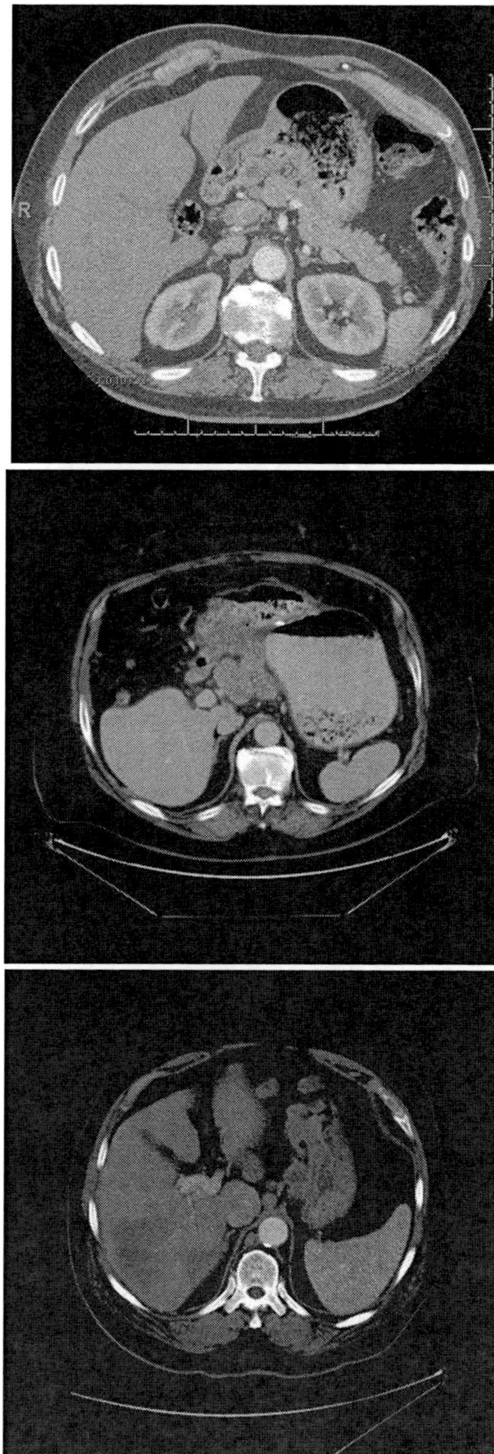

(a)

(b)

(c)

Figure 4. A: CT Abdomen showing gastric cancer (Stage IIA) involving the antrum. (Figure courtesy of Dr. John Hagen, University of Toronto), B: CT Abdomen demonstrating invasion of the neck of the pancreas. (Figure courtesy of Dr. Caitlin McGregor, University of Toronto), C: CT Abdomen demonstrating liver metastases (Figure courtesy of Dr. Caitlin McGregor, University of Toronto).

Most studies examining the utility of CT scan in diagnosing nodal positivity define it as enlarged LN, with heterogeneity of the definition, ranging from >6mm to >1cm [35]. Correlation of LN metastases with LN shape has also been examined. Irregularly shaped LN have been suggested to have a higher risk of malignancy than consistently shaped nodes. However, most benign and malignant appearing LN were round in shape, thus the shape of the LN does not often allow for correct differentiation between benign and malignant nodes [41, 42].

Reported sensitivities and specificities for determining nodal involvement range from 50 to 95% and 40 to 99%, respectively; typically, specificity is higher than sensitivity for nodal involvement, but this is not consistent between studies [43-45]. A recent meta-analysis by our group found MDCT with multi-planar reformation images has the highest overall accuracy in predicting LN status (71%) [33]. Inaccuracies in true nodal status make pre-operative determination of disease spread difficult and must be taken into account in reports of pre-operative staging for neoadjuvant and peri-operative treatments and treatment decision-making.

CT scan is perhaps most useful in the determination of M stage, allowing examination of the entire abdomen and evaluation for the presence of metastases to the liver, viscera, distant LN and malignant ascites. The addition of CT scan of the pelvis allows for the evaluation of drop metastases into the pelvis, as well as the presence of Krukenberg tumors in the ovaries. The accuracy of demonstrating metastases on a CT scan is 81.2%, with sensitivity of 71.8% to 88.9% and specificity of 82.6% to 100% [33].

CT evaluation of the chest may also play a role in the staging of some patients. For gastroesophageal junction cancers, a CT chest is important for full evaluation of local disease, and surgical planning of esophagogastrectomy. CT chest is also useful for examining mediastinal lymphadenopathy and pulmonary metastases. The incidence of lung metastases is infrequent, ranging from 0.5 to 16% in reported series [46]. Therefore, routine use of CT chest in the staging of gastric cancer is not specifically advocated by all guidelines [47-49].

Several published practice guidelines advocate for the use of CT scans in the preoperative evaluation of patients with gastric cancer. Guidelines from the Association of Upper Gastrointestinal Surgeons of Great Britain and Ireland (AUGIS)/British Gastroenterology Society (BGS) [47] recommend that initial staging should be performed with a CT including multi-planar reformation images of the thorax, abdomen and pelvis to determine the presence of metastatic disease.

The European Society Medical Oncology/World Congress Gastrointestinal Cancer (ESMO/WCGIC) 2010 meeting [48] concluded that CT scan is the method of choice for evaluation of local extension and distant metastases. Guidelines from the Scottish Intercollegiate Guidelines Network (SIGN) [50] recommend that CT chest and abdomen with IV contrast and gastric distention with oral contrast or water be performed routinely, and that the liver should be evaluated in the portal venous phase for any metastases.

Finally, the National Comprehensive Cancer Network (NCCN) [49] has recommended CT chest and abdomen be a part of the work up for the patient suspected of harboring gastric cancer, and CT pelvis in those where it is clinically indicated.

Although imperfect in terms of accuracy, CT scans are crucial in pre-operative staging. CT scans of the abdomen should be obtained in order to evaluate local disease, while CT scans of the chest and pelvis can give important information about distant metastases.

PET Scan

^{18}Fluorodeoxyglucose-positron-emission tomography (FDG-PET) scans have found a role in the staging of many cancers and have evolved as a promising metabolic imaging modality for demonstration of tumor morphology and pathological metabolic activity. This imaging modality takes advantage of the fact that tumor cells, which have uncontrolled growth and division, are generally a metabolically active tissue, with their primary energy source being glucose.

FDG, a radioactive detector molecule, is injected, phosphorylated by hexokinase, and then metabolized through normal aerobic respiration. In general, highly metabolically active cancer cells concentrate more FDG than normal tissues. The PET scanner detects pairs of gamma rays emitted by the ^{18}Fluoride isotope, and uses a semi-quantitative method, the standardized uptake value (SUV), to assess the uptake of FDG and localize the tumor [51]. When these tumor cells are located in tissues whose cells have a lower metabolic activity, FDG-PET (Figure 5) allows imaging based on the altered glucose metabolism in these tumor cells, and distinguishes the tumor from normal tissue. In tissues such as the brain and heart, which are highly metabolically active, it is difficult to distinguish the tumor from the surrounding normal tissue very well.

FDG-PET scans appear to have decreased diagnostic accuracy for GC compared to CT imaging. Unfortunately, the number of studies examining the use of FDG-PET in preoperative staging is small with low patient accrual. The overall accuracy with which FDG-PET can detect a primary gastric cancer ranges between 58.1% and 95.9% [44, 45, 52-55] with a pooled overall primary tumor detection rate of 80% [33]. FDG-PET has a poorer accuracy for detecting earlier stage gastric cancers (26-63%) than advanced gastric cancers (83-100%) [44, 52, 55]. Detection of early gastric carcinomas by FDG-PET can be complicated by background signaling secondary to high physiological uptake of FDG by the normal gastric wall [40]. There is also variability in its ability to detect the various histological subtypes. Overall accuracy for detecting intestinal type ranges from 65.5-83%, non-intestinal type 41-79% [53-55], poorly differentiated adenocarcinomas 61.5%-79% and signet ring cell carcinoma 0-78% [53, 55]. This reflects the variable metabolic utilization of the subtypes and appears to be directly related to overexpression of the glucose transporter-1 (GLUT-1) transmembrane transporter protein [40]. FDG-PET cannot differentiate depth of invasion, and thus cannot assign T stages [51].

As with N-staging for CT scan, FDG-PET leaves much to be desired with an overall accuracy of 60%, and a sensitivity of 40% for detecting N+ disease. In patients with large, or advanced cancers, enhancement of local LN may be obscured by a stronger signal from the primary [56]. However, the specificity of FDG-PET scans for N-staging is 98% [33], the highest of any imaging modality, suggesting that FDG-PET may find a role in clarifying true nodal positivity in pre-operative planning. M staging by FDG-PET boasts an overall accuracy of 75.5% to 100% [44, 57, 58], which is comparable to CT scan. Some authors suggest that, for the detection and confirmation of solid organ and distant metastases, FDG-PET may be a superior modality. One study found that FDG-PET had a higher sensitivity (90% (95% CI: 80-97%)) than U/S, CT or MRI for detecting hepatic metastases in a series of mixed gastrointestinal malignancies, including gastric cancer [59] However, another study of only gastric cancer patients reported that the sensitivity and specificity of FDG-PET were 85% and 74%, respectively for liver metastases, and 67% and 88% for lung metastasis [60].

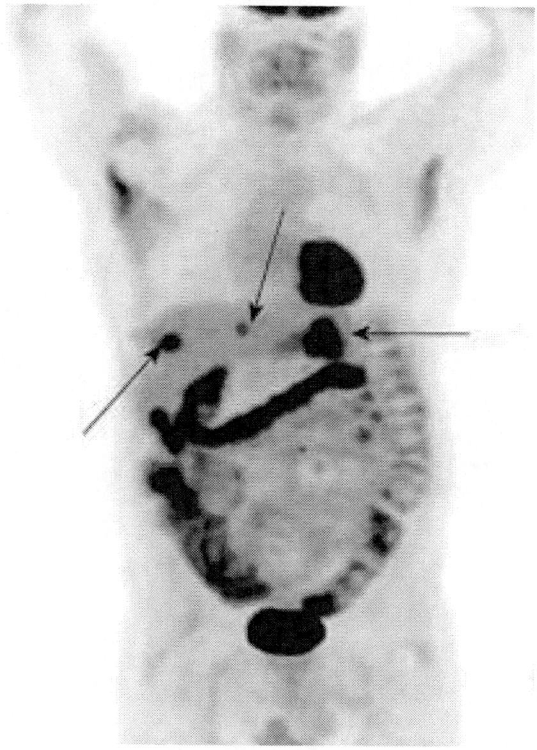

Figure 5. FDG-PET scan demonstrating proximal gastric cancer with liver metastasis. (From Smyth EC and Shah MA. *World J Gastroenterol* 2011;17(46): 5059-5074).

The ESMO/WCGIC guidelines state that FDG-PET may offer additional information for gastroesophageal junction tumors, but not gastric tumors [48]. NCCN guidelines state that FDG-PET alone is not an adequate diagnostic procedure in the detection and pre-operative staging of GC, but that it could be helpful when used in conjunction with CT scan [49]. AUGIS/BSG guidelines state that FDG-PET scans can be used in combination with endoscopic ultrasound and CT for esophageal and gastroesophageal junction cancers, but not necessarily for gastric cancer [47, 61]. With the high cost, need for specialized interpretation by nuclear medicine physicians and specialized radiologists and most importantly, its poorer overall accuracy when compared to CT scans, it is not used routinely as a primary radiologic staging modality. It may, however, be useful as an adjunct staging modality in selected cases.

MRI

Magnetic resonance imaging (MRI) is a powerful imaging tool and features high soft-tissue contrast, multi-planar imaging capability, provision of biochemical and anatomic information, versatility of sequence selection and modification, as well as an absence of ionizing radiation [56]. However, CT scan has traditionally been favored over MRI for the staging of gastric cancer (Figure 6) because of difficulty in obtaining clear images for stomach cancer with MRI due to variable distensibility, artifacts caused by active peristalsis, cardiovascular pulsation and respiration, lack of a suitable oral contrast medium, and high costs [56, 62-70].

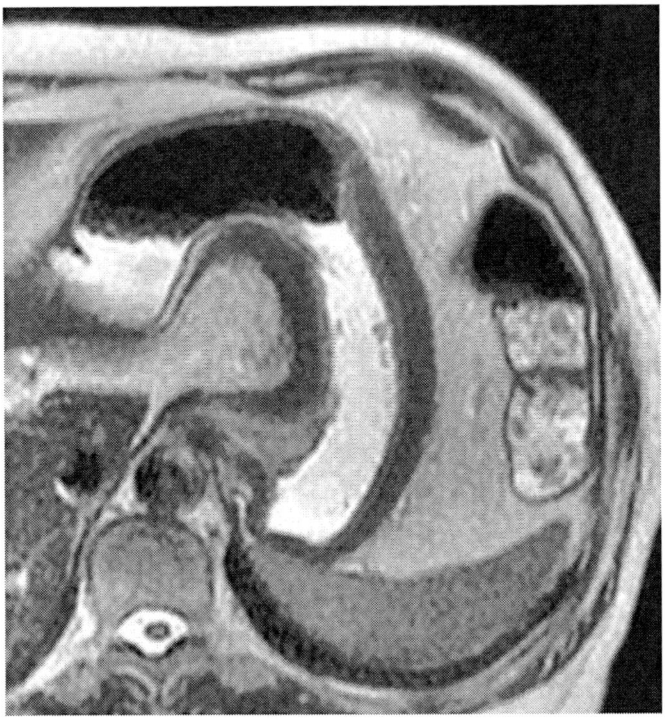

Figure 6. MRI demonstrating gastric cancer of the greater curvature. (Figure courtesy of Dr. John Hagen, University of Toronto).

Recent technological advances have improved gastric cancer imaging with MRI. First, faster MRI techniques allow image obtainment during a single breath-hold with less motion artifact than in the past [62]. This has, in turn, reduced motion artifacts [63] and improved image quality [56]. The rapid administration of intravenous contrast medium using an automatic power injector has improved the enhancement of the gastric wall and gastric tumors [63]. Administration of antiperistaltic agents has also allowed improved image quality [56]. Subtraction images can decrease signal intensities of perigastric fatty tissue, allowing potential demonstration of the different layers of the gastric wall [63]. Additionally, the use of phased array coils has increased the signal-to-noise ratio and has improved the spatial resolution of MR images [56]. Thus, MRI has become a more promising imaging modality for gastric cancer than in the past.

The ability of MRI to detect gastric cancers is strongly influenced by tumor size and morphology. Wang et al included no patients with flat or depressed type early gastric cancers. The spatial resolution of MR images prohibits it from detecting early gastric cancers [63], limiting the applicability of MRI. Advanced gastric cancers, on the other hand, are easily detectable on MRI because the infiltrated wall is well visualized with MR imaging as a thickened area, which is distinguished from the normal wall [62].

Arterial-dominant phase scanning is useful in detecting the tumor and evaluating tumor extent along the gastric wall [63]. Differing degrees of enhancement of the gastric wall can allow for layer differentiation. The inner mucosal layer shows rapid and marked enhancement, while the outer low-signal intensity submucosal and muscular layers have delayed enhancement [62]. Advanced gastric cancers show gradual enhancement from the inner mucosal side to the outer serosal side [63]. Therefore, depiction of the entire tumor is most clearly seen on the delayed images [63].

T staging has been possible with MR images. One study demonstrated that up to five layers of the gastric wall can be differentiated on MR images, as with endoscopic ultrasound [65]; however this was an ex vivo study, and no in vivo studies have recorded such visualization of the gastric wall [56]. Clinical studies have demonstrated that two [62] to three [63] layers of the normal gastric wall can be identified on dynamic MRI of the stomach. When two layers are identifiable, the first layer corresponds to the mucosa while the second layer corresponds to the submucosa and muscularis together. These layers are differentiated by degrees of enhancement [62]. When a third layer is visible, this allows differentiation of the submucosa and muscularis [63].

Identification of T4 lesions is important for surgical decision-making and planning for a multi-visceral resection or a neoadjuvant approach. Identification of pancreatic invasion is possible by observation of obscuring of the fat signals between the stomach and the pancreas [62]. Invasion of the transverse colon is suggested by arresting peristalsis with the administration of intravenous Buscopan [62], and observation of obscuring of the fat plane. Invasion of the left lobe of the liver can also be suggested by observing interruption of the low signal intensity between the liver and the stomach [62]. T staging performance of MRI has been examined by three studies [56, 62, 63] and was found to have an overall accuracy of 83% [33], which is comparable to MDCT scan. However, this data is based on only 3 studies examining a total of 109 patients [33], potentially representing a publication bias towards good results.

As with CT scan, determination of LN involvement by MRI is primarily based on size criteria. Accurate assessment of metastatic lymph nodes can be difficult when they are grouped together, or are in close proximity to the gastric mass [56]. Overall accuracy of N stage for MRI has been reported in only two studies, and is reported to be 52.2% to 55.2% [56, 62]. Only one study reported sensitivity and specificity, 85% and 75%, respectively [62], and while the sensitivity is the highest of the imaging modalities, this is reported in only one study. Therefore, MRI alone cannot reliably confirm or exclude the presence of LN metastases[33, 39].

The use of intravenous contrast may improve detection of LN by MRI. Tatsumi et al examined the identification of LN on MRI using ferumoxtran-10, a lymphotropic contrast agent for MRI with efficacy in detecting metastatic LN in a variety of other cancers. MRI findings were correlated with histopathologic findings in surgical specimens. The overall accuracy using ferumoxtran-10 was 94.8%, with sensitivity and specificity of 100% and 92.6%, respectively. The positive predictive value and negative predictive value were 85.5% and 100%, respectively. This suggests that use of newer contrast agents during MRI may improve identification of LN metastases in the future [71].

M staging for MRI have not been closely examined, and accuracy, sensitivity and specificity have not been reported. MRI is of limited utility for determination of an M stage as the entire abdomen is not routinely imaged. Additionally, some authors have found that peritoneal carcinomatosis without ascites is difficult to detect on staging MR images [56]. However, MRI may serve an important purpose for clarification of possible metastatic lesions found on CT or ultrasound in the liver or ovaries [56].

MRI may be a useful alternative to CT due to its high resolution of soft tissue, its multi-planar imaging capability and its lack of ionizing radiation [56]. While practice guidelines do not recommend the routine use of MRI in the staging of gastric cancer [47, 48], it may be a useful staging modality, reserved for patients who cannot undergo CT [50] because of renal impairment, pregnancy, or hypersensitivity to CT contrast materials [56], and for clarification of lesions found in the liver and ovaries.

AUS

Abdominal ultrasound (AUS) (Figure 7) has become a very versatile imaging technique. Cost effective and portable, AUS has found applicability in a wide variety of clinical settings. Furthermore, the presence of bowel gas can disrupt adequate examination. Specific to gastric cancer, AUS has difficulty accurately evaluating the fundus, greater curvature, lymph node basins [72, 73], the diaphragm and the splenic hilum [74].

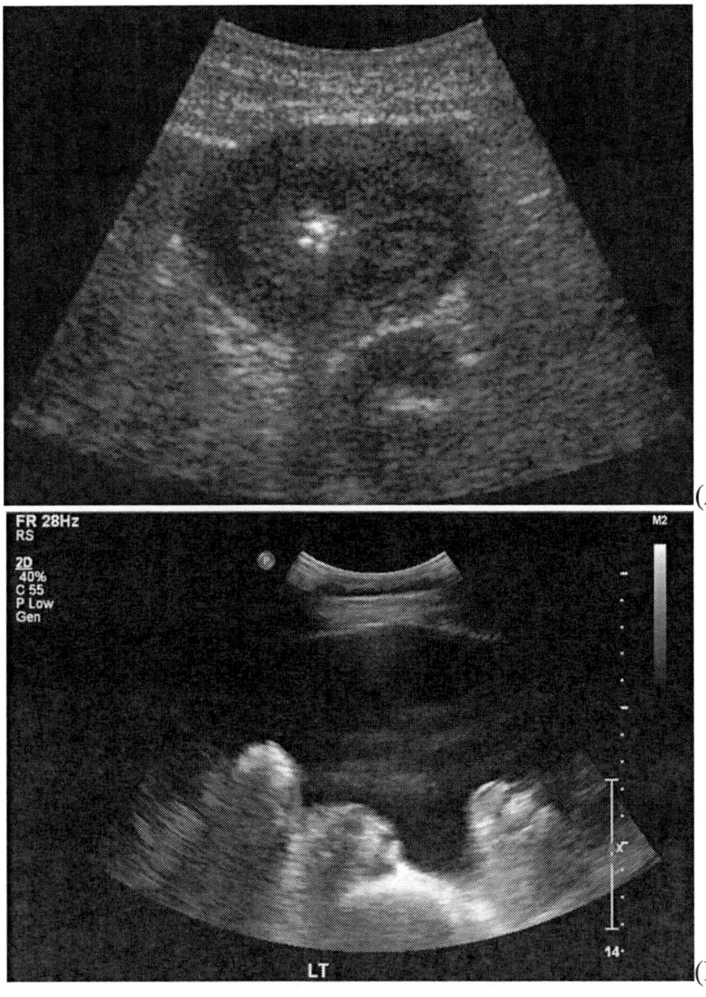

(A)

(B)

Figure 7. A: Abdominal ultrasound showing a 5 cm diameter stomach with its wall being abnormally thickened due to cancer. The bright area is gas in the stomach (Figure courtesy of Dr. John Hagen, University of Toronto). B: Abdominal ultrasound demonstrating ascites from gastric cancer. (Figure courtesy of Dr. Caitlin McGregor, University of Toronto).

The overall accuracy for T staging with AUS is 67.8% [33], which does not compare favorably to CT or MRI. Only two studies have evaluated the accuracies of each T stage [41, 74]; based on 168 patients, these studies suffer from low power. Accuracy of identifying T1 disease is 37.5% to 55.6%, 75.0% to 90.0% for T2, 56.2% to 87.3% for T3 and 0% to 71.1% for T4. Although identification of T1 lesions was least accurate, Liao et al described identification of T1 lesions in only 9 patients, 4 of which were overstaged. Three of these patients had ulcerative carcinoma. They found that in these cases, the normally hyperechoic submucosal layer becomes hypoechoic secondary to inflammation or edema around the tumor, giving it a similar echogenicity of the muscularis propria [41]. Therefore, T1 lesions are commonly overstaged by AUS [74].

Accuracy for identifying T2 and T3 lesions is better. The normal serosal layer is seen as a thin, smooth hyperechoic band. When the tumor remains below this hyperechoic band, it is diagnosed as T2. When the tumor histologically invades the serosa, interruption of this smooth hyperechoic band is visualized sonographically [41], and T3 status is assigned. AUS cannot reliably diagnose T4 lesions due to difficulty in visualizing perigastric organs [41]. However, a diagnosis of a T4 lesion may be made when there is interruption of the serosal layer of the gastric wall and it is indistinguishable from adjacent organs, the tumor and organs move synchronously, or there is no tumor movement with the patients breathing. In their study, Liao et al correctly identified invasion of the transverse colon with AUS in 1 out of 3 patients [41]. In the patient in whom invasion of the transverse colon was identified, there was circumferential involvement. When the tumor only invaded one luminal side of the transverse colon, luminal gas interfered with the diagnosis, suggesting that AUS will have difficulty in identifying this relationship.

N staging with AUS suffers from the same drawbacks as CT and MRI in that is based primarily on size of the LN. Overall accuracy for N staging by AUS is found to be 68.1% [33]. Again, this analysis is based on only two studies [41, 74] of 149 patients, suffering from low power. Overall sensitivity and specificity is 63.0% and 78.8%, respectively. While the specificity compares to CT and MRI, given the low number of cases evaluated, more studies are needed. Furthermore, MDCT, especially with multi-planar reformatted images has a higher specificity.

Irregularly shaped LN seen on AUS have been suggested to have a higher risk of malignancy than consistently shaped nodes. However, most benign and malignant appearing lymph nodes were round in shape and shape of the lymph node does not often allow for correct differentiation between benign and malignant nodes [41]. AUS can also evaluate echogenicity of LN. Some authors report that most malignant lymph nodes were hypoechoic, while most benign lymph nodes were isoechoic to slightly hyperechoic [75, 76]. On the other hand, Heinz et al state that echogenicity of nodes seen on endoscopic ultrasound does not allow for correct differentiation between benign and malignant lymph nodes [77]. Therefore, differentiation of benign and malignant nodes based on echogenicity remains unclear.

The overall accuracy for M staging by AUS is only 64.7% [33]. Kayaalp et al found that the sensitivity for detecting metastatic disease is unacceptably low. The sensitivity for detection of liver metastases, peritoneal metastases and ascites was 50%, 9% and 64%, respectively. Although low, the sensitivity of AUS for detecting ascites is with reported specificities for detecting liver metastases, peritoneal metastases, and ascites of 98%, 98% and 93%, respectively [78].

None of the published practice guidelines mention the use of AUS as a staging modality for gastric cancer given the limitations inherit in this technique.

Endoscopy

Upper endoscopy, or esophagogastroduodenoscopy (EGD) was first introduced in the 1970s and is one of the most commonly performed and important modalities in the diagnosis of gastric cancer (Figure 8). Upper endoscopy is frequently used in the screening of asymptomatic patients, as well as the diagnosis and work-up of patients with a variety of pathological processes of the upper GI tract [79]. The sensitivity and specificity of endoscopy for detection of gastric cancers is reported to be 93% and 100%, respectively [80] Despite the importance of endoscopy in the diagnosis of gastric cancer, the information obtained at endoscopy offers little in the oncologic staging of gastric cancer.

An advantage of endoscopy in the gastric cancer patient is its ability to directly visualize the luminal surface of the stomach, facilitating examination of the tumor appearance and allowing the endoscopist to biopsy the lesion. Endoscopy is important in surgical planning, as assessment of proximal and distant disease extent can facilitate anticipated need for resection of the duodenum or esophagus in order to obtain negative margins. As such, reporting for upper endoscopy should be done in a standard, systematic manner.

A complete upper endoscopy is recommended to include a thorough visualization from the upper esophageal sphincter to the second portion of the duodenum, including retroflexion [79]. Adequate documentation of the tumor size and appearance, description of the tumor location within the stomach relative to the gastroesophageal (GE) junction and/or duodenum, and description of any involvement of the esophagus, GE junction or duodenum constitutes a complete EGD report, which is necessary in the pre-operative planning of the patient with gastric cancer. If the above information is not clearly documented, it may be necessary to repeat the EGD prior to resection.

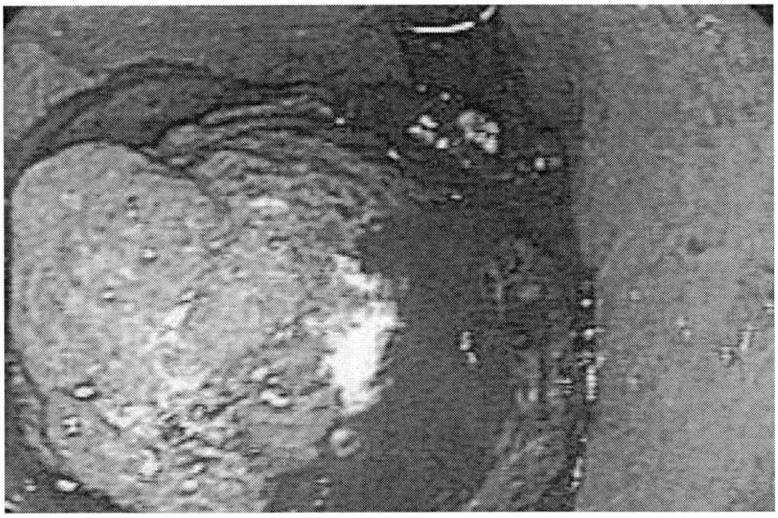

Figure 8. Esophagogastroduodenoscopy demonstrating a gastric mass on the greater curvature. (Figure courtesy of Dr. John Hagen, University of Toronto).

Endoscopic Ultrasound

Endoscopic ultrasound (EUS) was first introduced in the 1980s, providing a method for examining local tumor infiltration by allowing evaluation of the individual layers of the gastric wall [81, 82] without any interference from interposed fat, or bowel gas [83]. EUS is able to evaluate regional LN that may be enlarged, identify liver metastases, and detect ascites [84]. EUS, however, is not without its drawbacks. Like endoscopy, it is user dependent, and is a very demanding endoscopic procedure. As such, advanced training and extensive experience is required in order to obtain usable images with the echoendoscope [85]. Echoendoscopes provide frequencies at 5-12 MHz, while miniature probes are capable of ultra-high frequencies of 12-30 MHz. Higher frequencies yield higher resolution of the tumor at the expense of depth of penetration thus limiting nodal examination [50, 81]. The echoendoscope must be well positioned in order to obtain high quality images and permit full visualization of the tumor, which can be difficult, especially if the tumor causes strictures [37]. Furthermore, EUS is of limited usefulness in the overall assessment of more distant metastatic spread [37].

An important goal of performing EUS in gastric cancer is determining an accurate T stage for treatment decisions, such as whether the patient is a candidate for an endoscopic resection. The diagnostic accuracy for overall T staging by EUS and for each individual T stage is summarized in Table 9 For overall T stage, the diagnostic accuracy ranges from 56.9% to 87.7% with a pooled accuracy of 75%. The diagnostic accuracy for T1 cancer by EUS ranges from 14% to100% with a pooled accuracy of 77%. For T2 lesions, the diagnostic accuracy ranges from 24% to 90% with a pooled accuracy of 65% [85]. This low to moderate diagnostic accuracy for T staging in early gastric cancer, raises concerns as to whether or not this is in fact the ideal modality for T staging, especially for the identification of candidates for endoscopic resection. Kim et al found that early gastric cancer with undifferentiated histopathologic features was more frequently associated with an incorrect assessment of true tumor invasion depth by EUS [86].

Although of more limited clinical value, the pooled diagnostic accuracies for advanced gastric cancers (i.e. T3-4) is 79% to 85% [84]. Patients with such lesions, assuming they are candidates, would proceed to gastrectomy with or without peri-operative chemotherapy. Detection of invasion of adjacent organs could be important for clinical decision-making, as a multi-visceral resection, or neo-adjuvant approach could be planned.

N staging, to a certain degree, is also possible with EUS, as enlarged LN in the peri-gastric nodal basin (i.e. Group 1 nodes) can be visualized. More distant nodal basins (i.e. Group 2 or 3 nodes) are not within the range of tissue penetration for the EUS, and therefore may not be visualized. The range of accuracies for N staging in published studies was found to be 30% to 90% with a pooled accuracy of only 64% [84]. Therefore, while EUS can identify enlarged regional LN in the peritumoral area, N-staging by EUS is of limited value in the pre-operative assessment [87]. Similarly, although the left lobe of the liver can be assessed by EUS, the entire liver cannot be visualized, leaving a partial metastatic assessment.

Some practice guidelines have supported the optional use of EUS with or without fine needle aspiration of suspicious lymph nodes for further staging of esophageal and GEJ tumors prior to the administration of curative therapy [47, 49, 50], but this recommendation does not necessarily apply to gastric cancer.

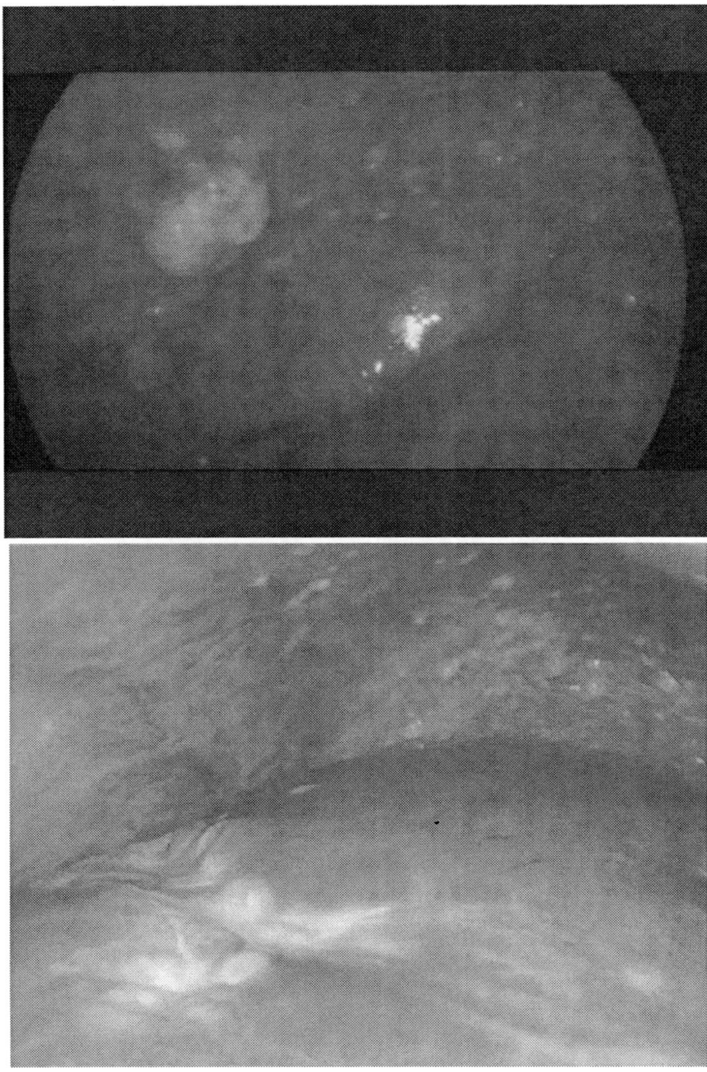

Figure 9. A: Peritoneal carcinomatosis of the underlying anterior abdominal wall found during staging laparoscopy for gastric cancer. A large lesion with multiple smaller lesions surrounding the larger lesion is identifiable. (Figure courtesy of Dr. John Hagen, University of Toronto), B: Liver metastases discovered during staging laparoscopy. Carcinomatosis is also seen on the inferior surface of the diaphragm. (Figure courtesy of Dr. Peter Stotland, University of Toronto).

Table 9. Summary of range of diagnostic accuracies and pooled accuracies for all T staging, and for each individual T stage asreported by Cardoso et al [84]

T stage	Range of Accuracy	Pooled Accuracy
Overall	56.9% to 87.7%	75%
T1	14% to 100%	77%
T2	24% to 90%	65%
T3	50% to 100%	85%
T4	25% to 100%	79%

NCCN guidelines state that EUS with FNA of suspicious lymph nodes (if it can be achieved without traversing an area of primary tumor or major blood vessels) is indicated for assessment for staging gastric cancer [49].

On the other hand, the Scottish Intercollegiate Guidelines Network states that other modalities may obviate the need for EUS in the staging of gastric cancer [50]. The ESMO/WCGIC guidelines for gastric cancer state that there is not a uniform consensus on the role of EUS in the staging of gastric cancer [48]. Therefore, routine use of EUS in staging of gastric cancer is likely indicated only in situations where the results will change clinical management.

Staging Laparoscopy

Since the inception of laparoscopic surgery, staging laparoscopy has evolved as a useful staging modality that aids in the accurate determination of M stage in patients before formal resection. Staging laparoscopy can identify metastatic disease too small to be detected on standard radiographic staging methods, avoiding an unnecessary laparotomy (Figure 9).

A complete staging laparoscopy should include a visual inspection of the stomach, diaphragm, liver and ovaries for the presence of any metastases. Using a thorough inspection, the accuracy for detecting intra-abdominal M1 disease by staging laparoscopy is 94% to 100% [88, 89].

However, with the improvement of image resolution of MDCT scans, the question of whether or not performing a staging laparoscopy is still relevant has been raised. Despite improvements in imaging accuracy, a recent study found that almost one third of patients who were identified by other staging modalities as M0, had radiologically occult intra-abdominal metastases, which were discovered by staging laparoscopy [90]. Another study found staging laparoscopy changed management in 25% to 54% of patients with advanced gastric cancer [89].

Therefore, even with the combined accuracy of performing multiple staging modalities in the work-up process, suboptimal identification of incurable disease by radiologic staging alone, results in high rates of unnecessary laparotomies in gastric cancer patients, with resultant morbidity and mortality.

The median hospital length of stay is shorter with staging laparoscopy compared to a negative laparotomy (2 days vs 10 days, $p < 0.001$) [91]. Furthermore, the in-hospital mortality of patients undergoing a staging laparoscopy is only 5.3%, compared to 13.1% for patients who underwent a futile laparotomy ($p<0.001$) [91].

Laparoscopy, however, should not be routinely performed on all patients. The diagnostic yield of performing a staging laparoscopy on a patient with early gastric cancer (i.e. T1-2) is low. As such, practice guidelines have recommended that staging laparoscopy be reserved for advanced gastric cancer (i.e. T3-4), where there is a higher likelihood of metastases [50, 92], Given its diagnostic accuracy, its ability to change management in appropriately selected patients, and the benefits to the patient in terms of reduction in hospital length of stay and mortality, staging laparoscopy should be utilized in the staging of all patients with advanced gastric cancer.

Peritoneal Washings

Peritoneal washings for cytological analysis have been advocated for the identification of free intraperitoneal cancer cells, despite the absence of any evidence of gross peritoneal disease. The etiology of these free intraperitoneal cancer cells is not fully understood, however, they are thought to arise from where the primary tumor invades the serosa [93]. Positive cytology is associated with advanced T stage, but not with N positivity [94].

Positive cytology of peritoneal washings is a poor prognostic indicator [95, 96] and a strong independent predictor of recurrence even after an R0 resection [94]. In gastric cancer, peritoneal dissemination is one of the most common patterns of metastasis and recurrence [97]. Reported recurrence rates for patients with positive cytology range from 11% to 100% [98], but appear to be dependent upon the method used to detect cancer cells in the peritoneal washings and the length of time that the patients are observed for recurrence.

Although the UICC/AJCC have defined positive peritoneal cytology as M1 disease [5], the treatment implications of this microscopic disease are debated. While some authors state that positive cytology is a contra-indication to resection [99, 100], others feel that positive peritoneal cytology is useful for identifying patients who are unlikely to benefit from resection alone, and would require additional treatment in order to improve survival [101]. Some authors have suggested that the early detection and eradication of intraperitoneal cancer cells may improve patient survival [102, 103]. Lorenzen et al reported that 37% of gastric cancer patients with positive peritoneal cytology were subsequently converted to negative after a minimum of 6 weeks of neoadjuvant chemotherapy. These patients had improved median survival (36.1 vs. 9.2 months; $p = 0.002$) and 2-year survival (71.4 vs. 25%; $p = 0.002$) compared to patients who had persistently positive cytology [104]. However, the 5-year survival of patients in whom peritoneal lavage was converted from positive to negative was only 14.3% [104]. Some groups have also suggested that the prognosis of patients with positive peritoneal cytology may be improved with intraperitoneal chemotherapy. The use of extensive peritoneal lavage followed by intraperitoneal therapy has been shown to improve 5-year survival of patients with positive peritoneal cytology over intraperitoneal therapy alone (43.8% vs 4.6%, $p < 0.0001$) [105]. Intraperitoneal chemotherapy has been demonstrated to be prophylactic against peritoneal recurrence and results in improved survival [106, 107]. Therefore, identification of intraperitoneal cancer cells may have an impact on management decisions with regards to peri-operative therapy.

Current guidelines are inconsistent in their recommendations for peritoneal washings. Obtaining peritoneal washings at the time of diagnostic laparoscopy is recommended by SAGES [92]. ESMO, on the other hand, does not consider obtaining peritoneal washings a necessary practice [48]. The NCCN guidelines do not explicitly incorporate peritoneal washings into the gastric cancer treatment algorithm, despite later considering positive peritoneal cytology a criterion of unresectability for cure [49]. An argument can be made for performing peritoneal washings at the time of staging laparoscopy because the length of time added to the procedure in order to obtain the washings is not significant. However, as there is no reliable mechanism for intra-operative assessment of cytology, performance of peritoneal washings must be planned several days prior to scheduled resection, necessitating two separate operations if resection is performed.

Conclusion

The importance of accurate staging of patients with gastric cancer cannot be overstated, and is the foundation for providing the most appropriate stage specific treatment. Understaging can lead to undertreating patients who are falsely diagnosed with highly aggressive local disease, while overstaging can lead to futile attempts at treatment with curative intent where palliation is the more appropriate.

Several investigative techniques for the staging of gastric cancer are available. Unfortunately, none of these techniques are perfect, and simply performing one of these techniques for the purposes of staging may be inadequate. However, the combination of several techniques will increase the chances of diagnosing the correct stage and allowing patients to be correctly allocated to appropriate treatment algorithms.

References

[1] Cunningham D, Allum WH, Stenning SP, et al: Perioperative chemotherapy versus surgery alone for resectable gastroesophageal cancer. *N Engl J Med* 2006;355:11-20.

[2] Macdonald JS, Smalley SR, Benedetti J, et al: Chemoradiotherapy after surgery compared with surgery alone for adenocarcinoma of the stomach or gastroesophageal junction. *N Engl J Med* 2001;345:725-30.

[3] Sakuramoto S, Sasako M, Yamaguchi T, et al: Adjuvant chemotherapy for gastric cancer with S-1, an oral fluoropyrimidine. *N Engl J Med* 2007;357:1810-20.

[4] Paoletti X, Oba K, Burzykowski T, et al: Benefit of adjuvant chemotherapy for resectable gastric cancer: a meta-analysis. *JAMA* 2010;303:1729-37.

[5] Chapter 11: Stomach. In: Edge SB, Byrd DR, Compton CC, et al. AJCC Cancer Staging Manual. 7th ed. New York, NY: Springer.

[6] JGCA. Japanese classification of gastric carcinoma: 3rd English edition. *Gastric Cancer* 2011;14:101-12.

[7] Soetikno R, Kaltenbach T, Yeh R, Gotoda T. Endoscopic mucosal resection for early cancers of the upper gastrointestinal tract. *J Clin Oncol* 2005;23(20):4490-8.

[8] Fang WL, Huang KH, Chen JH, et al. Comparison of the Survival Difference Between AJCC 6th and 7th Editions for Gastric Cancer Patients. *World J Surg* 2011;35(12): 2723-9.

[9] Brar SS, Seevaratnam R, Cardoso R, Yohanathan L, Law C, Helyer L, Coburn NG. Multivisceral resection for gastric cancer: a systematic review. *Gastric Cancer* 2011 Jul 23. [Epub ahead of print].

[10] Roberts P, Seevaratnam R, Cardoso R, Law C, Helyer L, Coburn N. Systematic review of pancreaticoduodenectomy for locally advanced gastric cancer. *Gastric Cancer* 2011 Aug 26. [Epub ahead of print].

[11] Jeong O, Choi W, Park Y. Appropriate selection of patients for combined organ resection in cases of gastric carcinoma invading adjacent organs. *J Surg Oncol* 2009;100 (2):115–20.

[12] Kitamura K, Tani N, Koike H, et al. Combined resection of the involved organs in T4 gastric cancer. *Hepatogastroenterology* 2000;47(36):1769–72.

[13] Hirose K, Onchi H, Iida A, Katayama K, Yamaguchi A, Nakagawara G. Surgical results of pancreaticoduodenectomy for carcinoma of the distal third of the stomach. *Int Surg* 1999;84(1): 18–24.

[14] Ajisaka H, Fujita H, Kaji M, et al. Treatment of patients with gastric cancer and duodenal invasion. *Int Surg* 2001;86(1):9–13.

[15] Boellaard R, Krak NC, Hoekstra OS, Lammertsma AA. Effects of noise, image resolution, and ROI definition on the accuracy of standard uptake values: a simulation study. *J Nucl Med* 2004;45(9):1519-27.

[16] UICC/AJCC. American Joint Committee on Cancer, Cancer Staging Manual. 1988-2002 [cited; Available from: http://www.cancerstaging.org/products/pasteditions.html]

[17] JGCA. Japanese Classification of Gastric Carcinoma - 2nd English Edition. *Gastric Cancer* 1998;1:10-24.

[18] Viera AJ, Garrett JM. Understanding interobserver agreement: the kappa statistic. *Fam Med* 2005;37(5):360-3.

[19] Bland JM, Altman DG. Multiple significance tests: the Bonferroni method. *BMJ* 1995;310(6973):170.

[20] Smith DD, Schwarz RR, Schwarz RE. Impact of total lymph node count on staging and survival after gastrectomy for gastric cancer: data from a large US-population database. *J Clin Oncol* 2005;23(28):7114-24.

[21] Bouvier AM, Haas O, Piard F, Roignot P, Bonithon-Kopp C, Faivre J. How many nodes must be examined to accurately stage gastric carcinomas? Results from a population based study. *Cancer* 2002;94(11):2862-6.

[22] Wagner PK, Ramaswamy A, Ruschoff J, et al. Lymph node counts in the upper abdomen: Anatomic basis for lymphadenectomy in gastric cancer. *Br J Surg* 1991;78(7):825-7.

[23] Onate-Ocana LF, Aiello-Crocifoglio V, Mondragon-Sanchez R, et al.: Survival benefit of D2 lympadenectomy in patients with gastric adenocarcinoma. Ann Surg Oncol 2000;7:210–7.

[24] de Gara CJ, Hanson J, Hamilton S: A population-based study of tumor-node relationship, resection margins, and surgeon volume on gastric cancer survival. *Am J Surg* 2003;186:23–7.

[25] Coburn NG. Lymph Nodes and Gastric Cancer. *J Surg Onc* 2009;99(4):199-206.

[26] Jamieson JK, Dobson JF. The lymphatic system of the stomach. *Lancet* 1907;169:1061–6.

[27] Coller FA, Kay EB, Mclntyre RS. Regional lymphatic metastases of carcinoma of the stomach. *Arch Surg* 1941;43:748–61.

[28] Hundahl SA, Phillips JL, Menck HR: The National Cancer Data Base Report on poor survival of U.S. gastric carcinoma patients treated with gastrectomy: Fifth Edition American Joint Committee on Cancer staging, proximal disease, and the "different disease" hypothesis. *Cancer* 2000;88:921-32.

[29] Wanebo HJ, Kennedy BJ, Chmiel J, Steele G Jr, Winchester D, Osteen R. Cancer of the stomach. A patient care study by the American College of Surgeons. *Ann. Surg* 1993;218(5):583-92.

[30] Powell FC, Cooper AJ, Massa MC, et al.: Sister Mary Joseph's nodule: A clinical and histologic study. *J Am Acad Dermatol* 1984;10:610–5.

[31] Baumgart DC, Fischer A. Virchow's node. *Lancet* 2007;370:1568.

[32] Mahar AL, Coburn NG, Singh S, Law C, Helyer LK. A systematic review of surgery for non-curative gastric cancer. *Gastric Cancer* 2011 Oct 28. [Epub ahead of print].

[33] Seevaratnam R, Cardoso R, McGregor C, et al. How useful is preoperative imaging for tumor, node, metastasis (TNM) staging of gastric cancer? A meta-analysis. *Gastric Cancer* 2011 Aug 12. [Epub ahead of print].

[34] Halvorsen RA. Which study when? Iodinated contrast-enhanced CT versus gadolinium-enhanced MR imaging. *Radiology* 2008;249(1):9-15.

[35] Chen CY, Wu DC, Kang WY, Hsu JS. Staging of gastric cancer with 16-channel MDCT. *Abdom Imaging* 2006;31(5):514-20.

[36] Kim AY, Kim HJ, Ha HK. Gastric cancer by multidetector row CT: preoperative staging. *Abdom Imaging* 2005;30(4):465-72.

[37] Kwee RM, Kwee TC. Imaging in local staging of gastric cancer: a systematic review. *J Clin Oncol* 2007;25(15):2107-16.

[38] Lim JS, Yun MJ, Kim MJ, et al. CT and PET in stomach cancer: preoperative staging and monitoring of response to therapy. *Radiographics* 2006;26(1):143-56.

[39] Kwee RM, Kwee TC. Imaging in assessing lymph node status in gastric cancer. *Gastric Cancer* 2009;12(1):6-22.

[40] Dassen AE, Lips DJ, Hoekstra CJ, Pruijt JF, Bosscha K. FDG-PET has no definite role inpreoperative imaging in gastric cancer. *Eur J Surg Oncol* 2009;35(5):449-55.

[41] Liao SR, Dai Y, Huo L, et al. Transabdominal ultrasonography in preoperative staging of gastric cancer. *World J Gastroenterol* 2004;10(23):3399-404.

[42] Takao S, Tadano S, Taguchi H, et al. Accurate analysis of the change in volume, location, and shape of metastatic cervical lymph nodes during radiotherapy. *Int J Radiat Oncol Biol Phys* 2011;81(3):871-9.

[43] Bhandari S, Shim CS, Kim JH, et al. Usefulness of threedimensional, multidetector row CT (virtual gastroscopy and multiplanar reconstruction) in the evaluation of gastric cancer: A comparison with conventional endoscopy, EUS, and histopathology. *Gastrointest Endosc* 2004;59:619–26.

[44] Chen J, Cheong JH, Yun MJ, et al. Improvement in preoperative staging of gastric adenocarcinoma with positron emission tomography. *Cancer* 2005;103:2383–90.

[45] Kim SK, Kang KW, Lee JS, et al. Assessment of lymph node metastases using 18F-FDG PET in patients with advanced gastric cancer. *Eur J Nucl Med Mol Imaging* 2006;33:148–55.

[46] Kemp CD, Kitano M, Kerkar S, et al. Pulmonary resection for metastatic gastric cancer. *J Thorac Oncol* 2010;5(11):1796-805.

[47] Allum WH, Blazeby JM, Griffin SM, Cunningham D, Jankowski JA, Wong R; On behalf of the Association of Upper Gastrointestinal Surgeons of Great Britain and Ireland, the British Society of Gastroenterology and the British Association of Surgical Oncology. Guidelines for the management of oesophageal and Gastric Cancer. *Gut* 2011;60(11):1449-72.

[48] Van Cutsem E, Dicato M, Geva R, et al. The diagnosis and management of Gastric Cancer: expert discussion and recommendations from the 12th ESMO/World Congress on Gastrointestinal Cancer, Barcelona, 2010. *Ann Oncol* 2011;22 Suppl 5:v1-9.

[49] Panel Members Gastric Cancer: NCCN Clinical guidelines in Oncology National Comprehensive Cancer Network 2011

[50] SIGN SIGN. Management of oesophageal and gastric cancer. Edinburg: Scottish Intercollegiate Guidelines Network 2006.
[51] Ozkan E, Araz M, Soydal C, Kucuk ON. The role of 18F-FDG-PET/CT in the preoperative staging and posttherapy follow up of gastric cancer: comparison with spiral CT. *World J Surg Oncol* 2011;9:75.
[52] Yun M, Lim JS, Noh SH, et al. Lymph node staging of gastric cancer using (18)F-FDG PET: a comparison study with CT. *J Nucl Med* 2005;46(10):1582-8.
[53] Mochiki E, Kuwano H, Katoh H, Asao T, Oriuchi N, Endo K. Evaluation of 18F-2-deoxy-2-fluoro-D-glucose positron emission tomography for gastric cancer. World J Surg 2004;28(3):247-53.
[54] Stahl A, Ott K, Weber WA, et al. FDG PET imaging of locally advanced gastric carcinomas: correlation with endoscopic and histopathological findings. *Eur J Nucl Med Mol Imaging* 2003;30(2):288-95.
[55] Mukai K, Ishida Y, Okajima K, Isozaki H, Morimoto T, Nishiyama S. Usefulness of preoperative FDG-PET for detection of gastric cancer. *Gastric Cancer* 2006;9(3):192-6.
[56] Sohn KM, Lee JM, Lee SY, Ahn BY, Park SM, Kim KM. Comparing MR imaging and CT in the staging of gastric carcinoma. *AJR Am J Roentgenol* 2000;174(6):1551-7.
[57] Lim JS, Kim MJ, Yun MJ, et al. Comparison of CT and 18F-FDG pet for detecting peritoneal metastasis on the preoperative evaluation for gastric carcinoma. *Korean J Radiol* 2006;7(4):249-56.
[58] Tian J, Chen L, Wei B, et al. The value of vesicant 18F-fluorodeoxyglucose positron emission tomography (18F-FDG PET) in gastric malignancies. *Nucl Med Commun* 2004;25(8):825-31.
[59] Kinkel K, Lu Y, Both M, Warren RS, Thoeni RF. Detection of hepatic metastases from cancers of the gastrointestinal tract by using noninvasive imaging methods (US, CT, MR imaging, PET): a meta-analysis. *Radiology* 2002;224(3):748-56.
[60] Yoshioka T, Yamaguchi K, Kubota K, et al. Evaluation of 18F-FDG PET in patients with advanced, metastatic, or recurrent gastric cancer. *J Nucl Med* 2003;44(5):690-9.
[61] Shoda H, Kakugawa Y, Saito D, et al. Evaluation of 18F-2- deoxy-2-fluoro-glucose positron emission tomography for gastric cancer screening in asymptomatic individuals undergoing endoscopy. *Br J Cancer* 2007;97:1493–8.
[62] Kang BC, Kim JH, Kim KW, et al. Value of the dynamic and delayed MR sequence with Gd-DTPA in the T-staging of stomach cancer: correlation with the histopathology. *Abdom Imaging* 2000;25(1):14-24.
[63] Wang CK, Kuo YT, Liu GC, Tsai KB, Huang YS. Dynamic contrast-enhanced subtraction and delayed MRI of gastric tumors: radiologic-pathologic correlation. *J Comput Assist Tomogr* 2000;24(6):872-7.
[64] Matsushita M, Oi H, Murakami T, et al. Extraserosal invasion in advanced gastric cancer: evaluation with MR imaging. *Radiology* 1994;192:87–91.
[65] Dux M, Roeren T, Kuntz C, et al. MRI for staging of gastric carcinoma: first results of an experimental prospective study. *J Comput Assist Tomogr* 1997;21:66–72.
[66] Paley MR, Ros PR. MRI of the gastrointestinal tract. *Eur Radiol* 1997;7:1387–97.
[67] Goldberg HI, Thoeni RF. MRI of the gastrointestinal tract. *Radiol Clin North Am* 1989;27:805–12.
[68] Werthmuller WC, Margulis AR. Magnetic resonance imaging of the alimentary tube. *Invest Radiol* 1991;26:195–200.

[69] Halvorsen RA Jr, Thompson WM. Primary neoplasm of the hollow organs of the gastrointestinal tract: staging and follow up. *Cancer* 1991;67:1181–8.

[70] Hahn PF, Stark DD, Glastad K. Biliary system, pancreas, spleen, and alimentary tract. In: Stark DD, Bradley WG Jr. *Magnetic resonance imaging* 2nd ed. St. Louis: Mosby,1992:1838–51.

[71] Tatsumi Y, Tanigawa N, Nishimura H, Nomura E, Mabuchi H, Matsuki M, Narabayashi I. Preoperative diagnosis of lymph node metastases in gastric cancer by magnetic resonance imaging with ferumoxtran-10. *Gastric Cancer* 2006;9(2):120-8.

[72] Lim JH, Ko YT, Lee DH. Transabdominal US staging of gastric cancer. *Abdom Imaging* 1994;19(6):527-31.

[73] Suk KT, Lim DW, Kim MY, et al. Thickening of the gastric wall on transabdominal sonography: a sign of gastric cancer. *J Clin Ultrasound* 2008;36(8):462-6.

[74] Lee DH, Ko YT, Park SJ, Lim JW. Comparison of hydro-US and spiral CT in the staging of gastric cancer. *Clin Imaging* 2001;25(3):181-6.

[75] Gimondo P, Mirk P, Messina G, Pizzi C. Abdominal lymphadenopathy in benign disease: sonographic detection and clinical significance. *J Ultrasound Med* 1996;15:353-9.

[76] Metreweli C, Ward SC. Ultrasound demonstration of lymph nodes in the hepatoduodenal ligament ('Daisy Chain nodes') in normal subjects. *Clin Radiol* 1995;50:99-101.

[77] Heintz A, Mildenberger P, Georg M, Braunstein S, Junginger T. Endoscopic ultrasonography in the diagnosis of regional lymph nodes in esophageal and gastric cancer-results of studies in vitro. *Endoscopy* 1993;25:231-5.

[78] Kayaalp C, Arda K, Orug T, Ozcay N. Value of computed tomography in addition to ultrasound for preoperative staging of gastric cancer. *Eur J Surg Oncol* 2002;28(5): 540-3.

[79] Cohen J, Safdi MA, Deal SE, et al. Quality Indicators for Esophagogastroduodenoscopy. *Am J Gastroenterol* 2006;101:886-91.

[80] Voutilainen ME, Juhola MT. Evaluation of the diagnostic accuracy of gastroscopy to detect gastric tumours: clinicopathological features and prognosis of patients with gastric cancer missed on endoscopy. *Eur J Gastroenterol Hepatol* 2005;17(12):1345-9.

[81] Puli SR, Reddy JBK, Bechtold ML, Antillo MR. How Good is Endoscopic Ultrasound for TMN Staging of Gastric Cancer? A Meta-Analysis and Systematic Review. *World J Gastroenterol* 2008;14(25):4011-9.

[82] Takedo T, Yanai H, Tada M, et al Application of ultrasonic probes prior to endoscopic resection of early gastric cancer. *Endoscopy* 1992;24(Suppl.1):329-33.

[83] Kelly S, Harris KM, Berry E, et al. A Systematic Review of Staging performance of Endoscopic ultrasound in gastro-oesophageal carcinoma. *GUT* 2001;49:534-9.

[84] Cardoso R, Coburn N, Seevaratnam R, Sutradhar R, Lourenco LG, Mahar A, Law C, Yong E, Tinmouth J. A systematic review and meta-analysis of the utility of EUS for preoperative staging for gastric cancer. *Gastric Cancer* 2012 Jan 12. [Epub ahead of print].

[85] Pollack B, Chak A, M SJ. Endoscopic Ultrasonography. *Semin Oncol* 1996;23:336-46.

[86] Kim JH, Song KS, Youn YH, et al. Clinicopathologic factors influence accurate endosonographic assessment for early gastric cancer. *Gastrointest Endosc* 2007;66(5):901-8.

[87] Bentrem D, Gerdes H, Tang L, Brennan M, Coit D. Clinical correlation of endoscopic ultrasonography with pathologic stage and outcome in patients undergoing curative resection for gastric cancer. *Ann Surg Oncol* 2007;14(6):1853-9.

[88] Burke E, Karpeh M, Conlon K, Brennan M. Laparoscopy in the managment of gastric adenocarcinoma. *Ann Surg* 1997; 225(3):262–7.

[89] Leake PA, Cardoso R, Seevaratnam R, Lourenco L, Helyer L, Mahar A, Law C, Coburn NG. A systematic review of the accuracy and indications for diagnostic laparoscopy prior to curative-intent resection of gastric cancer. *Gastric Cancer* 2011 Jun 11. [Epub ahead of print].

[90] Sarela AI, Lefkowitz R, Brennan MF, Karpeh MS. Selection of patients with gastric adenocarcinoma for laparoscopic staging. *Am J Surg* 2006;191(1):134-8.

[91] Karanicolas PJ, Elkin EB, Jacks LM, Atoria CL, Strong VE, Brennan MF, Coit DG. Staging Laparoscopy in the Management of Gastric Cancer: A Population-Based Analysis. *J Am Coll Surg* 2011;213(5):644-51

[92] Society of American Gastrointestinal and Endoscopic Surgeons Guidelines for Diagnostic laparoscopy. Available at: http://www.sages.org/publication/id/12/

[93] Abe N, Watanabe T, Toda H, Machida H, Suzuki K, Masaki T, Mori T, Sugiyama M, Atomi Y, Nakaya Y. Prognostic significance of carcinoembryonic antigen levels in peritoneal washes in patients with gastric cancer. *Am J Surg* 2001;181(4):356-61.

[94] Bentrem D, Wilton A, Mazumdar M, Brennan M, Coit D. The value of peritoneal cytology as a preoperative predictor in patients with gastric carcinoma undergoing a curative resection. *Ann Surg Oncol* 2005;12(5):1-7.

[95] Moore GE, Sako K, Kondo T, Badillo J, Burke E. Assessment of the exfoliation of tumor cells into the body cavities. *Surg Gynecol Obstet* 1961;112:469–74.

[96] Creasman WT, Rutledge F. The prognostic value of peritoneal cytology in gynecologic malignant disease. *Am J Obstet Gynecol* 1971;110(6):773–81.

[97] Boku T, Nakane Y, Minoura T, et al. Prognostic significance of serosal invasion and free intraperitoneal cancer cells in gastric cancer. *Br J Surg* 1990;77(4):436–9.

[98] Leake PA, Cardoso R, Seevaratnam R, et al. A systematic review of the accuracy and utility of peritoneal cytology in patients with Gastric Cancer. *Gastric Cancer* 2011 Aug 2. [Epub ahead of print]

[99] Badgwell B, Cormier JN, Krishnan S, et al. Does neoadjuvant treatment for gastric cancer patients with positive peritoneal cytology at staging laparoscopy improve survival? *Ann Surg Oncol* 2008;15(10):2684–91.

[100] Ajani JA, Barthel JS, Bekaii-Saab T, et al. Gastric cancer. *J Natl Compr Canc Netw* 2010;8(4):378–409.

[101] Burke EC, Karpeh MS Jr, Conlon KC, Brennan MF. Peritoneal lavage cytology in gastric cancer: an independent predictor of outcome. *Ann Surg Oncol* 1998;5(5):411-5.

[102] Vogel I, Kalthoff H. Disseminated tumour cells. Their detection and significance for prognosis of gastrointestinal and pancreatic carcinomas. *Virchows Arch* 2001;439(2):109–17.

[103] Mezhir JJ, Shah MA, Jacks LM, Brennan MF, Coit DG, Strong VE. Positive peritoneal cytology in patients with gastric cancer: natural history and outcome of 291 patients. *Ann Surg Oncol* 2010:17(12):3173-80.

[104] Lorenzen S, Panzram B, Rosenberg R, et al. Prognostic significance of free peritoneal tumor cells in the peritoneal cavity before and after neoadjuvant chemotherapy in patients with gastric carcinoma undergoing potentially curative resection. *Ann Surg Oncol* 2010;17(10):2733–9.

[105] Kuramoto M, Shimada S, Ikeshima S, et al. Extensive intraoperative peritoneal lavage as a standard prophylactic strategy for peritoneal recurrence in patients with gastric carcinoma. *Ann Surg* 2009;250(2):242–6.

[106] Yu W, Whang I, Suh I, Averbach A, Chang D, Sugarbaker PH. Prospective randomized trial of early postoperative intraperitoneal chemotherapy as an adjuvant to resectable gastric cancer. *Ann Surg* 1998;228(3):347–54.

[107] Yonemura Y, Ninomiya I, Kaji M, et al. Prophylaxis with intraoperative chemohyperthermia against peritoneal recurrence of serosal invasion-positive gastric cancer. *World J Surg* 1995;19(3):450–4 (discussion 5).

In: Gastric Cancer
Editors: A. D'Annibale, V. Pende and I. Monsellato
ISBN: 978-1-62081-294-5

Chapter III

Surgical Treatment of Early and Advanced Stage IV Gastric Cancer and Prognostic Factors

Ioannis Syrios[1], Elias Skopelitis[2*] and Nicolas Tsavaris[2]
[1]Metaxa Anticancer Hospital, Piraeus, Greece
[2]Laikon General University Hospital, Athens, Greece

Abstract

Most patients with gastric cancer present with locally advanced or metastatic disease on diagnosis, despite the availability of advanced imaging techniques. Gastrectomy in patients with stage II and III gastric carcinoma may contribute to a complete cure of the disease by total resection of the tumor and alleviation of overt metastatic or residual micrometastatic disease. Technically, this is achieved by allowing a 5cm resection disease-free margin. According to the "R" taxonomy, it is desirable to have a R0 stage post-gastrectomy. Generally, subtotal gastrectomy is more commonly used as it presents similar mortality and morbidity as total gastrectomy. The minimum number of lymph nodes required to be harvested during gastrectomy is 16, which usually allows a more accurate pathologic staging. The most appropriate method of lymph node resection, D1, D2, D3 or satellite node technique is a matter under extensive investigation in the literature.

The implementation of splenectomy together with gastrectomy depends on the location of the tumor and the suspected spleen infiltration intraoperatively. Similarly, if pancreas is infiltrated, a partial pancreatectomy should be undertaken.

In stage IV gastric carcinoma, gastrectomy serves only palliative purposes to alleviate symptoms, such as pain, hemorrhage, nausea and vomiting, dysphagia and obstruction; it might also reduce morbidity and hospitalizations. The most commonly types of operations used are bypasses, partial or sub-total gastrectomy and total gastrectomy. Clinical trials have shown that gastrectomy is more effective than the various bypasses in respect with duration of pain relief as well as survival. It is generally

* E-mail address: *iskopelitis@hotmail.com.*

accepted that for patients in stage IV M0 gastric cancer, surgery should be offered before the initiation of chemo- or radiotherapy.

For patients with unresectable disease at time of diagnosis and for those whose disease recurs after primary therapy, gastric cancer is incurable and therapy is palliative. This chapter will present the role of gastrectomy in advanced and/or metastatic gastric carcinoma and will specifically focus on a trial searching for potential prognostic factors of survival in such patients.

Introduction

Gastric cancer is an aggressive tumor, posing the second leading cause of cancer-specific mortality worldwide. The disease prevalence is higher in countries of northeast Asia (Japan, Korea, and China), intermediate in Europe, South America and lower in North America, Australia and New Zealand. The survival in Japan is good (52%) and has been attributed to early detection through nationwide implementation of screening programs [1]. However, in the United States, Europe and China, the overall survival is only 20-25%. In Greece, mortality rates for men and women have been reported to be 10.9 and 5.8 per 100000 population, respectively [2].

Surgery is considered the most appropriate treatment for gastric cancer, however only 36% of patients undergo curative resection as most patients present with locally advanced or metastatic disease, despite the progress in diagnostic modalities. Nevertheless, even patients with presumable resectable disease have relapse rates of 40-60% [3]. Therefore, palliative treatment with either surgery and / or chemotherapy is of great importance for gastric cancer patients. However, although a number of trials have reported that palliative chemotherapy improves survival compared to best supportive care [4], there is still insufficient evidence nowadays to recommend palliative gastrectomy in terms of survival benefit.

Treatment of Early Gastric Cancer

Early gastric cancer is limited to the gastric mucosa or submucosa regardless of whether regional lymph nodes are involved or not (T1) [5]. There are three different surgical approaches applied in the treatment of early gastric cancer: limited gastric resection, total gastrectomy and endoscopic mucosal resection (EMR) [6-8].

Limited gastric resection may be applied in patients with EGC smaller than 3 cm, limited to the gastric mucosa, and in those with non-ulcerated intramucosal tumors of any size. Given the low rate of nodal involvement in this setting, limited resection may be a reasonable alternative to gastrectomy. Limited resection should include a full-thickness mural excision and is often accompanied by intraoperative gastroscopy for tumor localization.

For patients with intramucosal tumors of high grade of histologic differentiation or size larger than 3 cm or who have tumor penetration into the submucosa, gastrectomy with lymph node dissection is preferred. As far as lymph node dissection is regarded, most centers favour dissection of level I lymph nodes as a reasonable minimum standard. Either subtotal or total gastrectomy is used, depending upon the tumor location. Total gastrectomy is performed for lesions in the upper third of the stomach and subtotal for lesions in the lower two-thirds.

Patients with well-differentiated, superficial type IIa or IIc lesions smaller than 2 cm in diameter or depressed lesions less than 1 cm without ulceration may be treated with endoscopic mucosal resection. This procedure involves submucosal injection of saline to raise the lesion and electrocautery for resection under endoscopic guidance. EMR-related complication rates are low and include bleeding and perforation. In one series of 308 patients, EMR successfully eradicated the cancer in 85% of cases and 5-year survival was 86% [9].

Other endoscopic modalities that may be used in the treatment of EGC are photodynamic therapy, Nd:YAG laser treatment, and argon plasma coagulation which are considered "tissue-destroying" therapies, since they do not allow tissue to be acquired en bloc for a detailed pathological examination [10-12].

Gastrectomy in Locally Advanced Gastric Adenocarcinoma

The best chances for long-term survival in stage II/III gastric adenocarcinoma are ensured by the surgical approach. Surgery in locally advanced gastric carcinoma should optimally remove all macroscopic lesions without leaving any microscopic residual disease. Technically, all macroscopic malignant lesions and adjacent lymph nodes are resected, along with allowing a 5 cm disease-free margin. Besides, according to the “R” taxonomy, it is desirable to have a R0 stage post-gastrectomy, which is achieved either by a total gastrectomy or a subtotal gastrectomy as well. The latter is preferable due to minor morbidity without a detrimental effect on survival [13-17].

Total gastrectomy is the method of choice for lesions located in the proximal stomach, while subtotal gastrectomy for lesions located in the distal stomach. However, patients with large mid-gastric lesions or diffuse, infiltrative disease (eg, linitis plastica) may also require total gastrectomy [16-19].

Lymph node dissection is an essential step of the surgical approach. In order to achieve high accuracy when determining the pathologic stage of the disease, at least 16 lymph nodes should be harvested [20,21]. The extent of lymphadenectomy is still a matter of debate in the literature. In the MRC study, survival rates of patients treated with D1 (perigastric lymph node resection) or D2 (resection of lymph nodes along the hepatic, left gastric, celiac and splenic arteries as well as those in the splenic hilum) lymphadenectomy were comparable (5-year survival 35% vs 33%, respectively), with major morbidity observed in D2 dissection (46% vs 28%, respectively, $P<0.001$); this fact may be attributed to the routine use of pancreatectomy and splenectomy during the D2 lymphadenectomy. Mortality following a D2 lymphadenectomy is higher in confronts with the D1 (13% vs 6%, respectively, $P<0.04$), however this procedure still remains a common approach in Japan. The authors of the MRC study concluded that D2 does not offer a survival benefit over D1 [22,23]. Moreover, the Dutch Gastric Cancer Group compared D1 with D2 lymphadenectomy in 711 patients who were treated with curative intent. Postoperative morbidity and mortality were higher in the D2 group (43% versus 25% and 10% versus 4%, respectively) and no survival advantage was observed in the radical dissection group [24-26]. Nevertheless, the update of the Dutch trial, after a 15-year follow-up period, revealed that survival curves had continued to separate, although the difference in overall survival was not statistically significant (22% versus 28% in the D1 and D2 arms, respectively, $p=0.34$). However, the gastric cancer-related death rate was significantly higher in the D1 arm (48% versus 37%). In the latest Dutch trial paper, D2 dissection is recommended in patients with potentially curable gastric cancer provided that the aggressive nodal dissection is performed in selected, well-experienced centers. Currently, National Comprehensive Cancer Network treatment guidelines recommend that D2 lymph node dissection should be performed in patients undergoing potentially curative resection of a gastric cancer [27,28].

D3 lymphadenectomy, which involves para-aortic lymph nodes dissection, does not confer any benefit and is not used any longer [29].

As far as sentinel lymph node evaluation is regarded, preliminary data suggest that lymph node dissection should not be abandoned, given that patients with gastric cancer may have multiple sentinel lymph nodes [30-34].

In the cases that neoplastic lesions involve the proximal gastric area, the greater curvature of the stomach or extend to the splenic hilum, splenectomy may be performed simultaneously. When pancreas is involved, a subtotal pancreatectomy may be warranted [35-38].

Gastrectomy in Stage IV Gastric Adenocarcinoma

The role of surgery in stage IV gastric adenocarcinoma is clearly palliative. In this setting, gastrectomy minimizes morbidity and the need for hospitalization. The aim of the surgical approach is to temporarily alleviate symptoms such as pain, bleeding, nausea, vomiting, dysphagia and obstruction. Practically, it can be achieved with a bypass (gastrojejunostomy), partial or subtotal gastrectomy, and total gastrectomy. Several studies reveal that gastrectomy confers higher response and survival rates in confronts with the bypass procedure. Some symptomatic patients may benefit from surgical resection, even in the presence of macroscopic residual disease. Moreover, in stage IV (M0) patients with a high performance status and a potentially resectable lesion, gastrectomy may precede radiotherapy and/or chemotherapy. Other modalities that are used to alleviate symptoms include the use of intraluminal stenting and endoscopic apply of laser therapy in case of obstruction [39,40].

Prognostic Factors

In current practice, the decision for surgery is individualized based on patient's clinical status and local surgical expertise aiming at symptom relief and maintenance of patient's independence and function. However, as chemotherapy and/or surgery could be associated with significant complications, there is a need to identify prognostic factors which may determine treatment response and survival in stage IV gastric cancer patients. Such an approach could refine palliative management according to the likelihood of clinical benefit. Since most patients with gastric cancer present with locally advanced or metastatic disease on diagnosis, prognostic factors should be studied that would identify the most appropriate and adequate treatment modality and the setting of patients who might benefit the most. Several potential prognostic variables, such as demographics, clinical parameters, biochemical markers and management modality have been examined.

Several studies revealed that liver metastases, local recurrence, abdominal and peritoneal metastases, grade III histology, poor performance status, increased tumor marker, LDH and

CRP values, blood transfusion requirements, low serum albumin, weight loss >10% of total body weight, and a high DNA ploidy index may be accompanied by increased risk of death [41-57]. Besides, therapeutic modalities, such as palliative gastrectomy and combination chemotherapy appear to favor survival. [41, 58-60]

In addition, it is anticipated that prognostic models, based on the above parameters or combinations of such parameters, may be applied that would facilitate individual risk stratification and assist in the design of future prospective studies. The aim of the study presented later in this chapter was to evaluate factors affecting survival in patients with advanced stage III or IV gastric adenocarcinoma receiving chemotherapy.

Patients and Methods

Patients and Data Sources

The medical records of 311 patients who received chemotherapy for histopathological confirmed stage IV gastric cancer between February 1997 and October 2007 were retrospectively reviewed. All were consecutive non-selected cases from a single Oncology Center and all patients were treated outside of clinical trials. Stage IV gastric cancer was defined based on American Joint Committee on Cancer (AJCC, 6th edition) as M1 or T4N1-3M0 [61]. Patients with Gastro-Esophageal junction tumors, small cell carcinoma, lymphoma, and squamous cell carcinoma were excluded. All patients included in the study had histological diagnosis of gastric adenocarcinoma and all demographic, clinical, imaging, laboratory and follow-up data were available. Metastatic disease was diagnosed by applying various imaging modalities, including chest X ray, ultrasonography and computed tomography. Tissue specimens were obtained by gastroscopy, surgery, or fine-needle aspiration biopsy from liver lesions. 218 (70%) had previously undergone palliative surgery (subtotal or total gastrectomy) at six different tertiary Greek hospitals from which primary evaluation and surgical treatment was performed and further referral to the oncology center was initiated. The indications for palliative gastrectomy were judged individually by attending surgeons based on patients' general health, performance status, symptoms, extend of disease, and feasibility of resection. Single-agent chemotherapy regimens were based on leucovorin modulated 5-Fluorouracil (5-FU, n= 135). Combination chemotherapy regimens included combination treatments based on Irinotecan, Oxaliplatin and Capecitabine according to established protocols (n=176) [4,62]. The primary end point of the study was Overall Survival (OS). The study protocol was approved by the Ethical Committee for Research Projects of Laiko Hospital, Athens, Greece.

Prognostic Variables

17 putative clinicopathological and therapeutic prognostic variables were selected, based on factors identified by previous studies, as well as our own clinical experience [63-71]. Patient-related factors included age (≤60 years or >60 years), gender, and pre-treatment performance status (PS) according to the Karnofsky Performance Status Scale Index.

Table 1. Patient Characteristics

		(n=311)	(%)
Age	≤60	137	44.2
	>60	173	55.8
Gender	Male	209	67.2
	Female	102	32.8
PS	60-70	117	37.6
	80	107	34.4%
	90-100	87	28.0%
Pain	No	176	56.6%
	Yes	135	43.4%
Weight Loss	No	73	23.5%
	0-5%	148	47.6%
	> 5%	90	28.9%
Blood Transfusion	No	183	58.8%
	Yes	128	41.2%
Tumor Location	Body	179	57.6%
	Antrum	132	42.4%
Histological Grade	I	14	4.5%
	II	179	57.6%
	III	118	37.9%
Metastases	Local invasion	163	52.4%
	Lymph nodes	247	79.4%
	Liver	162	52.1%
	Lung	26	8.4%
	Ovaries	29	9.3%
	Bone	12	3.9%
	Abdomen/Peritoneum	151	48.6%
CEA	≤ 5 ng/ml	158	50.8%
	> 5 ng/ml	153	49.2%
CA 19-9	≤30 U/ml	118	37.9%
	> 30 U/ml	193	62.1%
CA 72-4	≤7 U/ml	59	19.0%
	> 7 U/ml	251	81.0%
CRP	≤ 5 mg/dL	165	53.1%
	>5 mg/dL	146	46.9%
Albumin	>3.4 g/dL	171	55.0%
	< 3.4 g/dL	140	45.0%
LDH	<225 U/L	137	44.2%
	> 225 U/L	173	55.8%
Palliative gastrectomy	No	93	29.9
	Yes	218	70.1
Chemotherapy	single agent chemotherapy	135	43.5
	combination chemotherapy	176	56.5

PS: performance status.
CEA: Carcinoembryonic Antigen.
CA 19-9: Cancer Antigen 19-9.
CA 72-4: Cancer Antigen 72-4.
CRP: C-Reactive Protein.
LDH: Lactate Dehydrogenase.

Tumor-related factors included symptoms such as pain (yes vs. no), weight loss (no, 0 - 5%, >5%), and the necessity for blood transfusions (yes vs. no); location of primary tumor (body vs. antrum), histological grading according the World Health Organisation (WHO) system, location of metastases: Local invasion, lymph nodes, liver, lung, ovaries, bone abdomen/peritoneum; and biochemical parameters. For the latter, group categorizations were used: for carcinoembryonic antigen (CEA): normal ≤5 ng/dl vs. elevated >5 ng/dL; for cancer antigen 19 9 (CA 19 9): values ≤30 U/ml vs. >30 U/ml; for cancer antigen CA 72-4 (CA 72-4): normal ≤7 U/ml vs. elevated >7U/ml; for C reactive protein (CRP): normal <5 mg/dl vs. elevated >5 mg/dl; for Albumin: normal >3.4 g/dL vs. decreased <3.4 g/dL; and for Lactate Dehydrogenase (LDH): normal <225 U/L vs. elevated >225 U/L. Factors related to therapy included palliative gastrectomy (yes vs. no) and chemotherapy (single agent vs. combination chemotherapy).

Statistical Analysis

Descriptive statistics were calculated with the use of mean, median and standard deviation for quantitative measurements and counts/percentages for discrete factors.

Survival data were studied with the use of Kaplan-Meier method. Changes in survival between groups were recorded with the log-rank test. Prognostic models were established by searching all variables that significantly related OS at a level of P values ≤ 0.05 in the univariate analysis. Multivariate analysis was subsequently carried out using stepwise Cox proportional hazards modeling for OS. Best model selection for the factors that significantly affected OS factors were based on automated techniques.

Results of regression analyses were displayed in the form of regression estimates tables. Hazard ratios of outcomes under study were calculated for each parameter estimate as well as 95% confidence intervals. Categorical covariates are compared with a predefined reference category. All categorical variables were compared using a baseline category as reference. All analyses were conducted at a 5% significant level using SPSS v12.0 statistical package.

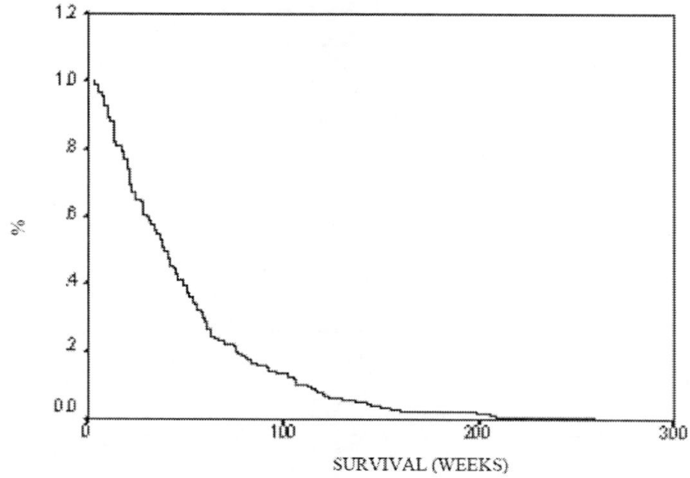

Figure 1. Overall Survival.

Table 2. Univariate Analysis for Survival

Variable			MST	1-year survival %	P-value
Age		≤ 60	39	37.2	0.536
		>60	40	34.1	
Gender		Male	40	35.4	0.728
		Female	36	32.4	
Chemotherapy		single agent	29	29.6	0.011
		combination chemotherapy	45	45.0	
PS		60-70	21	16.2	<0.001
		80	48	44.9	
		90-100	55	50.6	
Histological Grade		I	50	35.7	0.033
		II	42	39.1	
		III	34	29.7	
Metastases	Local	No	41	37.2	0.409
		Yes	33	34.4	
	Lymph nodes	No	36	21.9	0.110
		Yes	40	39.7	
	Liver	No	50	47.7	<0.001
		Yes	28	24.7	
	Lung	No	40	36.8	0.1547
		Yes	30	23.1	
	Ovaries	No	39	35.8	0.7155
		Yes	40	34.5	
	Bone	No	40	36.1	0.078
		Yes	17	25.0	
	Abdomen/Peritoneum	No	42	40.6	0.009
		Yes	33	27.8	
Blood Transfusion		No	53	50.3	<0.001
		Yes	21	15.6	
Weight Loss		No	51	48.0	<0.001
		0-5%	48	45.3	
		> 5%	12	8.9	
Palliative gastrectomy		Yes	53	51.4	<0.001
		No	16	0.0	
Albumin		>3.4 g/dL	50	46.2	<0.001
		< 3.4 g/dL	21	22.1	
LDH		<225 U/L	57	51.8	<0.001
		> 225 U/L	30	22.0	
CRP		≤ 5 mg/dL	48	44.9	<0.001
		>5 mg/dL	24	25.3	
Pain		No	45	43.2	<0.001
		Yes	22	25.9	
CA 19-9		≤30 U/ml	48	42.4	0.009

Variable			MST	1-year survival %	P-value
		> 30 U/ml	38	31.6	
CA 72-4		≤7 U/ml	50	44.1	0.007
		> 7 U/ml	38	33.5	
CEA		≤ 5 ng/ml	40	32.3	0.359
		> 5 ng/ml	37	39.2	
Location	Body	No	40	34.9	0.454
		Yes	38	34.1	
	Antrum	No	40	34.1	0.454
		Yes	38	34.9	

MST: median survival time.
PS: performance status.
LDH: Lactate Dehydrogenase.
CRP: C-Reactive Protein.
CA 19-9: Cancer Antigen 19-9.
CA 72-4: Cancer Antigen 72-4.
CEA: Carcinoembryonic Antigen.

Table 3. Multivariate Analysis of Survival

		P-Values	HR	95.0% CI	
				Low	High
Palliative Gastrectomy No vs. Yes		0.000	12.009	7.969	18.099
Chemotherapy single agent vs. combination		0.013	1.356	1.068	1.721
Liver metastases Yes vs. No		0.000	1.607	1.246	2.073
Abdominal/Peritoneal metastases Yes vs. No		0.024	1.335	1.039	1.715
Histological Grade	Grade III vs. Grade I	0.007	1.399	1.098	1.782
	Grade II vs. Grade I	0.889	0.959	0.528	1.741
CA72-4 >7 vs. ≤7		0.034	1.391	1.026	1.887
LDH Yes vs. No		0.000	1.728	1.336	2.236
Weight Loss	> 5% vs. 0-5%	0.599	0.923	0.685	1.244
	> 5% vs. No	0.000	1.964	1.352	2.853
Blood Transfusions Yes vs. No		0.001	1.589	1.213	2.082

HR: Hazard Ratio.
CI: Confidence Interval.
CA 72-4: Cancer Antigen 72-4.
LDH: Lactate Dehydrogenase.

Results

Patients

311 patients with Stage IV gastric cancer were included in this analysis. The median age was 62 years (mean: 60, range: 30-74, SD: 8.893) and the frequencies of the clinicopathological variables are shown in Table 1. Palliative surgery was performed in 70% of patients. All patients received chemotherapy; single agent and combination chemotherapy were administered in 43.5% and 56.5% of patients respectively.

Overall Survival

Survival data were collected for all patients. No patient was alive by the time of this analysis. The 1-year overall survival rate was 36%. Based on the Kaplan-Meier method, the mean survival time (MST) was recorded at 50 weeks [95% confidence interval (CI) 45- 55 weeks], with a median survival of 39 weeks (95% CI 34- 44 weeks) (Figure 1).

Univariate Analysis

In the univariate analysis the following parameters were found to adversely relate to survival (Table 2): Single agent chemotherapy (P=0.011), PS 60-70 (P<0.001), histology Grade III (P=0,033), presence of hepatic (P<0.001) and peritoneal/abdominal metastases (P=0.009) , need for blood transfusions (P<0.001), weight loss >5% (P<0.001), no previous palliative gastrectomy (P<0.001), albumin <3.4 g/dL (P<0.001), LDH >225 U/L (P<0.001), CRP >5 mg/dL (P<0.001), presence of pain (P<0.001), CA19-9 >30 U (P=0.009) and CA 72-4 >7 U/ml (P=0.007).

Multivariate Analysis

Factors that were found to be significantly related to OS were included in the multivariate analysis which is presented in Table 3.

Hazard Ratios of Risk Factors

Nine prognostic factors were found to independently affect survival. Two factors had a positive influence on survival including palliative gastrectomy and combination chemotherapy. In particular, patients who had undergone palliative gastrectomy had 12 times lower probability of death compared with those who had no surgery and patients who received combination chemotherapy had 1.35 lower probability of death compared to those received single agent chemotherapy. Seven factors were found to adversely affect survival including the presence of hepatic and abdominal/peritoneal metastasis (HRs 1.60 and 1.30 respectively), Grade III histology (HR, 1.40) CA 72-4 >7 U/L (HR, 1.39), LDH >225 U/L (HR, 1.72), weight Loss >5% (HR, 1.96), and the need for blood transfusions (HR 1.58) at presentation.

Prognostic Grouping

A prognostic grouping for the 311 patients was carried out according to the following criteria: low risk group = zero to two factors, intermediate risk group = three to six factors, high risk = seven to nine factors; the survival curves that were accordingly produced are depicted in Figure 2. One year survival rates for low, intermediate and high risk patients were calculated at 71%, 33% and 0%, respectively (Figure 2).

Discussion

We retrospectively analyzed data from 311 patients with Stage IV gastric adenocarcinoma who had undergone palliative chemotherapy. Our analysis demonstrated that factors associated with disease burden had a negative effect on survival. These included the presence of hepatic and abdominal/peritoneal metastases, histological grade III, elevated CA 72-4 levels, elevated LDH levels and poor functional status at the time of initial presentation as indicated by weight loss >5% and severe anemia necessitating blood transfusions.

Hepatic and abdominal/peritoneal metastases have been shown previously to adversely affect survival in a multivariate analysis of a large cohort of patients with locally advanced and metastatic esophago-gastric cancer with an estimated hazard ratio of 1.41 and 1.33 respectively [63]; similar results were subsequently reported by others [63,65,71].

The various histological indexes commonly used for grading gastric cancer have been extensively investigated with regards to their prognostic potential with conflicting results [72, 73]. The main difficulty in the histological classification of gastric cancer is the great variability of architectural and cytological features that may be present within the same tumor. Hence, the prognostic significance of the various histological indexes which are commonly used for grading gastric cancer is rather controversial [74].

Nevertheless, our study supports the prognostic significance of the WHO histological staging since Histology Grades I, II and III were associated with progressively decreasing survival time (MST 50, 42 and 34 weeks, respectively).

Tumor markers can be used clinically for the monitoring of recurrence, as well as prognostic factors. Our results demonstrate the prognostic significance of CA 72-4 in Stage IV gastric cancer, in accordance with previously published data. In a cohort of 95 patients who underwent surgical resection of gastric cancer, preoperative CA72- 4 levels were shown to be more frequently elevated in patients with lymph node (P=0.01), peritoneal (P=0.03) and liver involvement (P=0.001).

In the same study, elevated CA72-4 levels were associated with a 3.8-fold higher risk of death in multivariate analysis [75]. In the study published by Louhimo et al., sub- analysis of a group of patients with advanced gastric cancer (stages III and IV) revealed that CA 72. 4 is an independent prognostic factor for survival (HR 1.2) [68]. In addition, our study reinforces the prognostic significance of elevated LDH levels, a well-established prognostic indicator in terminally ill cancer patients [76].

The etiology of weight loss at presentation in patients with gastric cancer is complex and poorly characterized and implies a physical wasting process in excess of the degree of nutritional deficit. Decreased intake due to the anatomical location of tumor and cytokine induced anorexia may further aggravate the problem. The association of weight loss with poor survival, as well as with higher toxicity and lower chemotherapy response rates has already been described among patients with gastric cancer [77]. Similarly, in our study weight loss >5% evolved as an independent prognostic factor for decreased survival in patients with Stage IV gastric cancer.

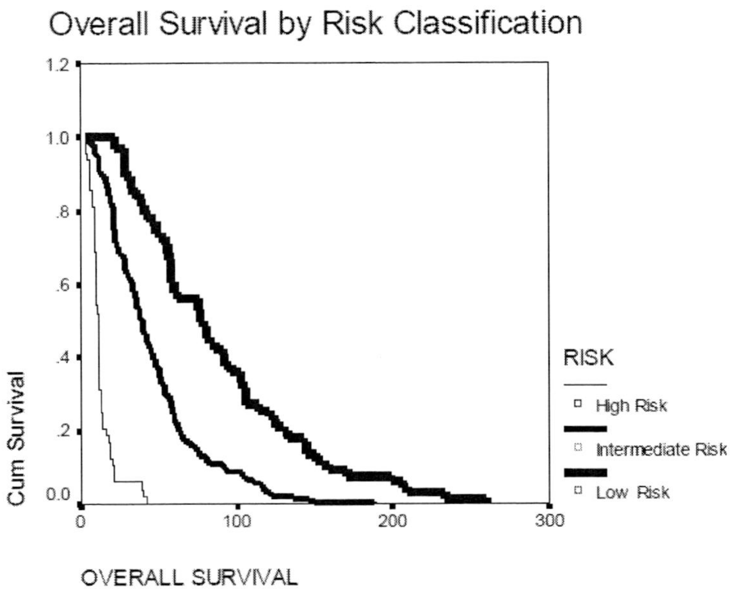

Figure 2. Survival data according to Risk Classification.

Risk Group	n (%)	Median survival	1-year OS	P-Value
Low	66 (21,2)	76	71%	<0.001
Intermediate	197 (63,3)	40	33%	
High	48 (15,4)	11	0%	

The relationship between blood transfusions and survival in gastric cancer remains controversial. A previous study by Kampschoer et al [78] showed no difference between 5-years survival rates in transfused and non-transfused patients grouped by stage and similar results were reported by others [79]. On the contrary, other reports [80,81], including an analysis of 1,710 patients with Stage III and IV gastric cancer by Hyung et al., showed that survival in transfused patients was clearly poorer than in non-transfused patients, in accordance with our findings.

On the other hand, our study highlights the importance of palliative gastrectomy and combination chemotherapy as modalities associated with improved survival. The value of palliative operations, including gastrectomy, in patients presenting with metastatic gastric cancer is still unsettled since palliative gastrectomy was associated in some early studies with significant postoperative morbidity, prolonged hospital stay and poor quality of life [69]. Moreover, the indications and the type of the appropriate palliative surgical treatment in such patients are rather based on clinical judgment, local surgical expertise and patient's arguments than on data from controlled studies [82].

The rationale for offering palliative gastrectomy to patients with unresectable or metastatic gastric cancer is to avoid tumor bleeding, perforation, obstruction, or complicated ascites and to possibly improve the outcome by reducing tumor burden rendering the patients more responsive to adjuvant modalities. It has been postulated that volume and tumor reduction diminishes the hypercatabolic state and may also confer immunological benefit by reducing the production of tumor derived immunosuppressive cytokines [70,83]. Although limited by a small number of patients, Saidi et al. demonstrated a significantly better survival in gastrectomised patients who received adjuvant chemotherapy as compared with a chemotherapy only group (mean survival 16.3 months versus 5.9 months, P= 0.01). In their study the mortality and morbidity of palliative gastrectomy was 8.7% and 33.3%, respectively, which was not statistically different from the mortality and morbidity of curative gastrectomy [70]. Similar results were obtained from subsequent analysis of larger cohorts, demonstrating improved survival in patients with advanced gastric adenocarcinoma after palliative gastric resection as compared to those who did not undergo the procedure [64-66]. In the current study, patients with previous palliative gastrectomy had clearly more favorable clinical course compared with those without gastrectomy (MST 53 vs 16 weeks).

Single agents used in the first line setting achieve only modest responses and are proffered for patients who are unable to tolerate combination chemotherapy [84]. Combination regimens are able to achieve better response rates at the expense of increased toxicity and are therefore preferred in appropriately selected patients. A meta-analysis comparing trials of systemic mono-therapy with those of multi-agent therapy, showed a significant increase in response with multi-agent therapy, with a hazard ratio of 0.83 (95% CI 0.74-0.93) and improvement in overall survival by about 1 month [4]. Nevertheless, no chemotherapy combination has been accepted as the gold standard in Stage IV gastric cancer. Both CF [cisplatin (CDDP/5) – 5-fluorouracil (5-FU)] and ECF (epirubicin – CDDP/5 – FU) are seen as regimens of reference, but the MST does not exceed 7-10 months [85]. Options have expanded as it has been shown that capecitabine is at least as good as 5-FU and that oxaliplatin at least as good as cisplatin in these combinations [62].

In our study, 135 patients were treated with single agent chemotherapy (leucovorin modulated 5-FU), while 176 patients had received combination chemotherapy and on multivariate analysis combination chemotherapy evolved as an independent prognostic factor for survival as compared to single agent chemotherapy (MST was 29 weeks for the single agent chemotherapy group and 45 weeks for the combination chemotherapy group, while 1-year survival was 29.6% and 45%, respectively). These results add further to the accumulation of data from other studies, suggesting a clear survival benefit when palliative gastrectomy is combined with postoperative chemotherapy [67,70]. In particular, Lin et al. have shown that the 1-year, 3-year and 5-year survival rate of those stage IV gastric cancer patients who were treated with palliative gastrectomy and postoperative chemotherapy were 85.7%, 32.1%, and 8.9%, which were far better for those who were not, whilst survival benefits were also apparent in patients with liver metastasis, peritoneal dissemination, and/or N3 lymph metastasis if treated with this multimodality approach.

Prognostic scoring systems have been defined in several cancer types and are being increasingly used in clinics to stratify patients into different risk groups. The nine factors which have been found by our analysis to independently affect survival in stage IV gastric cancer were further evolved into a prognostic model, which separates patients into three groups with distinct prognosis with 1-year survival rates for low, intermediate and high risk patients at 71%, 33% and 0%, respectively.

The limitations of this analysis is the retrospective setting, as well as the fact that the initial evaluation and decision for palliative gastrectomy was performed by different surgical teams, albeit in hospitals with adequate case volume [86], prior referring their patients to a specialized Oncology Center for postoperative chemotherapy. Subsequently, the surgery plan was individualized based on patient's clinical status and local surgical expertise, which, although depicts the routine clinical practice, hampers the results of survival analysis due to the lack of postoperative survival data from each individual surgical center. Nevertheless, all patients were consecutive, non-selected cases, and received chemotherapy in the same Oncology Center under the supervision of a specialist medical team and all were treated outside clinical trials, a fact which resembles a real life situation.

In conclusion a number of factors may independently influence survival in Stage IV gastric cancer patients. Factors associated with the severity of the disease, such as the presence of hepatic and abdominal/peritoneal metastases, histological grade III, elevated CA 72-4, elevated LDH and poor functional status at time of initial diagnosis, as indicated by weight Loss >5% and severe anemia necessitating blood transfusions, have a detrimental effect on survival, while therapeutic modalities, such as palliative gastrectomy and combination chemotherapy favor survival. In addition, it is anticipated that the prognostic model based on the above parameters will facilitate the individual risk stratification and help the design of future prospective studies.

References

[1] Hartgrink H. H. , Jansen E. P., van Grieken N. C., van de Velde C. J.: Gastric cancer. *Lancet* 2009;374:477-490.

[2] Ong S. H., Smithers M. B.: Gastric cancer in Australia. *Gastric Cancer* 2002;5: 118-121.

[3] D'Angelica M., Gonen M., Brennan M. F., et al.: Patterns of initial recurrence in completely resected gastric adenocarcinoma. *Ann. Surg.* 2004; 240:808-816.

[4] Wagner A. D., Grothe W., Haerting J., et al.: Chemotherapy in advanced gastric cancer: a systematic review and meta-analysis based on aggregate data. *J. Clin. Oncol.* 2006;24:2903-2909.

[5] Murakami, T. Pathomorphological diagnosis. Definition and gross classification of early gastric cancer. *Gann. Monogr. Cancer Res.* 1971; 11:53.

[6] Miyata M., Yokoyama Y., Okoyama N., et al. What are the appropriate indications for endoscopic mucosal resection for early gastric cancer? Analysis of 256 endoscopically resected lesions. *Endoscopy* 2000;32:773.

[7] Yamao T., Shirao K., Ono H., et al. Risk factors for lymph node metastasis from intramucosal gastric carcinoma. *Cancer* 1996;77:602.

[8] Brennan M. F., Karpeh M. S. Jr.: Surgery for gastric cancer: the American view. *Semin. Oncol.* 23 (3): 352-9, 1996.

[9] Takekoshi T., Baba Y., Ota H., Kato Y., Yanagisawa A., Takagi K., Noguchi Y.. Endoscopic resection of early gastric carcinoma: results of a retrospective analysis of 308 cases. *Endoscopy*. 1994;26(4):352.

[10] Mimura S., Ito Y., Nagayo T., Ichii M., Kato H., Sakai H., Goto K., Noguchi Y., Tanimura H., Nagai Y., Suzuki S., Hiki Y., Hayata Y. Cooperative clinical trial of photodynamic therapy with photofrin II and excimer dye laser for early gastric cancer. *Lasers. Surg. Med.* 1996;19(2):168.

[11] Oguro Y. J. Laser endoscopic treatment for early gastric cancer. *Gastroenterol.* 1994;29 Suppl. 7:91.

[12] Kitamura T., Tanabe S., Koizumi W., Mitomi H., Saigenji K. Argon plasma coagulation for early gastric cancer: technique and outcome. *Gastrointest Endosc.* 2006;63(1):48.

[13] Cady B. Subtotal gastric resection. In: Daly J. M., Cady B., Low D., eds. Atlas of surgical oncology. *St. Louis: Mosby-Year Book*, Inc., 1993:221.

[14] Lawrence J. W. Total gastrectomy. In: Daly J. M., Cady B., Low D., eds. Atlas of surgical oncology. *St. Louis: Mosby-Year Book*, Inc., 1993:241.

[15] Robertson C. S., Chung S. C., Woods S. D., et al. A. prospective randomized trial comparing R1 subtotal gastrectomy with R3 total gastrectomy for antral cancer. *Ann. Surg*. 1994;220:176.

[16] Gouzi J. L., Huguier M., Fagniez P. L., et al. Total versus subtotal gastrectomy for adenocarcinoma of the gastric antrum. A. French prospective controlled study. *Ann. Surg*. 1989;209:162.

[17] Bozzetti F., Marubini E., Bonfanti G., et al. Subtotal versus total gastrectomy for gastric cancer: five-year survival rates in a multicenter randomized Italian trial. Italian Gastrointestinal Tumor Study Group. *Ann. Surg*. 1999;230:170.

[18] Anderson I. D., MacIntyre I. M. Symptomatic outcome following resection of gastric cancer. *Surg. Oncol.* 1995; 4:35.

[19] Wu C. W., Chiou J. M., Ko F. S., et al. Quality of life after curative gastrectomy for gastric cancer in a randomised controlled trial. *Br. J. Cancer* 2008; 98:54.

[20] Karpeh M. S., Leon L., Brennan M. F. Lymph node staging in gastric cancer: is location more important than number? An analysis of 1,038 patients. *Ann. Surg.* 2000;232:362.

[21] Stomach. In: Greene F., Page D., Fleming I. D., et al., eds. *AJCC cancer staging manual.* New York: Springer-Verlag, 2002:99.

[22] Cuschieri A., Weeden S., Fielding J., et al. Patient survival after D1 and D2 resections for gastric cancer: long-term results of the MRC randomized surgical trial. Surgical Co-operative Group. *Br. J. Cancer* 1999;79:1522.

[23] Cuschieri A., Fayers P., Craven J., et al. Postoperative morbidity and mortality after D1 and D2 resections for gastric cancer: preliminary results of the MRC randomised controlled surgical trial. The Surgical Cooperative Group. *Lancet* 1996;347:995.

[24] Bonenkamp J. J., Hermans J., Sasako M., et al. Extended lymph-node dissection for gastric cancer. *N. Engl. J. Med.* 1999; 340:908.

[25] Hartgrink H. H., van de Velde C. J., Putter H., et al. Extended lymph node dissection for gastric cancer: who may benefit? Final results of the randomized Dutch gastric cancer group trial. *J. Clin. Oncol.* 2004; 22:2069.

[26] Petrelli N. J. The debate is over; it's time to move on. *J. Clin. Oncol.* 2004; 22:2041.

[27] Songun I., Putter H., Kranenbarg E. M., et al. Surgical treatment of gastric cancer: 15-year follow-up results of the randomised nationwide Dutch D1D2 trial. *Lancet Oncol.* 2010; 11:439.

[28] National Comprehensive Cancer Network (NCCN) guidelines *www.nccn.org.* (Accessed on February 04, 2011).

[29] Sano T., Sasako M., Nashimoto A., et al. Gastric cancer surgery: results of morbidity and mortality of a prospective randomized controlled trial (JCOG 9501) comparing D2 and extended para-aortic lymphadenectomy. *J. Clin. Oncol.* 2004.

[30] Aikou T., Higashi H., Natsugoe S., et al. Can sentinel node navigation surgery reduce the extent of lymph node dissection in gastric cancer? *Ann. Surg. Oncol.* 2001;8:90S.

[31] Kitagawa Y., Fujii H., Mukai M., et al. Radio-guided sentinel node detection for gastric cancer. *Br. J. Surg.* 2002;89:604.

[32] Ichikura T., Morita D., Uchida T., et al. Sentinel node concept in gastric carcinoma. *World. J. Surg.* 2002;26:318.

[33] Miwa K., Kinami S., Taniguchi K., et al. Mapping sentinel nodes in patients with early-stage gastric carcinoma. *Br. J. Surg.* 2003;90:178.

[34] Hayashi H., Ochiai T., Mori M., et al. Sentinel lymph node mapping for gastric cancer using a dual procedure with dye- and gamma probe-guided techniques. *J. Am. Coll. Surg.* 2003;196:68.

[35] Furukawa H., Hiratsuka M., Ishikawa O., et al. Total gastrectomy with dissection of lymph nodes along the splenic artery: a pancreas-preserving method. *Ann. Surg. Oncol.* 2000;7:669.

[36] Doglietto G. B., Pacelli F., Caprino P., et al. Pancreas-preserving total gastrectomy for gastric cancer. *Arch. Surg.* 2000;135:89.

[37] Schwarz R. E. .Spleen-preserving splenic hilar lymphadenectomy at the time of gastrectomy for cancer: technical feasibility and early results. *J. Surg. Oncol.* 2002;79:73.

[38] Csendes A., Burdiles P., Rojas J., et al. A prospective randomized study comparing D2 total gastrectomy versus D2 total gastrectomy plus splenectomy in 187 patients with gastric carcinoma. *Surgery* 2002;131:401.

[39] Ekbom G. A., Gleysteen J. J. Gastric malignancy: resection for palliation. *Surgery* 1980;88:476.

[40] Meijer S., De Bakker O. J., Hoitsma H. F. Palliative resection in gastric cancer. *J. Surg. Oncol.* 1983;23:77.

[41] Buonadonna A., Lombardi D., De Paoli A., Bidoli E., Frustaci S. Adenocarcinoma of the stomach: univariate and multivariate analyses of factors associated with survival. *Suppl. Tumori.* 2003 Sep.-Oct.;2(5):S3 1-4.

[42] Kubota H., Kotoh T., Dhar D. K., Masunaga R., Tachibana M., Tabara H., Kohno H., Nagasue N. Gastric resection in the aged (> or = 80 years) with gastric carcinoma: a multivariate analysis of prognostic factors. *Aust. N. Z. J. Surg.* 2000 Apr.;70(4): 254-7.

[43] De Vita F., Romano C, Orditura M., Galizia G., Martinelli E., Lieto E., Catalano G. Interleukin-6 serum level correlates with survival in advanced gastrointestinal cancer patients but is not an independent prognostic indicator. *J. Interferon Cytokine Res.* 2001 Jan.;21(1):45-52.

[44] Webb.A., Scott-Mackie P., Cunningham D., Norman A., Andrevev J., O'Brien M., Bensted J. The prognostic value of serum and immunohistochemical tumour markers in advanced gastric cancer. *Eur. J. Cancer.* 1996 Jan.;32A(1) :63-8.

[45] Dewys W. D., Begg C., Lavin P. T., et al. Prognostic effect of weight loss prior to chemotherapy in cancer patients. Eastern Cooperative Oncology Group. *Am. J. Med.* 1980;69:491.

[46] Park S. H., Lee J., Lee S. H., Park J. O., Kim K., Kim W. S., Jung C. W., Park Y. S., Kang W. K., Park K., Kim S., Bang S. M., Cho E. K., Shin D. B., Lee J. H. Anemia is the strongest prognostic factor for outcomes of 5-fluorouracil-based first-line chemotherapy in patients with advanced gastric cancer. *Cancer Chemother. Pharmacol.* 2006 Jan.;57(1):91-6. Epub 2005 Nov. 5.

[47] Onate-Ocana L. F., Aiello-Crocifoglio V., Mondragon Sanchez R., Ruiz Molina J. M., Gallardo-Rincon D. [Prognostic factors in 793 cases of gastric cancer in an oncologic referral center]. *Rev. Gastroenterol Mex.* 1999 Jul.-Sep.;64(3):114-21.

[48] Baba H., Okuyama T., Hiroyuki O., Anai H., Korenaga D., Maehara Y., Akazawa K., Sugimachi K. Prognostic factors for noncurative gastric cancer: univariate and multivariate analyses. *Surg. Oncol.* 1992 Oct.;51(2):104-8.

[49] Nekarda H., Gess C., Stark M., Mueller J. D., Fink U., Schenck U., Siewert J. R. Immunocytochemically detected free peritoneal tumour cells (FPTC) are a strong prognostic factor in gastric carcinoma. *Br. J. Cancer.* 1999 Feb.;79(3-4):611-9.

[50] Elahi M. M., McMillan D. C., McArdle C. S., Angerson W. J., Sattar N. Score based on hypoalbuminemia and elevated C-reactive protein predicts survival in patients with advanced gastrointestinal cancer. *Nutr. Cancer.* 2004;48(2):171-3.

[51] Grem J. The prognostic importance of tumor markers in adenocarcinomas of the gastrointestinal tract. *Curr. Opin. Oncol.* 1997 Jul.;9(4):380-7.

[52] Pectasides D., Mylonakis A., Kostopoulou M., Papadopoulou M., Triantafillis D., Varthalitis J., Dimitriades M., Athanassiou A. CEA, CA 19-9, and CA-50 in monitoring gastric carcinoma. *Am. J. Clin. Oncol.* 1997 Aug.;20(4):348-53.

[53] Sougioultzis S., Syrios J., Xynos I. D., Bovaretos N., Kosmas C., Sarantonis J., Dokou A., Tzivras D., Zografos G., Felekouras E., Papalambros E., Tsavaris N., Palliative gastrectomy and other factors affecting overall survival in stage IV gastric adenocarcinoma patients receiving chemotherapy: a retrospective analysis. *Eur. J. Surg. Oncol.* 2011 Apr.;37(4):312-8.

[54] Fujimaki, E., et al., DNA ploidy heterogeneity in early and advanced gastric cancers. *Cytometry*, 1996. 26(2): p. 131-6.

[55] Furuya, T., et al., Relationship between chromosomal instability and intratumoral regional DNA ploidy heterogeneity in primary gastric cancers. *Clin. Cancer Res.*, 2000. 6(7): p. 2815-20.

[56] Umehara, Y., et al., Metastatic mode and DNA ploidy in gastric carcinoma. *Surg. Today*, 1992. 22(5): p. 405-8.

[57] Ooiwa, H., et al., [Heterogeneity in gastric carcinoma with special reference to DNA content and mitotic activity: histopathologic differentiation*]. Gan To Kagaku Ryoho*, 1994. 21 Suppl. 1: pp. 17-20.

[58] Wang S., Sun Z., Wang S. Study on factors influencing survival in patients with advanced gastric carcinoma after resection by Cox's proportional hazard model. *Zhonghua Zhong Liu Za Zhi.* 1996 Nov.;18(6):433-5.

[59] Doglietto G. B., Pacelli F., Caprino P., Sgadari A., Crucitti F. Surgery: independent prognostic factor in curable and far advanced gastric cancer. *World J. Surg.* 2000 Apr.;24(4):459-63; discussion 464.

[60] Llanos O., Butte J. M., Crovari F., Duarte I., Guzman S. Survival of young patients after gastrectomy for gastric cancer. *World J. Surg.* 2006 Jan.; 30 (1):17-20.

[61] AJCC: "Cancer staging manual." Springer, New York 2003.

[62] Van Cutsem E., Van d. e. Velde C., Roth A., et al.: Expert opinion on management of gastric and gastro-oesophageal junction adenocarcinoma on behalf of the European Organisation for Research and Treatment of Cancer (EORTC)-gastrointestinal cancer group. *Eur. J. Cancer* 2008;44:182-194.
[63] Chau I., Norman A. R., Cunningham D., et al.: Multivariate prognostic factor analysis in locally advanced and metastatic esophago-gastric cancer--pooled analysis from three multicenter, randomized, controlled trials using individual patient data. *J. Clin. Oncol.* 2004;22:2395-2403.
[64] Hartgrink H. H., Putter H., Klein Kranenbarg E., et al.: Value of palliative resection in gastric cancer. *Br. J. Surg.* 2002;89:1438-1443.
[65] Kim J. G., Ryoo B. Y., Park Y. H., et al.: Prognostic factors for survival of patients with advanced gastric cancer treated with cisplatin-based chemotherapy. *Cancer Chemother Pharmacol.* 2008;61:301-307.
[66] Lee J., Lim T., Uhm J. E., et al.: Prognostic model to predict survival following first-line chemotherapy in patients with metastatic gastric adenocarcinoma. *Ann. Oncol.* 2007;18:886-891.
[67] Lin S. Z., Tong H. F., You T., et al.: Palliative gastrectomy and chemotherapy for stage IV gastric cancer. *J. Cancer Res. Clin. Oncol.* 2008;134:187-192.
[68] Louhimo J., Kokkola A., Alfthan H., et al.: Preoperative hCGbeta and CA 72-4 are prognostic factors in gastric cancer. *Int. J. Cancer* 2004;111:929-933.
[69] Ouchi K., Sugawara T., Ono H., et al.: Therapeutic significance of palliative operations for gastric cancer for survival and quality of life. *J. Surg. Oncol.* 1998;69:41-44.
[70] Saidi R. F., ReMine S. G., Dudrick P. S., Hanna N. N.: Is there a role for palliative gastrectomy in patients with stage IV gastric cancer? *World J. Surg.* 2006;30:21-27.
[71] Shiraishi N., Sato K., Yasuda K., et al.: Multivariate prognostic study on large gastric cancer. *J. Surg. Oncol.* 2007;96:14-18.
[72] Inoue K., Nakane Y., Michiura T., et al.: Histopathological grading does not affect survival after R0 surgery for gastric cancer. *Eur. J. Surg. Oncol.* 2002;28:633-636.
[73] Perrone G., Ruffini P. A., Catalano V., et al.: Intratumoural FOXP3-positive regulatory T. cells are associated with adverse prognosis in radically resected gastric cancer. *Eur. J. Cancer* 2008;44:1875-1882.
[74] Luebke T., Baldus S. E., Grass G., et al.: Histological grading in gastric cancer by Ming classification: correlation with histopathological subtypes, metastasis, and prognosis. *World J. Surg.* 2005;29:1422-1427; discussion 1428.
[75] Ucar E., Semerci E., Ustun H., et al.: Prognostic value of preoperative CEA, CA 19-9, CA 72-4, and AFP levels in gastric cancer. *Adv. Ther.* 2008;25:1075-1084.
[76] Suh S. Y., Ahn H. Y.: Lactate dehydrogenase as a prognostic factor for survival time of terminally ill cancer patients: a preliminary study. *Eur. J. Cancer.* 2007;43:1051-1059.
[77] Costa M. L., de Cassia Braga Ribeiro K., Machado M. A., et al.: Prognostic score in gastric cancer: the importance of a conjoint analysis of clinical, pathologic, and therapeutic factors. *Ann. Surg. Oncol.* 2006;13:843-850.
[78] Kampschoer G. H., Maruyama K., Sasako M., et al.: The effects of blood transfusion on the prognosis of patients with gastric cancer. *World J. Surg.* 1989;13:637-643.

[79] Moriguchi S., Maehara Y., Akazawa K., et al.: Lack of relationship between perioperative blood transfusion and survival time after curative resection for gastric cancer. *Cancer* 1990;66:2331-2335.

[80] Hyung W. J., Noh S. H., Shin D. W., et al.: Adverse effects of perioperative transfusion on patients with stage III and IV gastric cancer. *Ann. Surg. Oncol.* 2002;9:5-12.

[81] Ojima T., Iwahashi M., Nakamori M., et al.: Association of allogeneic blood transfusions and long-term survival of patients with gastric cancer after curative gastrectomy. *J. Gastrointest Surg.* 2009;13:1821-1830.

[82] Cunningham S. C., Schulick R. D.: Palliative management of gastric cancer. *Surg. Oncol.* 2007;16:267-275.

[83] Pollock R. E., Roth J. A.: Cancer-induced immunosuppression: implications for therapy? *Semin. Surg. Oncol.* 1989;5:414-419.

[84] Wesolowski R., Lee C., Kim R.: Is there a role for second-line chemotherapy in advanced gastric cancer? *Lancet Oncol.* 2009;10: 903-912.

[85] Cervantes A., Rosello S., Roda D., Rodriguez-Braun E.: The treatment of advanced gastric cancer: current strategies and future perspectives. *Ann. Oncol.* 2008;19 Suppl. 5:v103-107.

[86] Damhuis R. A., Meurs C. J., Dijkhuis C. M., et al.: Hospital volume and post-operative mortality after resection for gastric cancer. *Eur. J. Surg. Oncol.* 2002;28:401-405.

In: Gastric Cancer
Editors: A. D'Annibale, V. Pende and I. Monsellato
ISBN: 978-1-62081-294-5

Chapter IV

Clinical Usefulness of Intraoperative Sentinel-Node Biopsy in Gastric Cancer

A. E. Dassen, D. J. Lips* and K. Bosscha
Jeroen Bosch Ziekenhuis Hospital,
Hertogenbosch, The Netherlands

Abstract

Gastric cancer is one of the main causes of cancer-related deaths around the world. The prevalence of early gastric cancer is growing partly because of better diagnostics and screening programs. Possible treatment options for early gastric cancer treatment are expanded by the introduction of endoscopic mucosal resection and endoscopic submucosal dissection. Therefore, detailed knowledge about nodal metastatic risk is warranted. The role of sentinel lymph node biopsy in early gastric cancer has been investigated intensively for this and other purposes. Several detection substances and injection methods have been investigated. Whether sufficient sensitivity and accuracy percentages have been reported is subject of this chapter. The various methods are presented and their (dis)advantages discussed. Although large experience has been gained by several centers, the precise role of sentinel lymph node biopsy in gastric cancer is unclear. The implementation of such a procedure heavily depends on the local experience and manner of implementation. Further research is needed for the determination of sentinel lymph node biopsy in gastric cancer.

Introduction

Incidence and mortality rates for gastric cancer are, although declining, still high worldwide. In Europe it ranks fourth on the list of cancer incidence rates and fifth on the list of mortality rates [1]. There are differences between the West and East in incidence, survival

* E-mail address: *D.Lips@jbz.n.*

and treatment. Gastric cancer is endemic in Asian countries. Therefore, a screening program has been implemented to detect gastric cancer in an early stage [2]. In Europe, such a screening program is not cost-effective. Due to lack of pathognomonic signs, gastric cancer is detected in a late stage. Gastric cancer can be subdivided in early gastric cancer (EGC) and advanced gastric cancer (AGC). EGC is defined as tumour confined to the mucosa or submucosa, irrespective of nodal metastases (T1N0-2). EGC is found in 37-51%[3-5] of patients in Asia. In contrast, in Western countries this percentage does not surpass 7-28% [3]. In Asia, treatment of gastric cancer consists of (partial) gastric resection combined with an extended lymphadenectomy. In Europe, several studies have been conducted to evaluate the benefit of such an extended lymphadenectomy, e.g. D2 or more. The systematic review of McCulloch concluded that no advantage of a D2 over a D1 lymphadenectomy could be found due to high postoperative morbidity and mortality, probably as a result of the concomitant partial pancreatectomy and splenectomy in the hands of inadequately trained surgeons. There was no advantage in overall survival [6-8]. Therefore, in Europe, except for some (university) hospitals, (partial) gastric resection is accompanied by a regional lymph node dissection.

All patients with curable gastric cancer will undergo a (partial) gastric resection combined with a(n extended) lymphadenectomy, with associated morbidity and mortality risk. Not all patients with tumours confined to the mucosa or submucosa (EGC) will benefit from it, for only 2-23% have lymph node metastases (see table 1). In predicting lymph node metastases, non-invasive techniques such as computed tomography (CT), magnetic resonance imaging (MRI) and endoscopic ultrasound (EUS) have low sensitivity rates [9-11]. Sentinel lymph node biopsy (SLNB) could be a solution for this problem. In the East and West several studies have been conducted to evaluate the usefulness of SLNB in predicting lymph node metastases in EGC.

This chapter will review the results of those studies and give a recommendation whether to use SLNB in EGC [12].

Several methods have been described in literature to perform sentinel lymph node biopsy, using different kinds of detection substance, different injection methods, and different pathology protocols. The following paragraphs discuss some of these techniques.

Sentinel Node Handling

The sentinel lymph nodes are investigated with haematoxylin and eosin staining, either directly after surgery (fresh frozen sectioning) or after embedding in formalin. The number of sections of lymph nodes varies between two or multiple sections of 2-3 mm of thickness. Additional immunohistochemical staining for cytokeratin using various techniques is sometimes used to detect isolated tumour cells (i.e. clustered cells with maximal diameter <0.2 mm) or micrometastases (i.e. clustered cells with maximal diameter 0.2 – 2 mm and signs of stromal invasion) in case of a negative sentinel node. The prognostic significance of these latter nodal metastases is currently unknown.

Nowadays, new techniques are implemented and predominantly used in experimental setting. These new techniques constitute of immediate nodal investigation by full-automated reverse-transcriptase RNA modalities. Detection of isolated tumour cells and micrometastases is considered to be more effective with these methods.

Table 1. T-status and Observed Metastatic Lymph Node Involvement According to Depth of Tumour Invasion*

T-status	Depth of tumour invasion of gastric wall	Metastatic lymph node involvement	Reference
T_{is} T_{1a} T_{1b}	Intraepithelial tumour without invasion of lamina propria. Tumour invasion of mucosa and/or muscularis mucosa . Tumour invasion of submucosa.	 2 – 5% 6 – 23%	Gotoda, et al. Gastric Cancer 2000; Hohenberger P, Gretschel S. Lancet 2003.
T_2	Tumour invasion of muscularis propria or subserosa	10 – 41%	Hohenberger P, Gretschel S. Lancet 2003; Sasako, et al. Br J Surg 2005; Di Leo A, et.al. J Gastrointest Surg 2007
T_3	Tumour penetration of serosa	17-64%	Hohenberger P, Gretschel S. Lancet 2003; Di Leo A, et al. J Gastrointest Surg 2007
T_4	Tumour invasion of adjacent structures	84%	Di Leo A, et al. J Gastrointest Surg 2007

*Derived from International and Japanese Gastric Cancer Associations (Gastric Cancer 1998;1:10-24) and the International Union Against Cancer (UICC) TNM staging system (6th edn, 2002) Tis (carcinoma in situ). Early gastric cancer is defined as tumour invasion confined to the mucosa or submucosa, irrespective of nodal metastases, i.e. T1N0. The incidence of lymph node metastasis is low in early gastric cancer patients, with more than a 90% 5-year survival rate. The overall prognosis for patients with gastric cancer remains poor, with a 5-year survival rate of 5 to 15%. (Akoh, 1992; Itoh, 1989).

Sentinel Node Detection by Dye

Detection substances used are dye or radioactive colloid. Isosulphan blue, indocyanine green and Patent V blue are mainly used in case of a dye. The injection of the dye is performed in two different manners, either via an endoscopic procedure or during laparotomy. There are two methods described for the endoscopic procedure. The patient is firstly submitted to the endoscopic procedure immediately after anesthesia. Via the endoscope 0.25 ml-2 ml dye is injected submucosal at four points around the tumour (see table 2 for references). Five to 20 minutes after the injection the blue (or green) stained lymph nodes are either marked with a suture or taken out with the rest of the specimen, or are dissected immediately, considered being sentinel lymph nodes. The other method starts with surgery. After inspection of the abdomen (some describe mobilization of the stomach), dye is injected subserosal during endoscopy. In case of the subserosal technique the surgeon injects dye at four points around the tumour after laparotomy. Sometimes, prior to surgery, the surrounding of the tumour is clipped, in case the tumour might not be palpable.

Table 2. Results Sentinel Lymph Node (SLN) Procedures in Gastric Cancer

Reference	Method	TNM^	N	Detection succes-rate	SLN/pt (range)	SLN+[¶]	Sens	Spec	PPV	NPV	Acc SLN status	Acc frozen biopsy	Skip metastasis[†] (detected)	SLN micrometastasis[‡]
Hiratsuka M, et al. Surgery 2001	Indocyanine green; subserosal; laparotomy	T_{1-2}	74	98.6%	2.6 (1-9)	12.3%	90%	100%	100%	98.4%	98.6%	-	-	-
Kitagawa Y, et al. Br J Surg 2002	^{99m}Tc tin colloid; submucosal; endoscopically	T_{1-2}	145	95%	3.6 (1-8)	7.8%	91.7%	100%	100%	98.4%	98.6%	-	0.8% -100%	-
Hundley JC, et al. Am Surg 2002.	Isosulfan blue; subserosal, laparotomy	T_{1-3}	14	100%	2.8 (1-5)	28.2%	70%	75%	90%	50%	70%	-	-	0%
Ichikura T, et al. World J Surg 2002	Indocyanine green; submucosal; endoscopically	T_{1-2}	62	100%	4.5[#] (1-12)	24%	86.7%	100%	100%	95.7%	93.5%	-	1.6% 0%	-
Hayashi H, et al. J Am CollSurg 2003	^{99m}Tc tin colloid	T_{1-2}	28	90%	3.7	10.7%	85.7%	100%	100%	95.5%	96.4%	-	-	0%
	Patent blue; submucosal; endoscopically		28	90%	3.6	21.4%	71.4%	100%	100%	91.3%	92.9%	-	-	0%
	(cb)		31	100%	5,2	22.8%	100%	100%	100%	100%	100%			
Miwa K, et al. Br J Surg 2003	Patent blue; submucosal; endoscopically	T_{1-3}	211	96.2%	6 (1-16)	5.2%	88.6%	100%	100%	97.8%	98.1%	98.6%	1.4% -100%	-
Simsa J, et al. ActaChirBelg 2003	Patent blue; subserosal; laparotomy	T_{1-3}	13	100%		61.5%	100%	100%	100%	100%	100%	84.6%	-	0%
Ryu KW, et al. EJSO 2003	Isosulfan blue; subserosal; laparotomy	T_{1-2}	71	91.5%	2.5 (1-8)	28.2%	61.1%	100%	100%	87%	89.2%	-	10.8% 0%	-
*Tonouchi H, et al. Dig Surg 2003^*	^{99m}Tc tin colloid	T_1	17	82.4%	2.8 (1-9)									
	Patent blue; submucosal; endoscopically		17	88.2%	2.5 (1-6)									
	(cb)		17	100%	4.2 (2-9)	17.6%	100%	100%	100%	100%	100%	33.3%^^	11.8% (50%)	66%

Reference	Method	TNM^	N	Detection succes-rate	SLN/pt (range)	SLN+[¶]	Sens	Spec	PPV	NPV	Acc SLN status	Acc frozen biopsy	Skip metastasis[†] (detected)	SLN micrometas tasis[‡]
Uenosono U, et al. Canc Lett 2003	^{99m}Tc tin colloid; 500 nm 100 nm 50 nm submucosal; endoscopically (overall)	$T_{1\text{-}2}$	12 13 11 36	66.7% 100% 100% 88.9%	1.8 (0-4) 3.8 (1-6) 3.0 (1-7) 2.9 (0-7)	37.5% 7.7% 18.2% 18.8%	100% 100% 100% 100%	100% 100% 100% 100%	100% 100% 100% 100%	100% 100% 100% 100%	100% 100% 100% 100%	100% 100% 100% 100%	25% 0% 9.1% 9.4%	- - - -
Kim M-C, et al. Ann Surg 2004	^{99m}Tc tin colloid; submucosal; endoscopically	$T_{1\text{-}3}$	46	93.5%	2 (1-8)	25.6%	84.6%	100%	100%	93.8%	95.3%	97.7%	7% -100%	0%
Isozaki H, et al. Gastric Cancer 2004	Isosulfan blue; submucosal; endoscopically	$T_{1\text{-}3}$	144	97.2%	3.3 (1-9)	-	-	-	-	-	-	-	-	-
Song X, et al. Am J Surg 2004	Isosulfan blue; subserosal; laparotomy	$T_{1\text{-}3}$	27	96.3%	2.7 (1-6)	20%	100%	100%	100%	100%	100%	-	0	-
Nimura H, et al. Br J Surg 2004	Indocyanine green; submucosal; endoscopically	$T_{1\text{-}2}$	8	98.8%	5.5	8.4%	63.6%	100%	100%	94.7%	95.2%	-	-	-
	+ IREE		98.8%	10.5	13.3%	100%	100%	100%	100%	100%	-	-	-	
Zulfikaroglu B, et al. Surgery 2005	148 MBq ^{99m}Tc filtered sulfur colloid; submucosal; endoscopically	$T_{1\text{-}3}$	32	97%	2.4	18%	100%	95.5%	90%	100%	96.7%	97%	10%	0%
Gretschel S, et al. EJSO 2005.	^{99m}Tc colloidal rhenium sulphide;	$T_{1\text{-}3}$	15	93.3%	3 (1-5)	57.1%	88.9%	100%	100%	83.3%	92.9%	-	11.1% (0%)	
	Patent blue; submucosal; endoscopically		19	100%	3 (1-6)	73.4%	100%	100%	100%	100%	100%	-	7.1% (0%)	
Lee JH, et al. EJSO 2005	Isosulfan blue; subserosal (laparotomy)	$T_{1\text{-}2}$	71	91.5%	2.5	16.9%	61.1%	100%	100%	87%	89.2%	-	-	-
	versus submucosal (endoscopically)		50	94%	2.9	10.6%	45.5%	100%	100%	85.7%	87.2%	-	-	-
Park DJ, et al. EJSO 2006	Indocyanine green; subserosal; laparotomy	$T_{1\text{-}2}$	100	94%	4.4	11.7%*	78.6%*	100%*	100%*	96.4%*	96.8%*	-	-	4.3%
Mochiki E, et al. Am J Surg 2006	^{99m}Tc colloidal rhenium sulphide; submucosal; endoscopically	$T_{1\text{-}3}$	59	96.6%	3.8\ (1-10)	35.1%	83.3%	100%	100%	89.2%	93%	-	-	-

Table.2. (Continued)

Reference	Method	TNM	N	Detection succes-rate	SLN/pt (range)	SLN+¶	Sens	Spec	PPV	NPV	Acc SLN status	Acc frozen biopsy	Skip metastasis† (detected)	SLN micrometas tasis‡
Gretschel S, et al. Ann SurgOncol 2007	^{99m}Tc colloidal rhenium sulphide;		35	97%	3 (1-10)	64.7%	91.7%	100%	100%	83.3%	94.1%	-	-	31.8%
	Patent blue; submucosal; endoscopically	T_{1-3}	35	97%	3 (1-6)	47.1%	66.7%	100%	100%	55.6%	76.5%	-	-	31.3%
	(cb)		35	97%	3 (1-10)	64.7%	91.7%	100%	100%	83.3%	94.1%	-	-	31.8%
Cozzaglio L et al. ESJO 2010	Patent blue dye technique	T_{1-2}	29	96,5%	1.6 (1-3)	61%	75%	75%	88%	55%	75%	-	-	18%
Tonouchi H, et al. W J Surg	^{99m}Tc tin colloid; submucosal; endoscopically; Patent blue; submucosal; endoscopically	T_{1-2}	37	94,6%	4	8,1%	75%	100%	100%	96,9%	97,1%	97,1	-	
Rino Y, et al. Surg Endosc 2006	Patent blue; submucosal; endoscopically	T_1	38	92,1%	2,5	5,30%	100%	100%	100%	100%	100%	100%	-	
Saikawa Y et al. W J Surg	^{99m}Tc tin colloid; submucosal; endoscopically; Isosulphan blue; submucosal; endoscopically	T_1	35	94,3%	3,9	2,90%	50%	100%	100%	96,9%	97%	97%	-	
Saikawa Y et al. W J Surg	^{99m}Tc tin colloid; submucosal; endoscopically; Isosulphan blue; submucosal; endoscopically	T_1	35	94,3%	3,9	2,90%	50%	100%	100%	96,9%	97%	97%	-	
Lee YJ et al. J Lap End SurgTechn 2008	^{99m}Tc tin colloid; submucosal; endoscopically; Indocyanine green; submucosal; endoscopically	T_{1-2}												
	Pick-up method		42	54,8%	2,1	17,4%	66,0%	100%	100%	89,5%	91,3%	91,3%	-	

Reference	Method	TNM	N	Detection succes-rate	SLN/pt (range)	SLN+¶	Sens	Spec	PPV	NPV	Acc SLN status	Acc frozen biopsy	Skip metastasis† (detected)	SLN micrometastasis‡
	Lymph node bassin method		50	96,0%	3,5	25%	85,7%	100%	100%	94,4%	95,8%	95,8%	-	
Lee HJ et al. J SurgOncol 2008	^{99m}Tc tin colloid; submucosal; endoscopically; Isosulphan blue; submucosal; endoscopically	T_1	21	95,2%	7	10%	100%	94,4%	67%	100%	95,0%	95,0%	-	
Tajima Y et al. Ann Surg Onc 2010	Indocyanine green; submucosal; endoscopically + IREE	T_{1-2}	77	94,8%	7,5	18%	76,5%	100%	100%	93,3%	94,5%		-	
Miyashiro I et al. Surg Endosc 2011	Indocyanine green; submucosal; endoscopically + EM-CCD + Xenon lamp	T_1	10	100,0%	3,1 (1-6)	30%	100%	100%	100%	100%	100%	100%	-	
Park DJ et al. Ann SurgOncol 2011	^{99m}Tc tin colloid	T1	68	73,5%	2,5		81,3%	100%	100%	100,0%	91,9%	91,9%	-	
	Patent blue; submucosal; endoscopically			80,9%	3,1		93,8%	100,0%	100%	97,5%	98,2%	98,2%	-	
	(cb)			91,2%	3,3		100%	100%	100%	100%	100%	100%	-	

Abbreviations: Acc accuracy; cb combination; IREE infrared ray electronic endoscopy; EM-CCD electron multiplier charge-coupled device; NPV negative predictive value; PPV positive predictive value; Sens sensitivity; Spec specificity; SLN sentinel lymph node.

^The actually observed T-status is mentioned; all studies excluded patients with metastatic disease. SLN positivity (+) for metastasis is calculated by the equation: patient with SLN positive for tumour/total patients with SLNs found.

†Skip metastases are defined as lymph node metastases in D2 or D3 compartments, without involvement of the perigastric D1 compartment. Percentage calculated by the equation: patient with skip metastasis/total patients studied.

‡SLN micrometastasis detection rate is defined by the equation: SLN micrometastasis positive/total SLN metastasis positive.

#Based on the results of group patients injected with 4 ml 1.25% indocyanine green, excluding the group injected with 8ml 0.63% indocyanine green, as the former is the preferred method to identify SLNs according to the investigators.

^Study investigating laparoscopic gastrectomy with lymphatic mapping.

^^In the SNs of 2 of 3 patients with positive lymph nodes micrometastasis were found in frozen-sections by immunohistochemistry staining, not in the frozen-section examination by hematoxylin and eosin staining (diagnostic accuracy frozen biopsy 1 out of 3, 33%).

*and**Results of respectively hematoxylin and eosin and immunohistochemistry staining on final pathological non-frozen examination.

The rest of the procedure is followed as described above. The detection rates of SLNB with the use of dye are currently 88.2-100%. Combining the injection of indocyanine green with IREE (infrared ray electronic endoscopy) results in a SLN detection rate of 94.8-100%. Detection rates do not differ very much between the submucosal and subserosal technique (94 vs 91.5%).

Sentinel Node Detection by Radiocolloid Substance

In case of radioactive colloid, the use of 99mTc tin colloid and 99mTc colloidal rhenium sulphide are mainly used (see table 2 for references). The substance is injected submucosal at 4 points around the tumour mostly 16-24 hours prior to surgery during endoscopy. The injection can also be performed 2-4 hours prior to surgery with adjustment of the amount of colloid injected. The quantities used are ranging from 0.5 ml - 2 ml. Sentinel lymph nodes are detected with a hand-held gamma probe, either during surgery, postoperative on the specimen or both. Sentinel nodes are the first echelon nodes draining from the tumour, which primarily absorb the radioactive substance. The gamma probe detects the nodes with radioactivity and thereby discriminates them from non-sentinel nodes. When activity is 10 times the surrounding activity, they are considered to be sentinel lymph nodes. Sentinel node detection preoperative has the advantage of intact anatomy. Postoperative sentinel node detection has the advantage of a freely movable en-block tissue specimen. The precise technique is however not different. After gastric resection and lymph node dissection a check-up is performed for residual activity. The radiocolloid particle size is of influence on detection rate. In case of 99mTc tin colloid detection rates are fairly low with 500 nm particle size. 50 and 100 nm particle size give a significant higher detection rate[13]. Excluding the detection rate with a 500 nm particle, SLN detection rates range from 82.4-100%.

Sentinel Node Detection by Dye and Radiocolloid Substances Combined

The combined procedure of using of radiocolloid and submucosal dye is currently giving a detection range of SLN of 97-100%. Methods of injection are as described above.

Sentinel Node Detection and Laparoscopy

Mostly the method combining dye and radiocolloid is used. Both detection substances are injected submucosal during endoscopy either a day before or during surgery. After introducing the trocars into the abdomen, the greater omentum is divided near the transverse colon to expose the lesser sac, the posterior stomach wall and the pancreas head. After occluding the proximal jejunum near the ligament of Treitz with a laparoscopic intestinal clamp, the endoscope is introduced. Dye is injected round the tumour and after 5-20 minutes the colored lymph nodes are assigned as sentinel lymph nodes. The radioactive nodes are identified using a gamma probe as described above. Either a pick-up method or a sentinel lymph node basin dissection method is used. During the pick-up method lymph nodes assigned as sentinel nodes are dissected, compared to dissection of the surrounding tissue during the sentinel node basin dissection. The colored and/or 'hot' nodes are depicted extra corporally and sent to the pathologist accordingly.

SLN detection rate is 54.8-100%, with the least percentage described in the earlier mentioned pick-up method, and the highest in indocyanine green combined with EM-CCD and a Xenon lamp.

Value of SLNB in Gastric Cancer

Sensitivity is defined as the number of patients with true positive SLNs divided by the number of patients with true positive SLNs and false negative SLNs. Sensitivity rates are fairly high when combining dye and colloid substances (table 2), although overall sensitivity is still very low (85.5%, range of 45.5-100%). This means that if a patient has lymph node metastases these will be detected by SLNB in only 85.5% of patients.

In case of specificity higher rates were found (98.2%). Specificity is defined as the number of patients with negative SLNs divided by the number of patients with true negative SLNs and false positive SLNs. This high specificity means in case of a patient without lymph node metastases that the chance is very high that the SLN is negative.

Positive predictive value, defined as the number of patients with true positive SLNs divided by the number of patients with true positive SLNs and false positive SLNs, is 99%. The chance of having lymph node metastases is very high in case of a positive result. The chance of not having lymph node metastases in case of a negative SLN is lower, as negative predictive value is 90.7%. This is defined as the number of patients with negative SLNs divided by the number of patients with negative lymph nodes and false negative lymph nodes.

In laparoscopic assisted gastrectomy and SLNB sensitivity ranges from 66-100%. The SLN basin method seems to have higher sensitivity rates compared to the pick-up method. Specificity of approximately 100% is high.

The Future of Sentinel Node Detection in Gastric Cancer

In patients with gastric cancer confined to the mucosa and muscularis propria without lymph node metastases a(n extended) lymphadenectomy could be omitted, resulting in less morbidity and mortality rates without withholding benefit to the patients. The current imaging techniques are not useful in detecting lymph node metastases. Therefore, several studies investigated the role of SLNB in gastric carcinoma, but based on the current results, not enough proof was found to implement SLNB in gastric cancer. A mean sensitivity rate of 88.5% is too low to justify the use of SLNB. A sensitivity rate of >95% should be achieved before implementing this method in gastric cancer.

The results described above were extracted from a review of the literature[12] on sentinel lymph node biopsy in gastric cancer. These studies show a high heterogeneity, with different kinds of detection methods, implementation methods and pathologic examination. Some studies included patients with T3 tumours, with a risk of lymph node metastases in 70%. No clear distinction was made in those studies between T1 and T2 vs T3 tumours. Therefore, not all results are comparable.

Laparoscopic sentinel lymph node detection rates are comparable to open SN detection rates. Regarding sensitivity rates these are still too low to justify implementation of SLNB.

Detection rate of sentinel lymph nodes and sensitivity are suggested to grow with experience[14,15]. Some proclaim a learning curve of less than 10 patients, although the exact amount is not clear14. As soon as one reaches sensitivity rates of 95% in SLNB, it can be argued that the surgeon has enough experience to perform this procedure. Most studies were held in Asian countries. It is not known if the results of those studies can be extrapolated to Western countries. In Japan a screening program for detecting gastric cancer leads to a higher percentage of T1 and T2 tumours. Experience in Western countries will be less compared to endemic regions with high incidence of EGC, and therefore the lack of experience might influence the results of SLNB. Furthermore, patients in Western countries are more obese, which makes it more difficult to find the SLN's.

Based on the current knowledge, in theory, prophylactic lymph node dissection could be omitted in patients with EGC with negative SLNB, if the sensitivity of SLNB is around 95%. When positive SLN is found, the patient will receive an additional lymphadenectomy, preferentially during the procedure. A fresh frozen sectioning is therefore mandatory. This type of pathological examination is only described in some studies in literature[16]. Investigation of fresh sentinels is performed by fresh frozen histology, or by RT-PCR techniques. Much about sensitivity and accuracy is currently unknown. Therefore, the results described above are not completely reliable. As all of these studies have been performed in Asian countries, more studies in Western countries should be performed investigating the role of SLNB in EGC before implementation. As the best results are found using the combination of dye and radiocolloid, it is recommended to use these two methods in further studies. The SLN's should be send to the pathologist for fresh frozen sectioning, because when implementing SLNB, it is preferable to perform the lymphadenectomy together with the gastric resection compared to a second separate surgery. The latter is less patient friendly. As current investigative methods are unpredictable at the moment, it is wise to perform an adequate lymphadenectomy aside of a sentinel node procedure during one surgical session. Moreover, the role of micrometastases and isolated tumour cells is even more obscure in gastric cancer. As laparoscopic (assisted) gastrectomy is gaining ground, the role of SLNB in laparoscopy should be further investigated. Lastly, it is recommended to perform SLNB before initiating the study to prevent bias in the result due to lack of experience.

References

[1] Ferlay J., Parkin D. M., Steliarova-Foucher E. Estimates of cancer incidence and mortality in Europe in 2008. *Eur. J. Cancer* 2010; 46(4):765-781.

[2] Hamashima C., Shibuya D., Yamazaki H., Inoue K., Fukao A., Saito H. et al. The Japanese guidelines for gastric cancer screening. *Jpn. J. Clin. Oncol.* 2008; 38(4): 259-267.

[3] Yuasa N., Nimura Y. Survival after surgical treatment of early gastric cancer, surgical techniques, and long-term survival. *Langenbecks Arch. Surg.* 2005; 390(4):286-293.

[4] Maeda H., Okabayashi T., Nishimori I., Sugimoto T., Namikawa T., Dabanaka K. et al. Clinicopathologic features of adenocarcinoma at the gastric cardia: is it different from distal cancer of the stomach? *J. Am. Coll. Surg.* 2008; 206(2):306-310.

[5] Tajima Y., Yamazaki K., Makino R., Nishino N., Masuda Y., Aoki S. et al. Differences in the histological findings, phenotypic marker expressions and genetic alterations between adenocarcinoma of the gastric cardia and distal stomach. *Br. J. Cancer* 2007; 96(4):631-638.

[6] Cuschieri A., Weeden S., Fielding J., Bancewicz J., Craven J., Joypaul V. et al. Patient survival after D1 and D2 resections for gastric cancer: long-term results of the MRC randomized surgical trial. Surgical Co-operative Group. *Br. J. Cancer* 1999; 79(9-10):1522-1530.

[7] Hartgrink H. H., van d., V., Putter H., Bonenkamp J. J., Klein K. E., Songun I. et al. Extended lymph node dissection for gastric cancer: who may benefit? Final results of the randomized Dutch gastric cancer group trial. *J. Clin. Oncol.* 2004; 22(11):2069-2077.

[8] McCulloch P., Nita M. E., Kazi H., Gama-Rodrigues J. Extended versus limited lymph nodes dissection technique for adenocarcinoma of the stomach. *Cochrane Database Syst. Rev.* 2004;(4):CD001964.

[9] Dassen A. E., Lips D. J., Hoekstra C. J., Pruijt J. F., Bosscha K.. FDG-PET has no definite role in preoperative imaging in gastric cancer. *Eur. J. Surg. Oncol.* 2009; 35(5):449-455.

[10] Puli S. R., Batapati Krishna R. J., Bechtold M. L., Antillon M. R., Ibdah J. A. How good is endoscopic ultrasound for TNM staging of gastric cancers? A meta-analysis and systematic review. *World J. Gastroenterol* 2008; 14(25):4011-4019.

[11] Chen C. Y., Hsu J. S., Wu D. C., Kang W. Y., Hsieh J. S., Jaw T. S. et al. Gastric cancer: preoperative local staging with 3D multi-detector row CT--correlation with surgical and histopathologic results. *Radiology* 2007; 242(2):472-482.

[12] Lips D. J., Schutte H. W., van der Linden R. L., Dassen A. E., Voogd A. C., Bosscha K. Sentinel lymph node biopsy to direct treatment in gastric cancer. A systematic review of the literature. *Eur. J. Surg. Oncol.* 2011; 37(8):655-661.

[13] Uenosono Y., Natsugoe S., Higashi H., Ehi K., Miyazono F., Ishigami S. et al. Evaluation of colloid size for sentinel nodes detection using radioisotope in early gastric cancer. *Cancer Lett.* 2003; 200(1):19-24.

[14] Nimura H., Narimiya N., Mitsumori N., Yamazaki Y., Yanaga K., Urashima M. Infrared ray electronic endoscopy combined with indocyanine green injection for detection of sentinel nodes of patients with gastric cancer. *Br. J. Surg.* 2004; 91(5): 575-579.

[15] Park D. J., Lee H. J., Lee H. S., Kim W. H., Kim H. H., Lee K. U. et al. Sentinel node biopsy for cT1 and cT2a gastric cancer. *Eur. J. Surg. Oncol.* 2006; 32(1):48-54.

[16] Tonouchi H., Mohri Y., Tanaka K., Konishi N., Ohmori Y., Kobayashi M. et al. Lymphatic mapping and sentinel node biopsy during laparoscopic gastrectomy for early cancer. *Dig. Surg.* 2003; 20(5): 421-427.

In: Gastric Cancer
Editors: A. D'Annibale, V. Pende and I. Monsellato
ISBN: 978-1-62081-294-5

Chapter V

The Standard D2 Gastrectomy for Advanced Gastric Cancer

***Maurizio Degiuli**[*1], **Fabio Forchino**[1], **Alessandra Marano**[1], **Mitsuru Sasako**[2] and **Alessandro Vendrame**[1]*

[1]Department of Surgery, Division of Surgical Oncology, ASO S Giovanni Battista, Molinette, Turin, Italy

[2]Tokio National Cancer Institute, Tokyo, Japan

Abstract

During the last decade the developments of gastric surgery have been focused on the technical viability and the oncological meaning of D2 nodal dissection. Two recent randomized trials, one from the Netherlands and the other from England, have showed a significantly higher rate of complications after D2 gastrectomy compared to the standard D1 dissection, without highlighting main survival benefits. The Italian Gastric Cancer Study Group one arm – phase two multicenter prospective trial on D2 node dissection has documented mortality and morbidity rates comparable to those shown by eastern authors also in western patients. Moreover, preliminary results of the new IGCSG randomized trial on D2 versus D1 gastrectomy, have documented that the D2 gastrectomy can be a feasible and safe procedure also in western world, with low morbidity and mortality rates as compared to the classic D1 dissection, whenever it is performed in specialized high-volume centers by well-trained surgeons and if the pancreas is preserved during total gastrectomy requiring splenectomy.

Most of the research on gastric cancer treatment is based on the evidence that while it is clear that gastric cancer develops distant metastasis rather seldom until the primary tumor becomes a T3 tumor, on the other hand the incidence of lymph node metastasis is already evident in early stages of the disease.

Therefore, local control of lymph node metastases through extended and super-extended node dissection during gastrectomy appears essential in order to cure the

[*] E-mail address: *alvendra@libero.it.*

disease. It has been proved to prevent the metastatic spread of the disease, avoid the abdominal relapse and improve patient's survival.

Nowadays, after a long debate concerning the indications to total gastrectomy de principe, most reference centers involved in the surgical treatment of gastric cancer have agreed that, according to the principles of the Japanese Research Society for the Study of Gastric Cancer, the indication to a subtotal (distal) or a total gastrectomy should depend on the site of the gastric cancer and on its macroscopic appearance, detected through the preoperative assessment (Borrmann Type). Following the criteria firstly described by the JRSGC and then assumed by the Italian Gastric Cancer Association (IGCA), a subtotal dissection is oncologically adequate when the proximal edge of the tumor is further than 3 cm from the cardia in case of early gastric cancer and well-circumscribed advanced gastric cancer (Bormann type 1 and 2) or further than 6 cm in case of advanced gastric cancer of infiltrative type (Bormann type 3). On the opposite, a total gastrectomy is required whenever those conditions are not respected or in case of linitis plastica (Borrmann type 4), even if it seems mainly located in the lower gastric area. A total gastrectomy is also necessary in case of tumors located close to the greater curvature and above the Demel's point (watershed), because of the specific intestinal- and diffuse-type cancers, some authors recommend to increase routinely the length of the proximal margin to at least 8 cm in case of diffuse cancer and to reduce it to 4 cm in case of intestinal type.

Introduction

During the last decade, the developments of gastric surgery have been focused on the technical viability and the oncological meaning of D2 nodal dissection. Two randomized trials, one from the Netherlands [1] and the other one from England[2], have showed a significantly higher rate of complications after D2 dissection as compared to the standard D1 gastrectomy, without highlighting main survival benefits. The Italian Gastric Cancer Study Group (IGCSG)3 one arm – phase two multicenter prospective trial on D2 node dissection has documented, for the first time in western patients, mortality and morbidity rates comparable to those shown by eastern authors. Moreover, preliminary results of the new IGCSG randomized trial on D2 versus D1 gastrectomy (5-years follow-up on December 2011), have documented that the D2 gastrectomy can be a feasible and safe procedure also in western world, with low morbidity and mortality rates as compared to the classic D1 dissection, whenever it is performed in specialized high-volume centers by well-trained surgeons, and if the pancreas is preserved during total gastrectomy requiring splenectomy. Interim analysis of this series has also shown a survival benefit for advanced cancers (T2-T3 and/or node positive patients) treated by D2 nodal dissection as compared to D1 procedure.

Most of the research on gastric cancer treatment is based on the evidence that while it is clear that gastric cancer develops distant metastasis rather seldom until the primary tumor becomes a T3 tumor, on the other hand the incidence of lymph node metastasis is already evident in early stages of the disease; in National Cancer Center Hospital series (1972-1991) lymph node metastasis is evident in 63% of T2 cancers (Table. 1-I) [4].

Therefore, local control of lymph node metastases through extended and super-extended node dissection during gastrectomy appears essential in order to cure the disease. It has been proved to prevent the metastatic spread of the disease, to avoid the abdominal relapse and to improve patient's survival.

Table 1.1. Incidence of nodal, hepatic, and peritoneal metastases in % (A) and pathologic N-stage distribution (B) according to the tumor depth among 4683 patients who underwent laparotomy at NCCH in Tokyo between 1972 and 1991 (mm: mucosal and muscolaris mucosa; sm: submucosal; mp: muscolaris propria; ss: subserosal; se: serosal; si: surrounding organ invasion. Reproduced with permission of the author from Sasako [4]

A				
Depth	Lymph node	Liver	Peritoneum	No. of patients
T1 mm	3.3	0.0	0.0	1,063
T1 sm	17.5	0.1	0.0	881
T2 mp	46.8	1.1	0.5	436
T2 ss	63.7	3.4	2.2	325
T3 se	79.9	6.3	17.8	1,232
T4 si	89.8	15.5	41.6	724
Total	47.7	4.5	11.5	4,683

a)

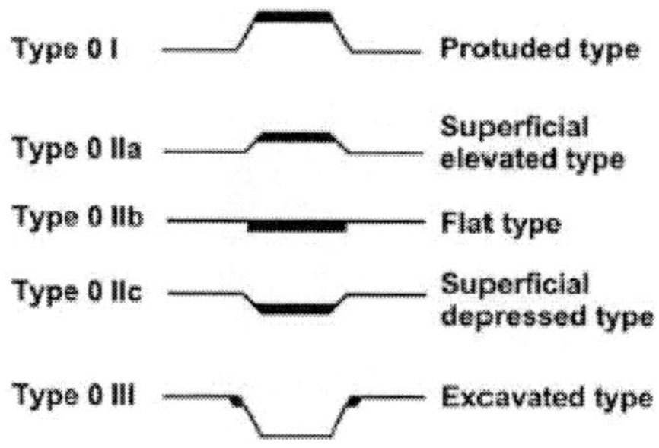

b)

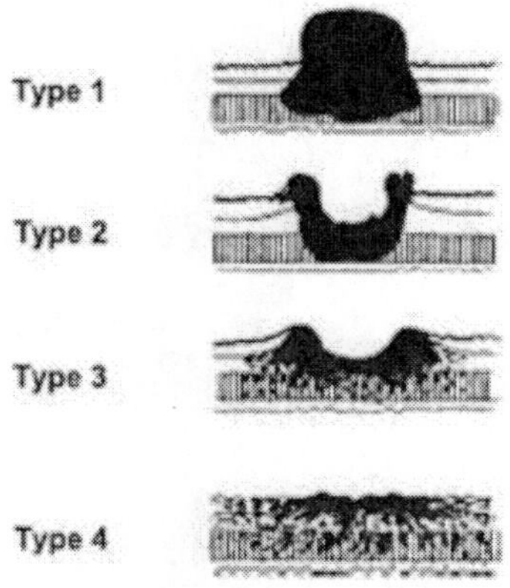

Figure 1.1. A) Subtypes of type 0 of Bormann's Classification: I: Protruded type; IIa: Superficial elevated type; IIb: Flat type; IIc: Superficial depressed type; III: Excavated type. B) Type 1: Polypoid tumors, sharply demarcated from the surrounding mucosa, usually attached on a wide base. Type 2: Ulcerated carcinoma with sharply demarcated and raised margins. Type 3: Ulcerated carcinoma without definite limits, infiltrating the surrounding wall. Type 4: Diffusely infiltrating carcinoma in which ulceration is usually not a marked feature. Type 5: Not-classifiable carcinoma. Reproduced with permission: "Japanese Classification of Gastric Carcinoma - 2nd English Edition", Gastric Cancer, 1998,1:10-24.

Surgical Technique

Extent of Resection: Distal or Total Gastrectomy?

Nowadays, after a long debate concerning the indications to total gastrectomy (TG) *de principe* [5,6], most reference centers involved in the surgical treatment of gastric cancer have agreed that, according to the principles of the Japanese Research Society for the Study of Gastric Cancer, the indication to a subtotal (distal) or a total gastrectomy should depend on the site of the gastric cancer and on its macroscopic appearance, detected through the preoperative assessment (Borrmann's Type, Figure 1.1). Following the criteria firstly described by the JRSGC and then assumed by the Italian Gastric Cancer Association (IGCA), a subtotal dissection is oncologically adequate when the proximal edge of the tumor is further than 3 cm from the cardia in case of early gastric cancer and well-circumscribed advanced gastric cancer (Bormann's type 1 and 2) or further than 6 cm in case of advanced gastric cancer of infiltrative type (Bormann's type 3). On the opposite, a total gastrectomy is required whenever those conditions are not respected or in case of linitis plastica (Borrmann's type 4), even if it seems mainly located in the lower gastric area. A total gastrectomy is also necessary in case of tumors located close to the greater curvature and above the Demel's point (watershed), because of the specific lymphatic drainage feeding into the splenic *hilum* and flowing along the splenic artery.

The main problem arising from the routine indication to partial gastrectomy in case of cancer of the lower part of the stomach is the quality of preoperative assessment of the proximal extension (mucosal or sub-mucosal) of the tumor. Despite the value of stepwise biopsy in detecting mucosal invasion and the usefulness of endoscopic ultrasonography in evaluating sub-mucosal or deeper extension of the tumor, the correct assessment of the proximal edge of the cancer is still under debate. Furthermore, consequently to the different biological pattern of intestinal and diffuse-type cancers, some authors recommend to increase routinely the length of the proximal margin to at least 8 cm in case of diffuse cancer and to reduce it to 4 cm in case of intestinal type [7-9].

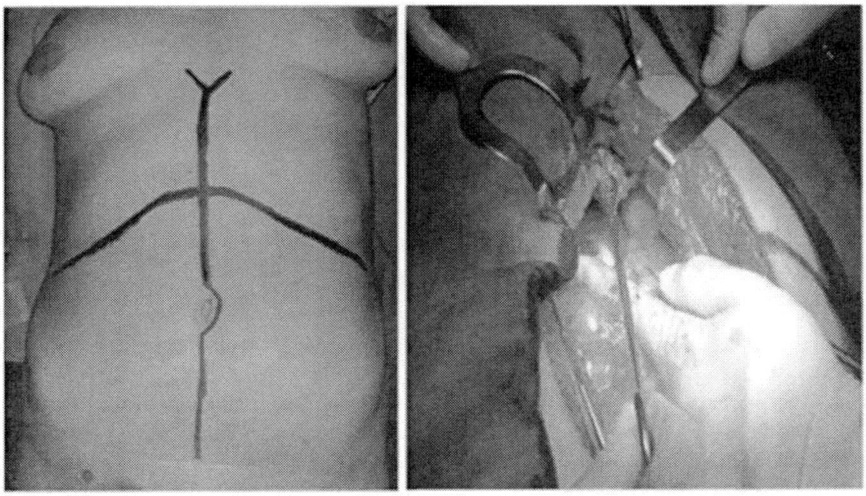

Figure 1.2. Abdominal incision and removal of xiphoid process.

Total D2 Gastrectomy

Incision and Evaluation

In most IGCSG reference centers the upper midline incision (from the xiphoid process to 2-3 cm above the umbilicus) is the preferred choice by the majority of surgeons. The bilateral sub-costal incision and the so-called Mercedes incision (a bilateral sub-costal incision associated to an upper midline incision above the xiphoid process) are other incisions performed in western countries and in Japan [10]. In order to improve the access to the cardia and the sub-phrenic area, the xiphoid process should be removed (Figure 1.2).

Evaluation of the Peritoneal Cavity and Peritoneal Washing

A careful exploration of the peritoneal surface should be performed at the opening of the abdomen in order to exclude peritoneal spread of the cancer both on visceral and parietal peritoneal layers. The whole liver should be carefully examined also by intraoperative ultrasonography in order to exclude hidden metastases. At the end of the intraoperative stage evaluation, the abdominal cavity is washed out with 100 mL of saline solution, while the stomach is carefully manipulated; the peritoneal lavage is then collected and sent to the pathologist for cytological sample (Figure 1.3).

16B1 Lymph Node Station Sampling

The first surgical procedure starts with the Kocher maneuver (Figure 1.4) in order to access the para-aortic area (Figure 1.5). This dissection allows a lymph node sampling of the group 16B1 (inferior para-aortic lymph nodes) for a frozen section analysis; the evidence of neoplastic cells at this level make the disease classified as M1 and any surgical treatment could not have a curative aim. Whenever a frozen section reveals no distant metastasis, a curative-intent procedure can be performed.

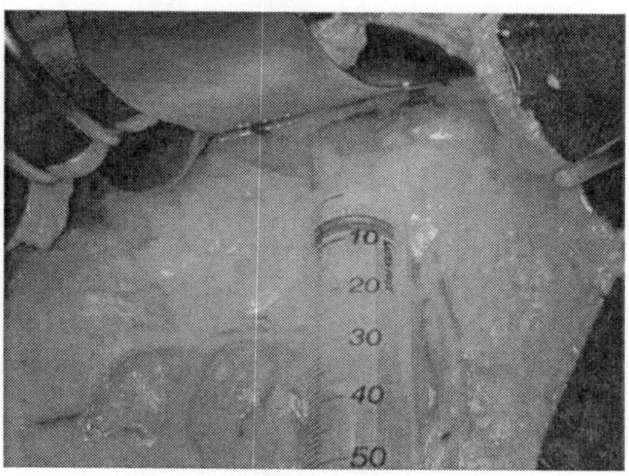

Figure 1.3. Peritoneal washing.

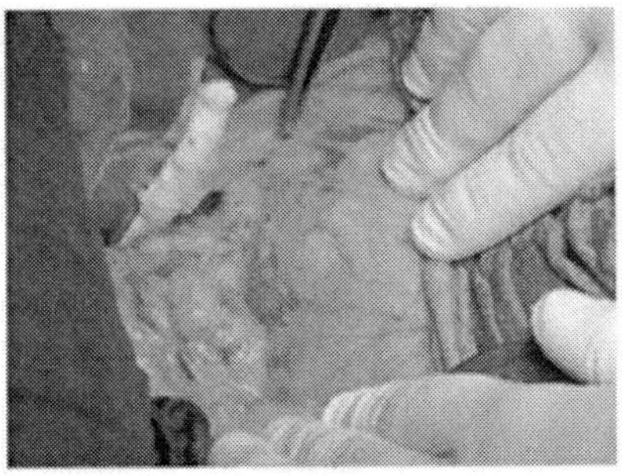

Figure 1.4. Kocher maneuver.

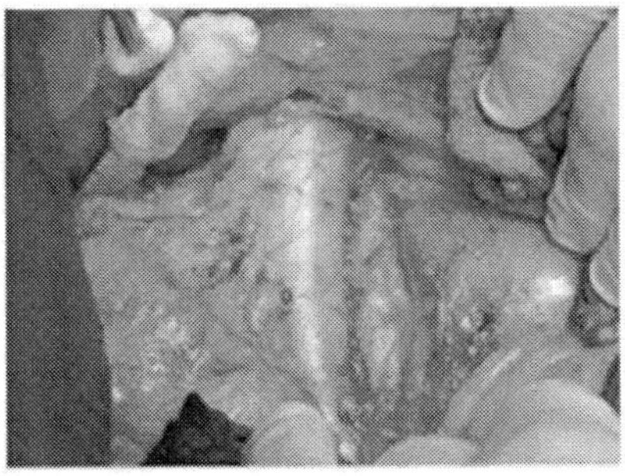

Figure 1.5. Interaorto-caval space: lymph node group 16B1.

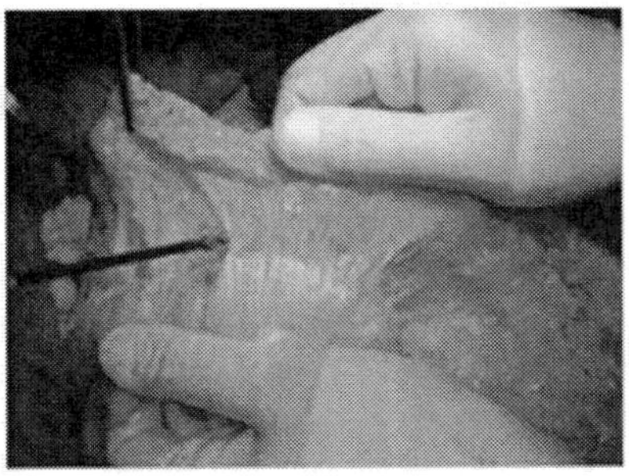

Figure 1.6. Dissection of the greater omentum and the anterior sheet of the transverse mesocolon.

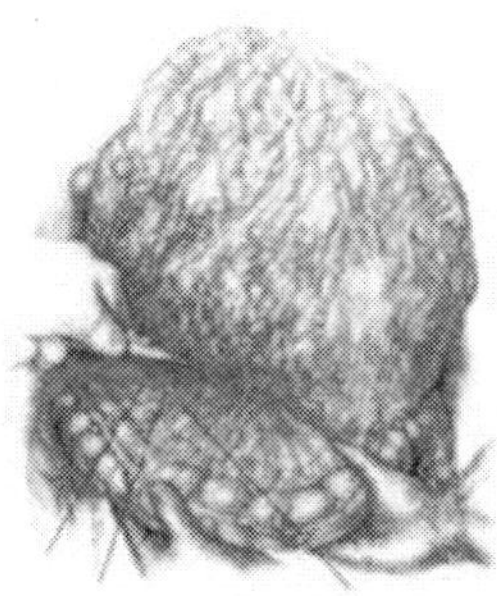

Figure 1.7. Dissection of the anterior leaf of mesocolon with omentum toward the pancreas. (Reproduced with permission of the author from Sasako11).

Dissection of the Greater Omentum from the Transverse Colon

The greater omentum is dissected from the transverse colon together with the anterior layer of the mesocolon (lesser sac) (Figures. 1.6, 1.7). It is not sure that a complete removal of the greater omentum (omentectomy) and of the lesser sac (bursectomy) is necessary for T2 cancers; however it is absolutely necessary for T3 cancers which can involve the lesser sac. Many cancers invading or adherent to the anterior layer of the mesocolon can be completely removed simply with the resection of the anterior layer without resecting the transverse colon. The omentum is pulled up, while the first assistant counter-extends the transverse colon so that the operator can easily dissect the anterior layer from the underlying tissue. This dissection is conducted from the hepatic flexure of the colon to the splenic one. The dissection continues cranially from the colon toward the pancreatic body and tail, close to the inferior border of the pancreas. On the right side, the anterior layer of the mesocolon continues on the duodenum and the head of the pancreas.

Dissection of the Right Gastro-Epiploic Vein and Pancreatic Capsule

The dissection of the anterior layer of the transverse mesocolon continues toward the right side in order to find and control the right accessory colic vein on its course until it joins Henle's trunk and the origin of the right gastro-epiploic vein (Figure 1.8). This vein is ligated and divided at its origin. The middle colic vein, which is clearly visible on the mesocolon, (Figures. 1.7-1.9) can lead this dissection towards Henle's trunk. A correct cranial traction of the omentum and the anterior layer of the transverse mesocolon plays a fundamental role in this procedure (Figure 1.10).

As the mesocolon contains vessels emerging from behind the pancreas, the dissection of the anterior layer of the mesocolon towards the pancreas leads to a plane behind it; therefore, at this point, the layer of dissection has to change from the posterior to the anterior surface of the pancreas. Several small vessels arising from behind the pancreas should be ligated and divided. The anterior layer of the transverse mesocolon continues into the "pancreatic capsule" which may contain lymphatic vessels and therefore should be dissected from the underlying pancreatic parenchyma and removed.

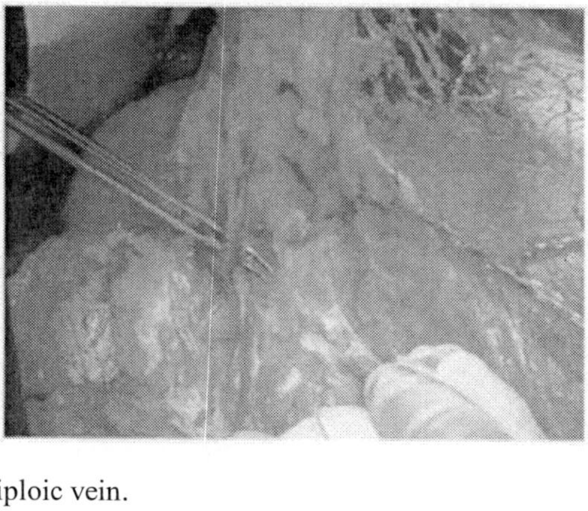

Figure 1.8. Right gastro-epiploic vein.

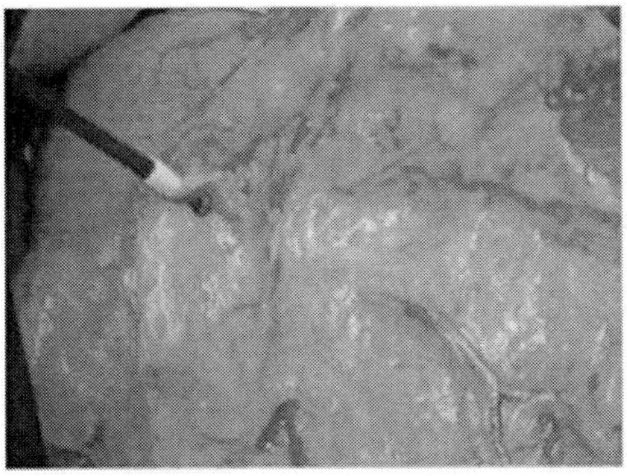

Figure 1.9. Colic vessels and Henle's trunk.

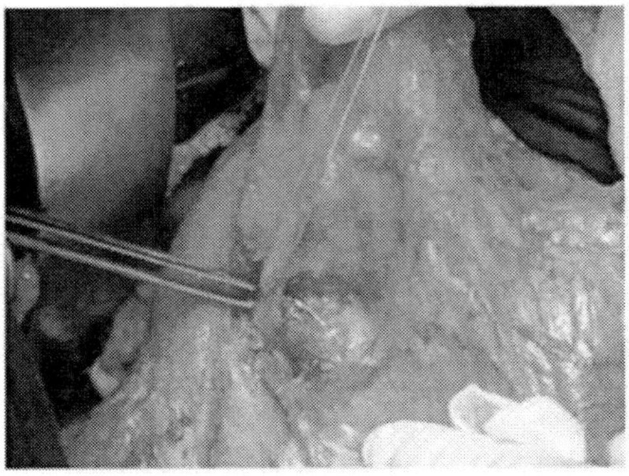

Figure 1.10. Right gastro-epiploc artery.

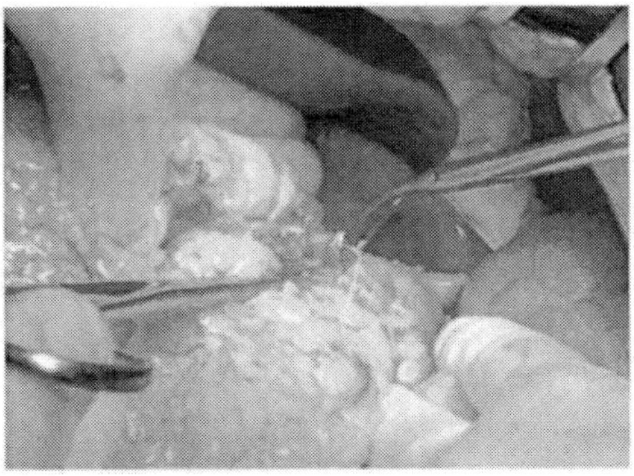

Figure 1.11. Left gastro-epiploic vessels at their origin.

Dissection of the Right Gastro-Epiploic Artery

The dissection of the pancreatic capsule is performed from the inferior to the superior border of the pancreas and from the middle of the pancreas body towards its head and the duodenum. The gastro-duodenal artery is found close to the duodenum. The course of this artery is followed caudally until the origin of the right gastroepiploic artery, which is ligated and divided at its origin (Figure 1.10). This dissection includes the removal of infra-pyloric lymph nodes (group 6).

Dissection of the Left Gastro-Epiploic Vessels

The dissection of the omentum and the anterior layer of the transverse mesocolon continues to the left until the origin of the left gastroepiploic vessels at the inferior border of the pancreatic tail. The left gastro-epiploic vessels are accurately isolated, ligated and divided at their origin (Figure 1.11). This dissection allows a complete removal of the left compartment of the lymph nodes of the greater curvature (group 4sb).

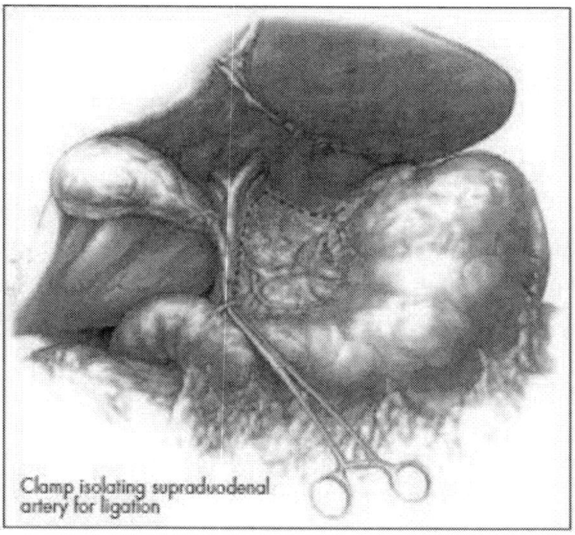

Figure 1.12. Incision line on lesser omentum. (Reproduced with permission [11]).

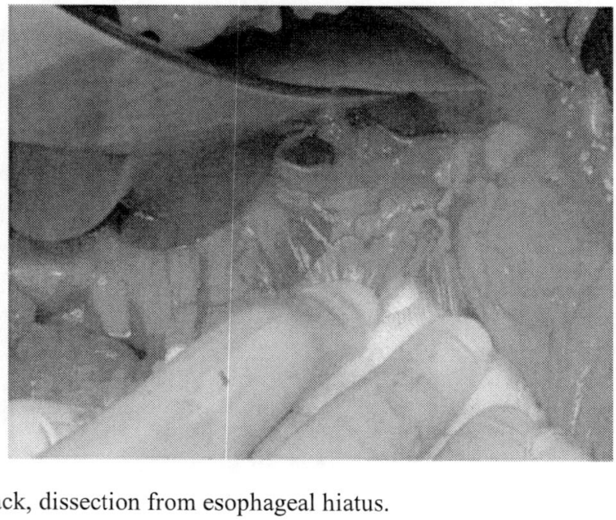

Figure 1.13. Lesser sack, dissection from esophageal hiatus.

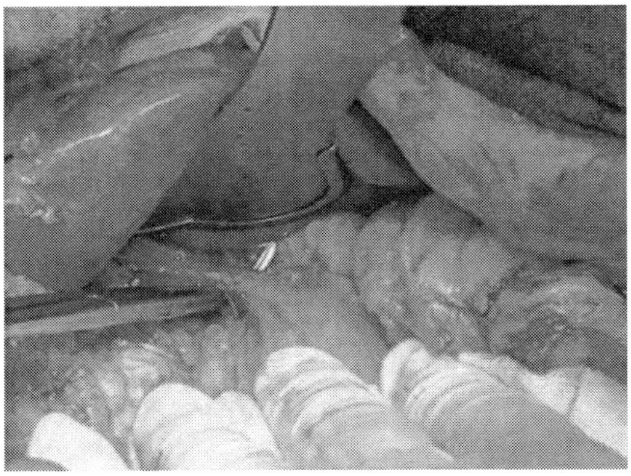

Figure 1.14. Left hepatic artery branching off from left gastric artery.

Dissection of the Lesser Omentum

The dissection of the lesser omentum is a main step for a correct D2 lymphadenectomy. After the gastro-epiploic artery is divided, the gastro-duodenal artery is controlled on its cranial course until the common and proper hepatic arteries are recognized. There is usually a large lymph node lying in the space between the gastroduodenal and common hepatic artery and the superior border of the pancreas. Recent studies have documented that this lymph node constitutes one of the sentinel lymph nodes from tumors of the distal third of the stomach. The stomach is pulled down by the first assistant so that the lesser omentum and the serosa covering the esophageal hiatus are extended. The lesser omentum is then divided 1 cm caudal to the attachment to the lateral sector of the liver (Figures. 1.12, 1.13), starting from the hiatus. In many cases an accessory left hepatic artery arising from the left gastric artery is found, (Figure 1.14). In these cases it is necessary to preserve the accessory artery whenever it is possible, removing all the lymphatic tissue around the origin of the left gastric artery over the celiac trunk (station 7).

The dissection of the peritoneal layer of the lesser (Figure 1.15) should be continued over the hepato-duodenal ligament, proceeding on the left side of the bile duct. The serosa of the ligament is then incised caudally toward the duodenum in order to find the common hepatic artery at the level of its bifurcation into the proper hepatic and the gastro-duodenal arteries (Figure 1.12).

Right Gastric Vessels Isolation

The proximal ends of supra-duodenal arteries are ligated at their origin from the gastro-duodenal artery. Dissection of the hepato-duodenal ligament continues to the bifurcation of the proper hepatic artery, close to the hepatic hilum. The right and left hepatic arteries are identified at this level and the surrounding fatty connective tissue is dissected caudally and from the right to the left. The right gastric artery is found at this level, arising from either the gastro-duodenal or proper hepatic artery in most of the cases. Alternatively, the right gastric artery can arise from the left hepatic artery, especially in case of low bifurcation of the proper hepatic artery (Figures. 1.12-1.17).

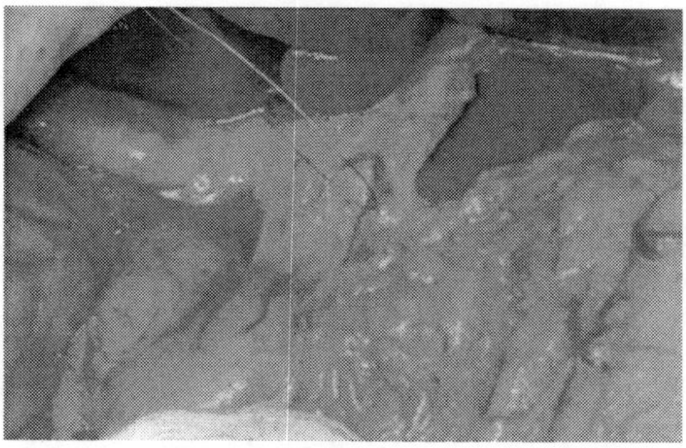

Figure 1.15. Lesser sack, dissection from the hiatus to the hepatoduodenal ligament.

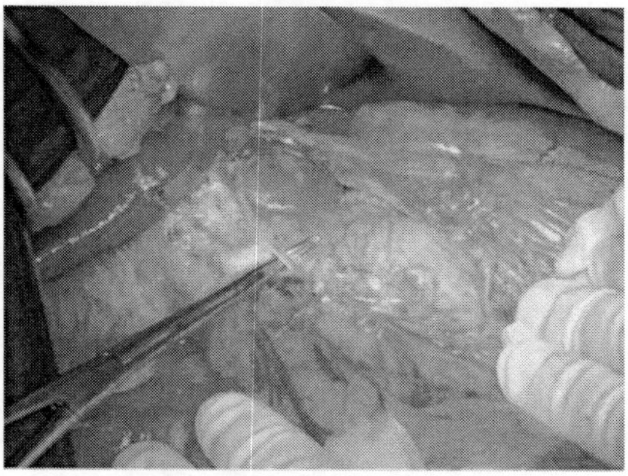

Figure 1.16. Dissection of the right gastric vessels.

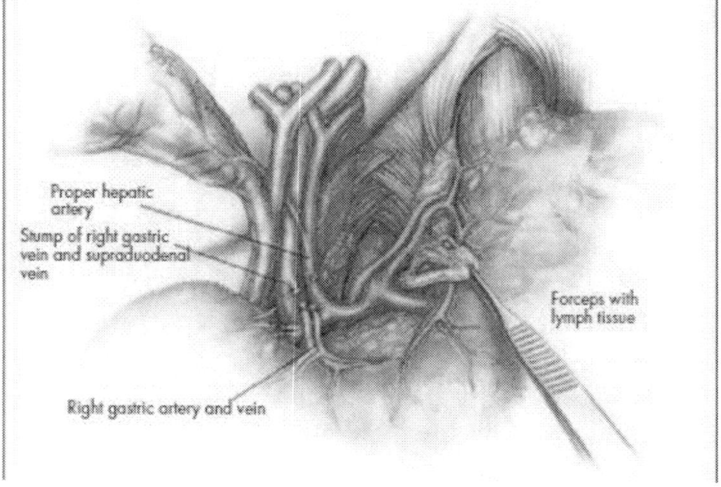

Figure 1.17. Division of the right gastric vessels. (Reproduced with permission [11]).

The first portion of the duodenum must be carefully dissected and divided in order to obtain a complete mobilization of the stomach (Figures. 1.18, 1.19). This maneuver exposes the pancreatic surface and the loco-regional vascular structures originated from the celiac trunk. The pancreatic capsule has to be completely removed together with the specimen (Figures. 1.20, 1.21), exposing the pancreatic parenchyma and the vascular and lymphatic tissue of the superior margin of the pancreas.

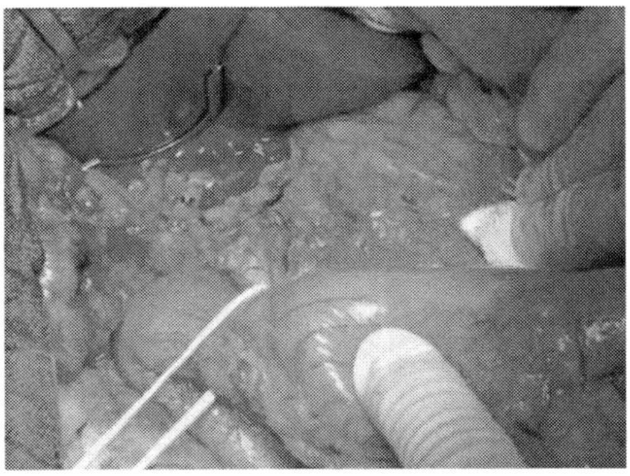

Figure 1.18. Duodenal dissection.

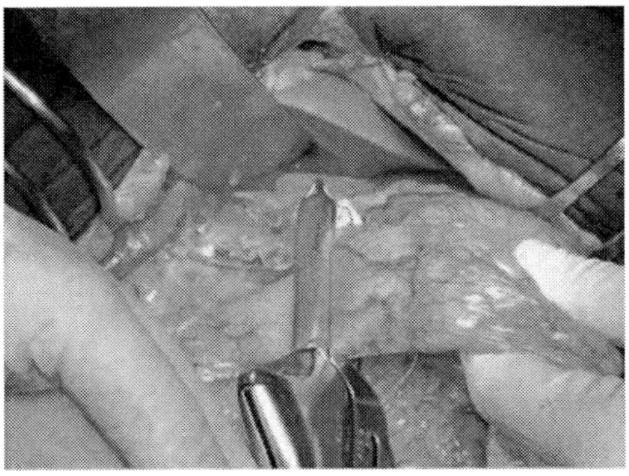

Figure 1.19. Duodenal division with a GIA device (Tyco).

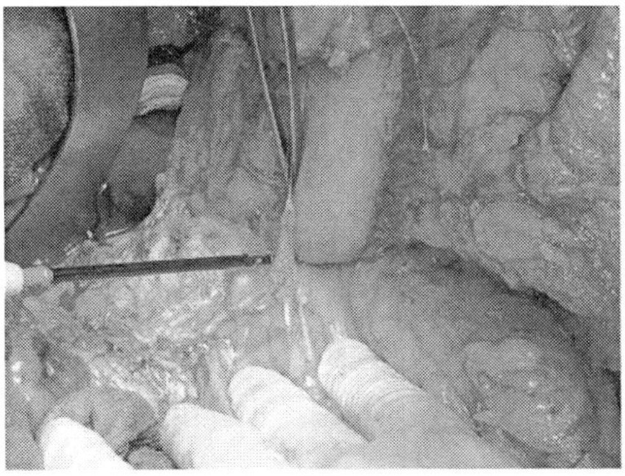

Figure 1.20. Removal of pancreatic capsule.

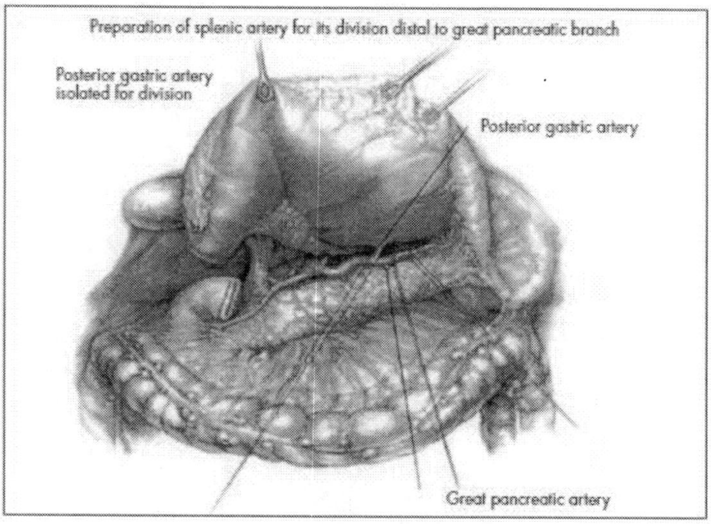

Figure 1.21. Removal of the pancreatic capsule (Reproduced with permission [11]).

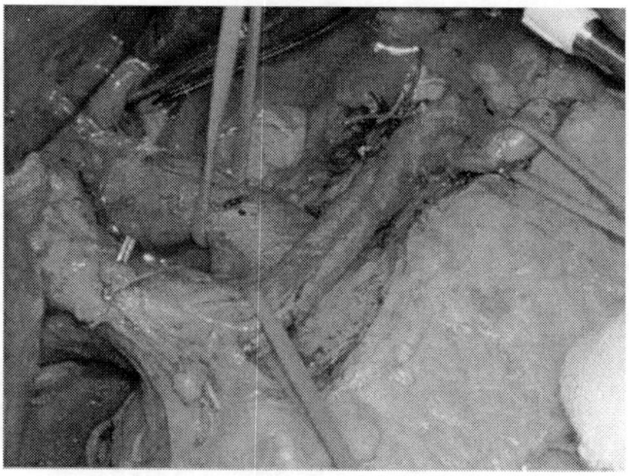

Figure 1.22. Final result of lymphatic dissection.

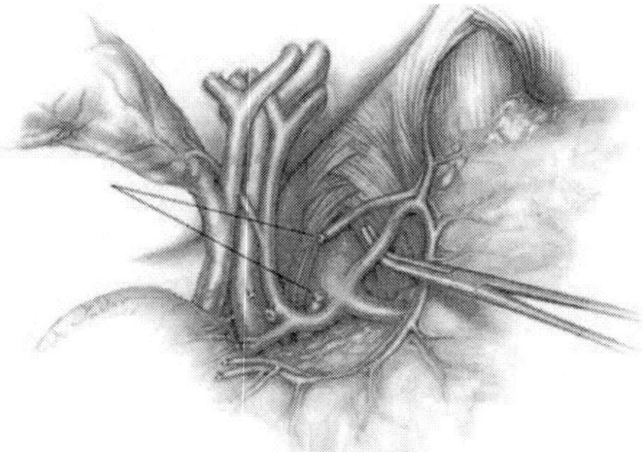

Figure 1.23. Dissection of left gastric vessels. (Reproduced with permission [11]).

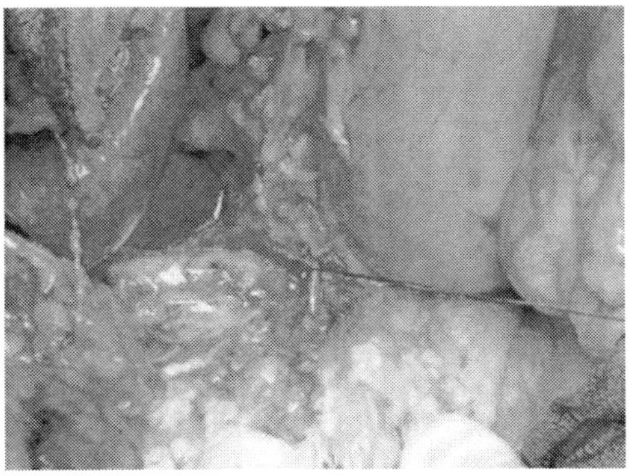

Figure 1.24. Left gastric vein.

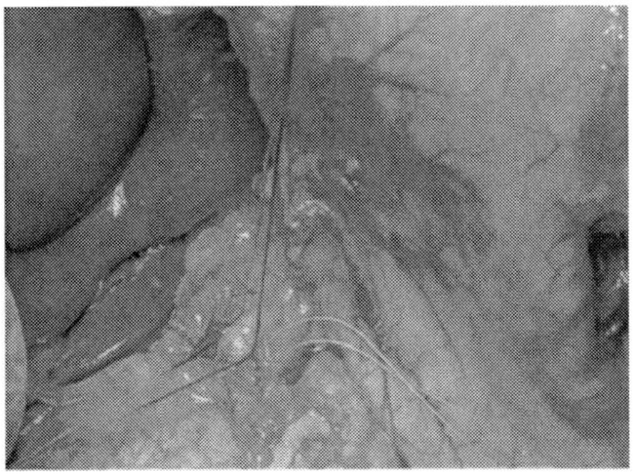

Figure 1.25. Left gastric artery.

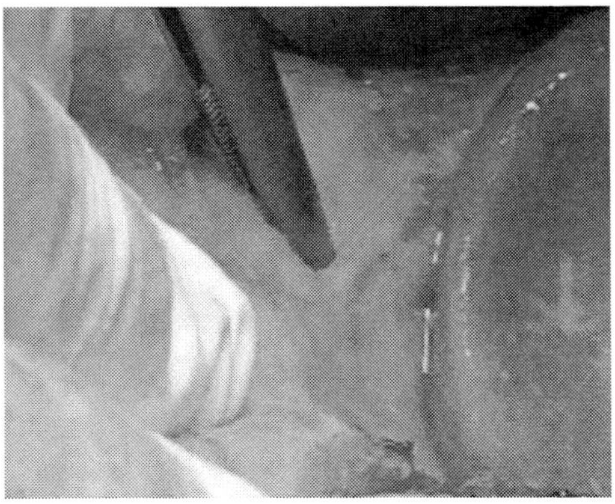

Figure 1.26. Cardio-esophageal branch of the inferior left phrenic artery.

Lymph nodes along the left side and behind the portal vein are dissected, exposing the left and the posterior sides of the portal vein. Dissection of the supra-pancreatic lymph nodes (common hepatic, coeliac, left gastric and splenic artery nodes) is now performed from the right to the left, from the portal vein to the middle of the splenic artery. The fatty tissue cranial to the pancreas contains many lymph nodes. This tissue is softly attached to the pancreatic parenchyma in most of the cases so it can be easily separated from the pancreas. In patients with a history of pancreatitis, however, dissection of supra-pancreatic fatty tissue is difficult and the pancreas can be easily damaged, resulting in pancreatic leakages.

Dissection of the Left Gastric Vessels

A left gastric vein crossing over the common hepatic artery or the splenic artery and joining the splenic vein may be encountered during this step of the procedure in about 30% of the cases (Figure 1.22). This vein should be ligated and divided near the superior border of the pancreas. The fatty tissue containing lymph nodes in this area is carefully dissected from the arteries and the surrounding nerves with a cranial direction. The nervous structures surrounding the arteries and including bilateral celiac ganglia should be preserved in absence of nodal metastases. The posterior border of this fatty tissue consists of the left and right diaphragmatic crus on each side of the celiac artery.

In about two thirds of the cases the left gastric vein anastomoses with the portal vein close to the spleno-portal junction. The vein is then ligated and divided (Figures. 1.23, 1.24). After dissection of this tissue from the right crus, the right side of the celiac artery and the root of the left gastric artery can be recognized from their right side. The left gastric artery is surrounded by thick nerve tissue, mainly celiac branches of the vagal nerves. The artery is ligated and divided at its origin. (Figures. 1.23-1.25).

Spleen Preserving D2 Total Gastrectomy (IGCSG Technique)

Since the critical analysis of the two European randomized trials [1,2] showed the increase of mortality and morbidity observed in the D2 arm was related to the pancreatectomy and splenectomy, several centers developed a different technique in order to preserve the pancreas and the spleen, in selected cases, when performing a total gastrectomy.

Currently, there is no evidence of survival benefit of performing a splenectomy during a total gastrectomy for cancer and data from JGCA randomized trial are not available. However, Japanese authors consider pancreas preserving D2 total gastrectomy with splenectomy as described by Maruyama (see below) the standard procedure for gastric cancer requiring total removal of the stomach. Recently, the Italian Gastric Cancer Study Group has developed a technique of total D2 gastrectomy, which consists of the preservation of the spleen in all cTNM T1 tumors, and in T2 and T3 cancers of the right part of the stomach, requiring splenectomy in all T4 cancers and in T2 and T3 tumors of the left part of the stomach.

After completing the lymphadenectomy on the left side of the celiac trunk, the dissection along the anterior surface of the splenic artery continues to the posterior gastric vessels (Figure 1.21). In total gastrectomy this artery should be dissected, ligated and divided at its origin. All the lymph nodes along the splenic artery must be removed, starting from the proximal lymph nodes (group 11p). The dissection along the splenic artery continues until the pancreas tail, allowing the removal of all the lymph nodes of the distal group (group 11d).

Therefore, at the splenic hilum, dissection continues with the ligation and division of the left gastroepiploic vessels, exposing the gastrosplenic ligament containing the short gastric vessels. In the spleen-preserving technique, the procedure continues with the dissection of the short gastric vessels in order to completely remove all the lymph nodes of group 4sa. The dissection ends at the left pericardial area. The stomach now can be further pulled up, exposing the left pericardial lymph nodes which should be completely removed by dissection of the cardio-esophageal branch of the inferior left phrenic artery (Figure 1.26), directed to the left side of the cardia.

Lifting the stomach up by the first assistant (Figure 1.21) allows exposing the different structures to dissect, correctly.

The abdominal esophagus is then sectioned with a safe oncological margin (Figure 1.27) and the stomach is removed "en bloc" with the loco-regional lymph node stations.

Alternatively, if splenectomy is performed (Figure 1.28), the splenic artery should be divided distal to the origin of the great pancreatic artery (arteria pancreatica magna), which branches off at the same point of the posterior gastric artery, in order to improve blood supply to the tail of the pancreas as suggested by Sasako's modification of the original Maruyama's pancreas preserving D2 total gastrectomy. The splenic vein is preserved all along the surface of the pancreas and is ligated at pancreas tip of the tail, necessary for the venous blood supply of the gland (see *pancreas preserving D2 total gastrectomy technique*).

This kind of surgical treatment includes the removal of the following lymph nodes stations (according to the Japanese Gastric Cancer Association guidelines):

- group 1: right para-cardial lymph nodes;
- group 2: left para-cardial lymph nodes;
- group 3: lymph nodes along the lesser curvature;
- group 4 d, sb, sa: lymph nodes of the greater curvature (along the right and left gastro-epiploic vessels and the short gastric vessels);
- group 5: suprapyloric lymph nodes;
- group 6: infrapyloric lymph nodes;
- group 7: lymph nodes along the left gastric artery;
- group 8a: lymph nodes along the common hepatic artery (anterosuperior group);
- group 9: lymph nodes around the celiac artery;
- group 10: lymph nodes of the splenic hilum (only in case of splenectomy);
- group 11p and d: lymph nodes along the proximal and distal splenic artery;
- group 12 a + b: lymph nodes in the hepato-duodenal ligament, along the proper hepatic artery and the common bile duct.

Reconstruction of the Alimentary Tract

The alimentary tract is reconstructed preferably with a stapled Roux-en-Y esophago-jejunal anastomosis (Figures. 1.29-1.31). Usually the Roux limb (jejunum) should be placed through an opening of the mesocolon just to the right of the middle colic vessels. The length of jejunum above the mesocolon should be not too long (as short as 10 cm) and straight, in order to avoid kinking and adhesions to the dissected surface. Usually it is preferable an end-to-side esophago-jejunal anastomosis for safety, being careful to leave a very short jejunal stump to avoid a "blind loop" syndrome and stasis of food. The Roux limb is fixed to the transverse mesocolon with closure of the opening.

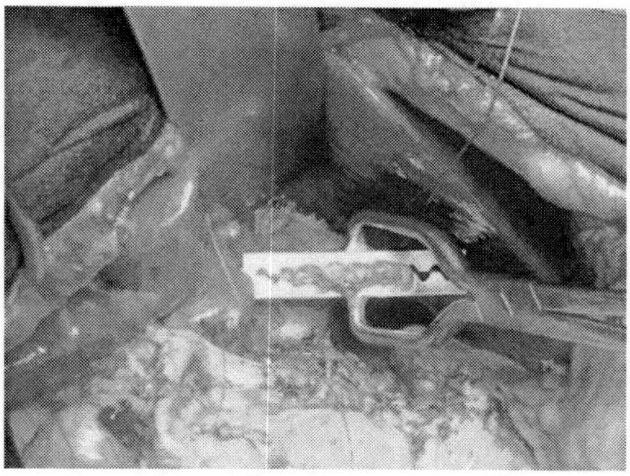

Figure 1.27. Esophageal section.

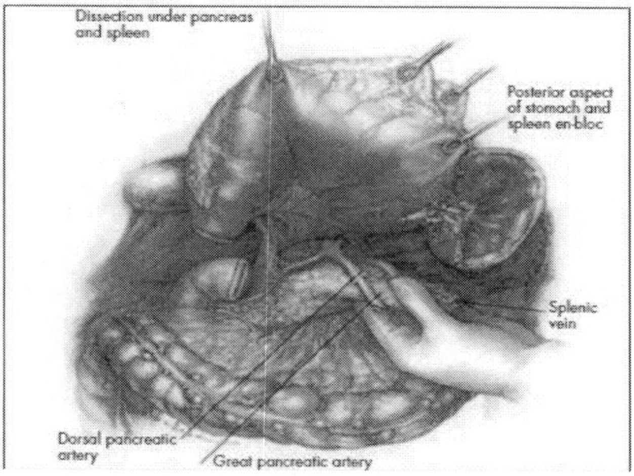

Figure 1.28. Vascular dissection at the body of the pancreas. (Reproduced with permission [11]).

Pancreas-Preserving D2 Total Gastrectomy (Maruyama's Technique)

Maruyama's technique represents the standard D2 gastrectomy with splenectomy and preservation of the pancreas for proximal cancer of the stomach.

Since the 60s, Japanese reference centers for gastric surgery performed D2 total gastrectomy with splenectomy and distal pancreatectomy for proximal and middle third gastric cancer. This procedure consists of the complete removal of loco-regional lymph node stations, including peri-pancreatic (lymph nodes along the upper border of the pancreas) and splenic hilum lymph nodes. The procedure was followed, however, by a high rate of complications such as pancreatic fistulas, left sub-phrenic abscesses, serious pancreatitis and postoperative diabetes [11]. Even in recent studies, the mortality rate after splenectomy and distal pancreatectomy during total gastrectomy for proximal cancer is very high [12].

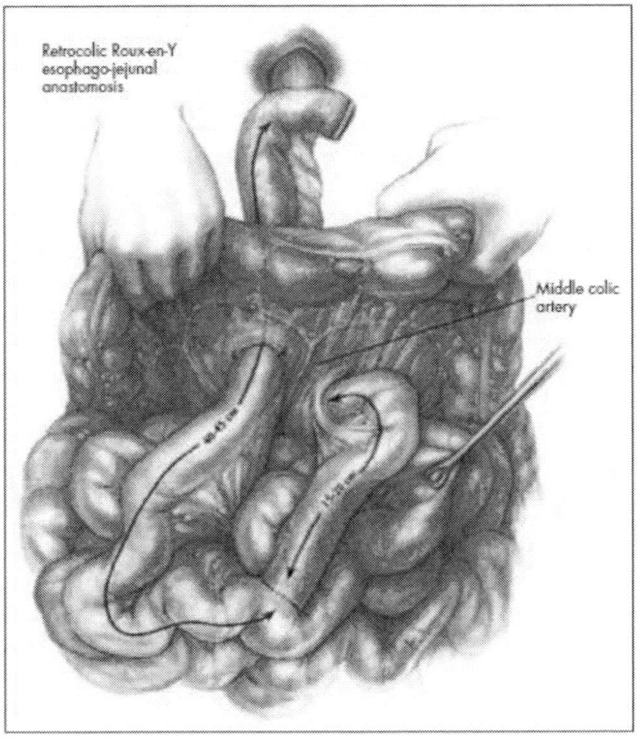

Figure 1.29. Reconstruction of the alimentary tract. (Reproduced with permission [11]).

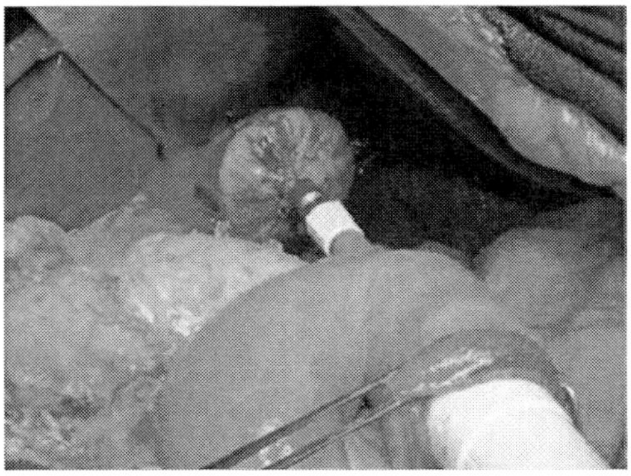

Figure 1.30. Cardio-esophageal branch of the inferior left phrenic artery.

Japanese Authors studied how to preserve the pancreas in proximal and middle third cancers, in order to avoid the increase of mortality and morbidity related to this procedure. Lymphatic drainage from the stomach, lymph node metastasis around the pancreas, blood supply of the pancreas and techniques of mobilization of the spleen and distal pancreas were studied.

Endoscopic and intraoperative lymphography documented that lymphatic channels were located only in the subserosal space of the pancreas but never inside the parenchyma. This demonstration could theoretically support D2 total gastrectomy with pancreas preservation as a curative procedure for cancer [13, 14].

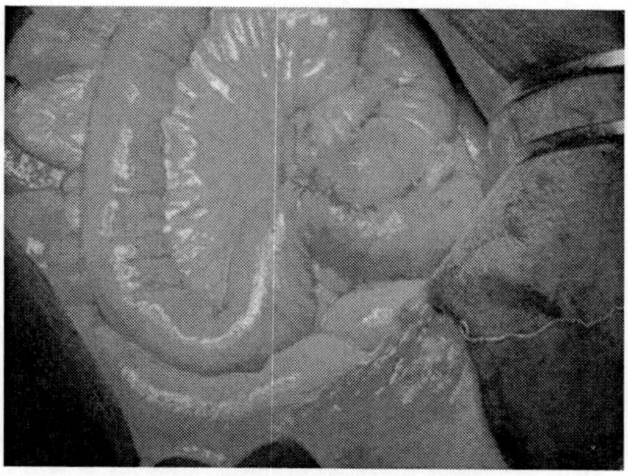

Figure 1.31. Jejuno-jejunal end to side anastomosis (trans-mesocolic Roux-en-y).

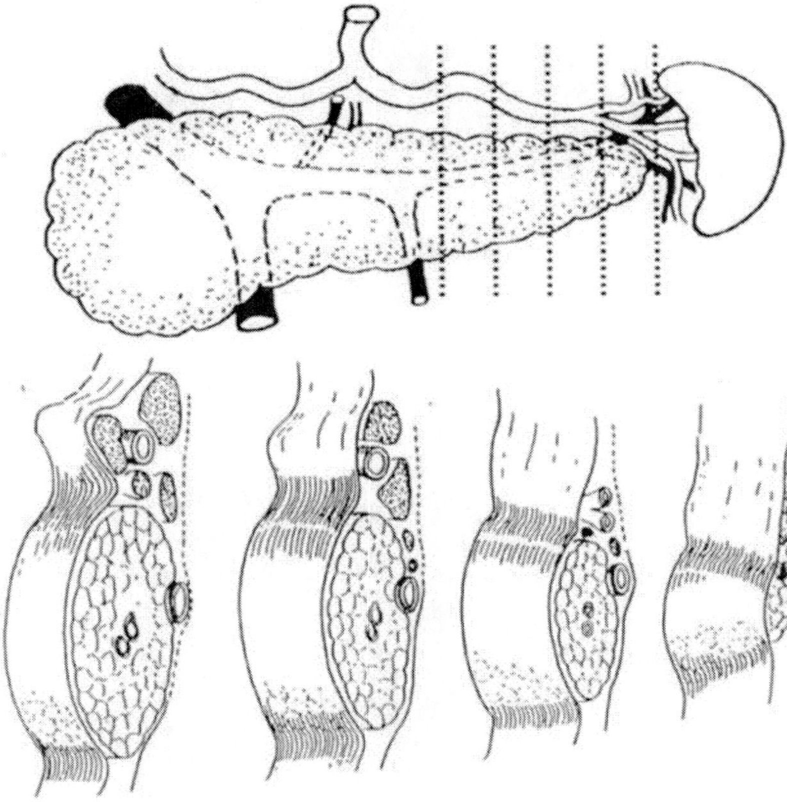

Figure 1.32. Lymphatic nodes and pancreas parenchyma (reproduced with permission [12]).

Histopathological studies [12] using resected and autopsy materials from gastric cancer patients, in addition, revealed that lymph nodes are present only in the subserosal fatty connective tissue of the pancreas, particularly along the splenic artery and at the splenic hilum. This result supported data from lymphography, confirming that lymph node metastasis does not occur in pancreas parenchyma and survival results should not be negatively affect by preservation of the pancreas (Figure 1.32).

As lymph node metastasis are located along the splenic artery which usually is removed during D2 pancreas preserving total gastrectomy with splenectomy, the blood supply of the preserved pancreas has been investigated. Anatomical studies and celiac angiography have clearly demonstrated that distal pancreas receives blood supply through the transverse pancreatic artery (along the pancreatic duct) branching off from the dorsal pancreatic artery and that the dorsal pancreatic artery branches 2 cm off the origin of the splenic artery from the celiac trunk.

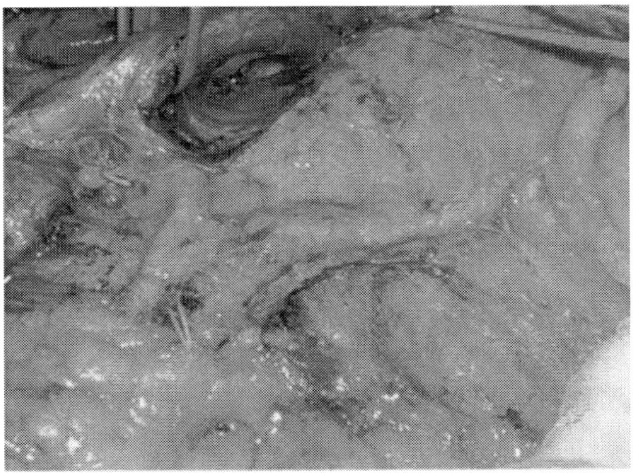

Figure 1.33. Peripancreatic dissection and removal of lymph nodes along the origin of the superior mesenteric vessels.

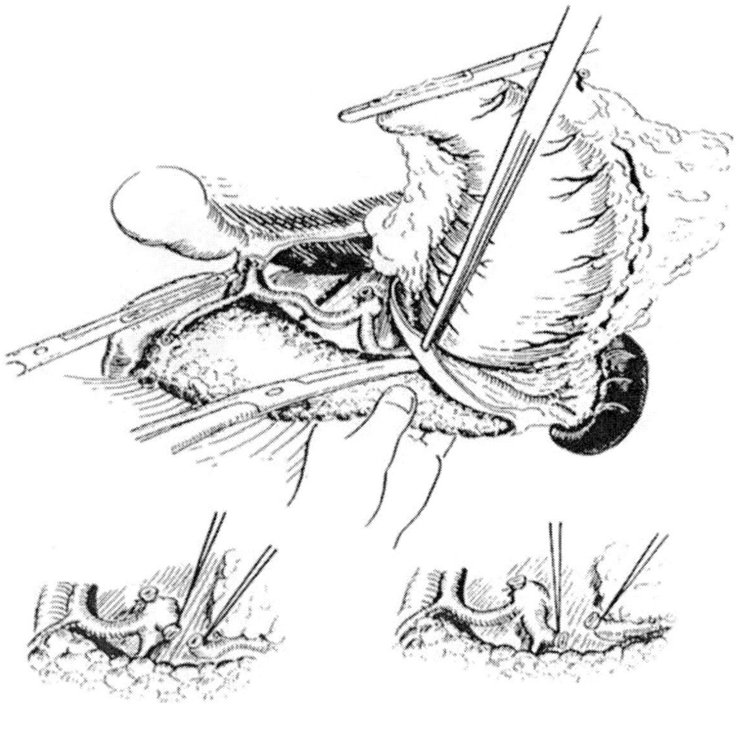

Figure 1.34. Preservation of dorsal pancreatic artery (reproduced with permission [12]).

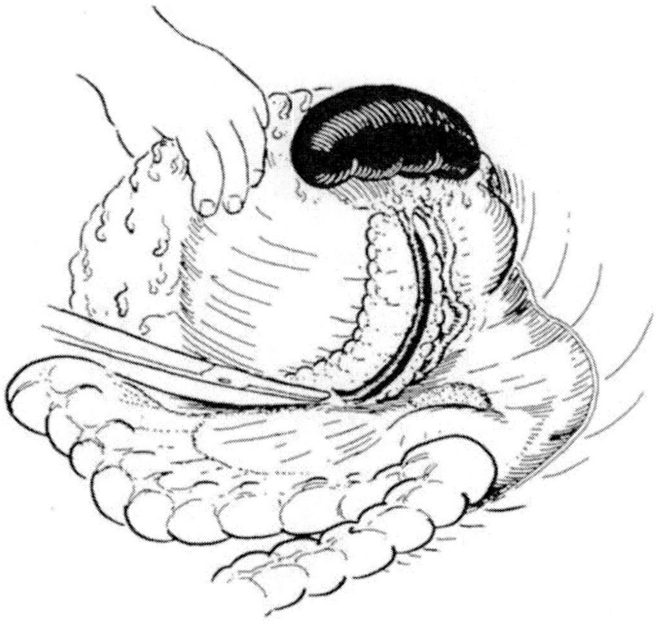

Figure 1.35. Mobilization of spleen and pancreas (reproduced with permission [12]).

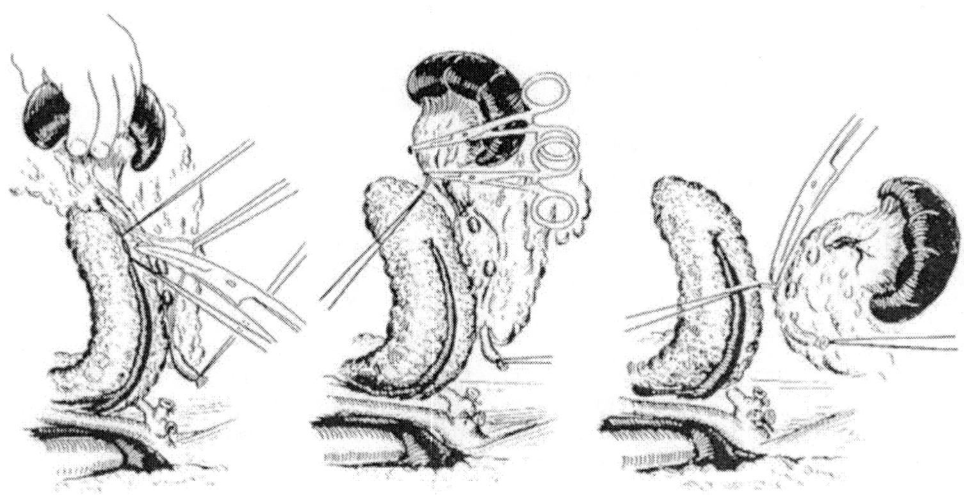

Figure 1.36. Splenectomy with splenic vein preservation (reproduced with permission [12]).

Therefore the division of the splenic artery distal to the origin of the dorsal pancreatic artery can preserve blood supply to the body and tail of the pancreas, as documented by celiac angiography [12] of patients submitted to D2 pancreas preserving total gastrectomy with splenectomy.

The splenic vein is adherent to the pancreas and it is not surrounded by lymphatic tissue. It can be preserved all along the pancreas parenchyma and divided at the tip of the tail of the pancreas, without affecting the oncological accuracy of the procedure and the venous blood drainage of the pancreas.

Surgical Technique

The aim of pancreas preservation technique is to completely remove the serosa and all the fatty connective tissue containing lymphatic channels and lymph nodes from pancreatic parenchyma (Figure 1.33).

After the completion of all the standard surgical procedure the pancreas preserving procedure is started. The serosa is carefully peeled off from the distal pancreas and all the fatty connective tissue including splenic artery lymph nodes is completely removed. Then the splenic artery is ligated and divided at about 2 cm from its origin preserving the dorsal pancreatic artery whenever it branches off from the splenic artery (Figure 1.34).

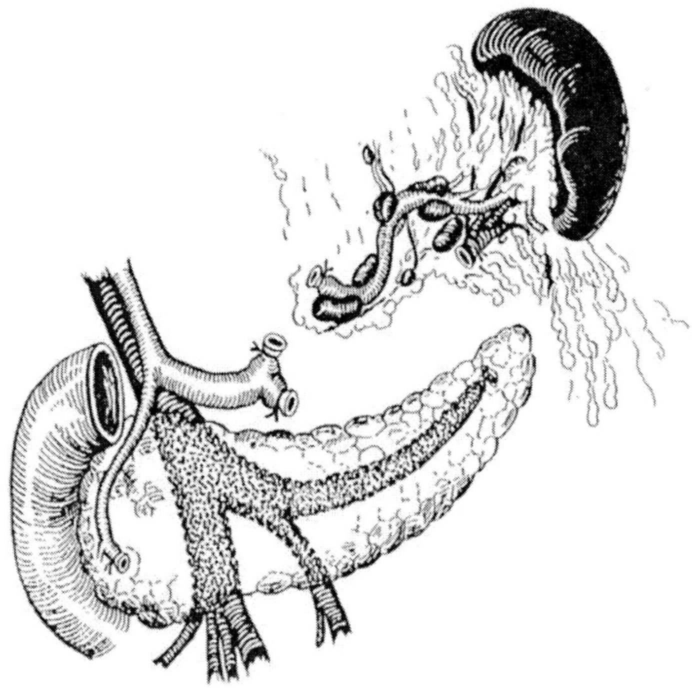

Figure 1.37. Splenectomy with removal of splenic artery (reproduced with permission [12]).

Afterwards, a mobilization of the spleen and the distal pancreas is mandatory (Figure 1.35). By an embryological point of view, indeed, the spleen and the pancreas are located in the dorsal mesogastrium which has no vascular connection with the retro-peritoneum. The spleen and the pancreas can therefore be easily mobilized with safety and without bleeding following the ideal layer between the posterior surface of the pancreas and the anterior surface of the retroperitoneum.

The mobilization continues along the posterior surface of the splenic vein. The spleen is pulled up, the serosa is removed from the posterior surface of distal pancreas and the tail of the pancreas is carefully exposed by removing the connective tissue from the gland. The splenic vein is ligated and divided at the tip of the tail of the pancreas (Figuress. 1.36, 1.37). Fatty connective tissue is carefully removed from the upper border of the pancreas with the distal part of the splenic artery. The pancreatic parenchyma and splenic vein are preserved.

Comments

Maruyama *et al.* demonstrated that pancreas preserving D2 total gastrectomy with splenectomy reduces complications related to pancreas resection such as pancreatic juice leakage, left subphrenic abscesses, severe pancreatitis and postoperative diabetes, without affecting the oncological accuracy of the procedure [12]. The procedure is performed in patients affected by adenocarcinoma of the proximal and middle third of the stomach without direct involvement of the pancreas and/or large macroscopic metastasis along the upper border of the pancreas.

D2 Distal Gastrectomy

The surgical steps of total gastrectomy are reproduced for a partial gastrectomy: careful exploration of the abdominal cavity, peritoneal washing for intraoperative cytology, and removal of the lymph nodes of the group 16B1 for intraoperative frozen section.

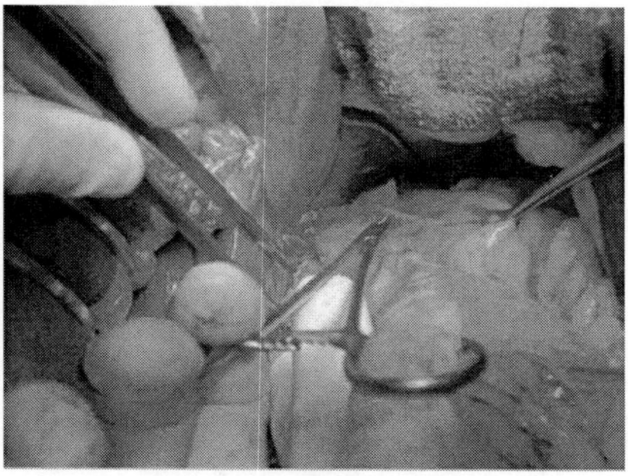

Figure 1.38. Dissection of right paracardial lymph nodes.

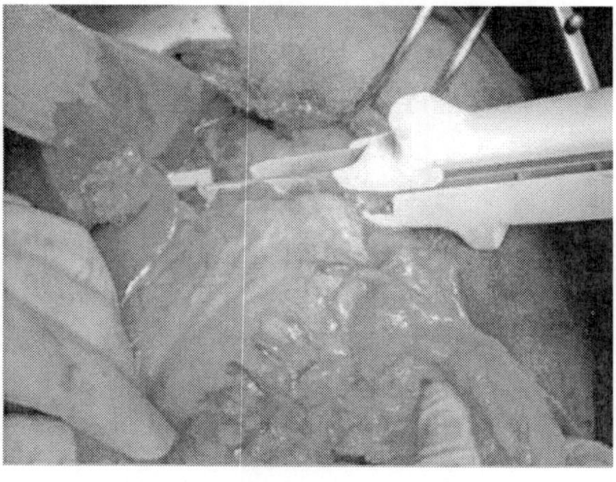

Figure 1.39. Division of the stomach between its proximal and middle third.

Lymph node dissection continues with the removal of lymph node stations of the proximal part of the splenic artery (group 11p). It is important not to damage the splenic artery during this dissection in order to absolutely preserve the spleen and the pancreas. The posterior gastric artery must be preserved in order to guarantee an efficient blood supply to the remnant stomach.

The right paracardial lymph nodes (station 1) should be removed (Figure 1.38) even if the proximal third of the stomach is preserved while left paracardial nodes (station 2) should not be dissected.

All the branches to the gastric wall emerging from the superior gastro-oesophageal branch of the left gastric artery should be ligated and divided in order to remove the right paracardial lymph nodes (Figure 1.38). Lymph node stations 3 (lesser curvature) and 5 (suprapylorics – right gastric artery) are removed "en bloc" with the specimen.

Lymph node dissection should preserve the short gastric vessels along the greater curvature, in order to guarantee an efficient blood supply to the proximal third of the stomach.

Lymphadenectomy includes also lymph nodes of the hepatoduodenal ligament, common hepatic artery, coeliac trunk, left gastric artery, as well as the splenic artery until the origin of the posterior gastric artery.

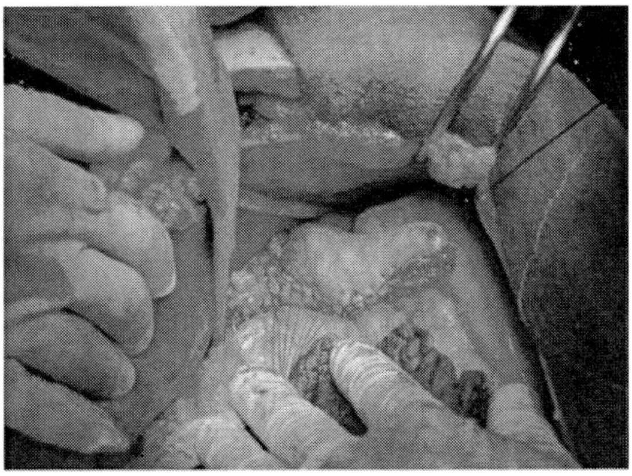

Figure 1.40. Manual seromuscolar reinforcement of stapled suture of gastric stump.

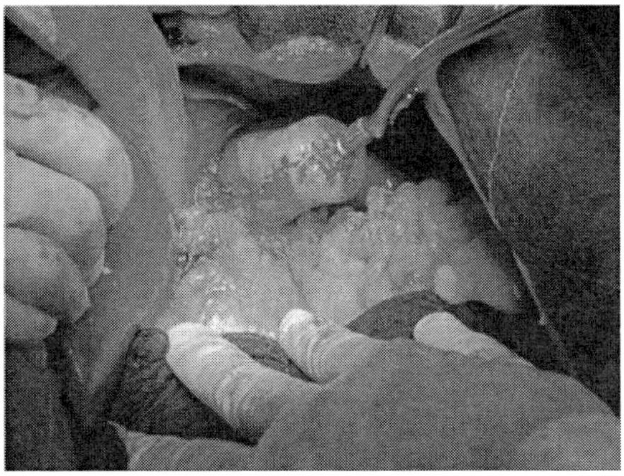

Figure 1.41. Introduction of the anvil into the gastric stump.

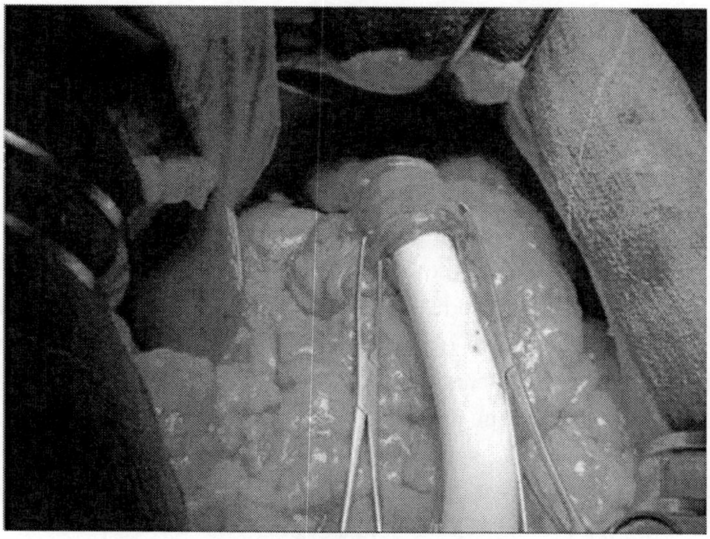

Figure 1.42. End-to-side stapled gastro-jejunal anastomosis with CEEA.

A complete D2 distal gastrectomy involves the removal of the lymph nodes surrounding the superior mesenteric vein at the inferior pancreatic border (Figure 1.33, station 14v). All the fatty tissue above the anterior face of the superior mesenteric vein, from the inferior margin of the pancreas until its first branch of division should be dissected and removed.

The following lymph node stations (according to the Japanese Gastric Cancer Association) should be removed:

- group 1: right paracardial lymph nodes;
- group 3: lymph nodes along the lesser curvature;
- group 4sb, d: lymph nodes along the greater curvature (along the left gastro-epiploic vessels, along the right gastro-epiploic vessels);
- group 5: suprapyloric lymph nodes;
- group 6: infrapyloric lymph nodes;
- group 7: lymph nodes along the left gastric artery;
- group 8a: lymph nodes along the common hepatic artery, anterosuperior group;
- group 9: lymph nodes around the celiac artery;
- group 11p: lymph node along the proximal splenic artery, until the branching off of the posterior gastric artery;
- group 12a: lymph nodes in the hepatoduodenal ligament (along the proper hepatic artery);
- group 14v: lymph nodes along the superior mesenteric vein.

The stomach is resected with a linear stapler (Figure 1.39). A continous suture is performed in order to guarantee the complete blood control of the suture line.

The reconstruction technique usually performed by the IGCSG surgical team is a trans-mesocolic end-to-side Roux-en-Y gastro-jejunostomy, performed with a mechanical stapler (Figures. 1.40-1.42).

Diffuse Cancers

Total D2 gastrectomy is the treatment of choice for diffuse tumors. In these cases, lymphadenectomy includes the removal of the following stations:

- group 1: right paracardial lymph nodes;
- group 2: left paracardial lymph nodes;
- group 3: lymph nodes along the lesser curvature;
- group 4 sa, sb, d: lymph nodes along the greater curvature (along the short gastric vessels, along the left gastro-epiploic vessels, along the right gastro-epiploic vessels);
- group 5: suprapyloric lymph nodes;
- group 6: infrapyloric lymph nodes;
- group 7: lymph nodes along the left gastric artery;
- group 8a: lymph nodes along the common hepatic artery, anterosuperior group;
- group 9: lymph nodes around the celiac artery;
- group 10: lymph nodes at the splenic hilum;
- group 11p: lymph node along the proximal splenic artery, until the branching off of the posterior gastric artery;
- group 12a: lymph nodes in the hepatoduodenal ligament (along the proper hepatic artery);
- group 14v: lymph nodes along the superior mesenteric vein.

References

[1] Bonenkamp J. J., Hermans J., Sasako M., et al.: Extended lymph-node dissection for gastric cancer. *N. Engl. J. Med.* 1999;340:908-14.

[2] Cuschieri A., Weeden S., Fielding J, et al.: Patients survival after D1 and D2 resections for gastric cancer: longterm results of the MRCrandomized surgical trial. *Br. J. Cancer* 1999;79:1522-30.

[3] Degiuli M., Sasako M., Ponti A., et al.: Morbidity and mortality after D2 gastrectomy fo gastric cancer: results of the Italian Gastric Cancer Study Group prospective multicentric surgical study. *J. Clin. Oncol.* 1998;16:1490-3.

[4] Sasako M.: Surgical management of gastric cancer: the Japanese experience. In: Daly J. M., Hennesy T. P. H., Reynolds J. Veditors. *Management of upper gastrointestinal cancer*. London: W. B. Saunders; 1999, p.107-22.

[5] Lindahl A. K., Harbitz T. B., Liavåg I: The surgical treatment of gastric cancer: a retrospective study with special reference to total gastrectomy. *Eur. J. Surg. Oncol.* 1988;14:55-62.

[6] Bozzetti F.: Total versus subtotal gastrectomy in cancer of the distal stomach: facts and fantasy. *Eur. J. Surg. Oncol.* 1992;18:572-9.

[7] Hermanek P.: Microcarcinoidosis of the stomach. *Dtsch. Med. Wochenschr.* 1985;110:1233.

[8] Hermanek P.: Limits of pathohistologic evaluation in surgical oncology. *Fortschr. Med.* 1985;103:567-70.

[9] Gall F. P., Hermanek P.: New aspects in the surgical treatment of gastric carcinoma – a comparative study of 1636 patients operated on between 1969 and 1982. *Eur. J.urg. Oncol*. 1985;11:219-25.

[10] Sasako M.: D2 nodal dissection. *Operative techniques in general surgery*. 2003;5: 36-49.

[11] Sasako M.: Complication after surgical tretment of gastric cancer. *In post-operative complications*. Tokyo: Kanehara Shuppan; 1990. p. 39-53.

[12] Maruyama M., Sasako M., Kinoshita T., et al.: Pancreas preserving total gastrectomy for proximal gastric cancer. *World J. Surg*. 1995;19:532-6.

[13] Hagiwara A., Takahashi T., Sawai K., et al.: Lymph nodal vital staining with newer carbon particle suspensions compared with India ink: experimental and clinical observations. *Lymphology* 1992;25:84-9.

[14] Maruyama K., Okabayashi K., Kinoshita T.: Progress in gastric cancer surgery in Japan and its limits of radicality. *World J. Surg*. 1987;11:418-25.

[15] Delaney H. M., Carnevale N., Garvey J. W., et al.: Postoperative nutritional support using needle catheter feeding jejunostomy. *Ann. Surg*. 1977;186:165-70.

[16] Witzel O.: Zur Technik der Magenfistelalegung. *Zbl. Chir*. 1891;18:601-4.

In: Gastric Cancer
Editors: A. D'Annibale, V. Pende and I. Monsellato
ISBN: 978-1-62081-294-5

Chapter VI

Laparoscopic Total and Subtotal Gastrectomy for Gastric Cancer

Giusto Pignata[1], Umberto Bracale[1,2], Cesare Stabilini[3], Giovanni Merola[2] and Marco Barone[4]

[1]General and Minimally-Invasive Surgical Unit, San CamilloHospital, Trento, Italy
[2]Department of General, Thoracic and Vascular Surgery, University "Federico II" of Naples, Italy
[3] Department of Surgical Science, University of Genova, Italy
[4]Department of General and Minimally-Invasive Surgery, San Polo Hospital, Monfalcone, GO, Italy

Abstract

Laparoscopic gastrectomy (LG) for malignancy has not fully entered into daily clinical practice. Since 1994, when Kitano performed the first laparoscopic gastrectomy with Billroth I anastomosis for early gastric cancer, there was not a wide acceptance of laparoscopic approach as in other procedures such as laparoscopic colectomy for both benign and malignant conditions, fundoplication and cholecystectomy. Technical and instrumental developments in laparoscopic surgery, however, allowed a more aggressive surgery for gastric cancer and improvedits diffusion.

Several studies have been conducted in order to define the adequacy of laparoscopic approach in gastrectomies for malignant disease in terms of short, long and oncological outcomes.

The aim of this chapter is to make a review of literature, about laparoscopic approach for gastric malignant disease versus the open approach, and describe the laparoscopic technique of total and subtotal gastrectomies for malignant disease.

Introduction

Laparoscopic surgery is rapidly emerging as the new standard for many surgical procedures and a wide scientific literature supporting its effectiveness and efficiency is present to date. Literature data showed that laparoscopic procedures overcome open surgery in post-operative pain, hospital stay, and return to work. This is also the case of laparoscopic colectomy for both benign and malignant conditions, fundoplication or cholecystectomy [1,2]. Laparoscopic gastrectomy for malignancy, however, has not fully entered into daily clinical practice.

Kitano et al [3] first reported laparoscopic gastrectomy with Billroth I anastomosis for early gastric cancer (EGC) in 1994. They described a technique of laparoscopy-assisted Billroth I gastrectomy under an abdominal wall-elevating method.

The first totally laparoscopic gastric resection for malignant disease was performed in 1993 by Azagra et al. [4] and was described later on, together with their series of laparoscopically assisted gastrectomies for malignant diseases. They reported that although laparoscopic gastrectomy could remain a challenging procedure, it appeared to be oncologically adequate. They believed that a pure laparoscopic approach should be reserved for low-stage lesions (N0, up to T2), while a combined approach was preferable for locally advanced cancer (N1 or higher, T3 or higher).

They concluded that much work was still needed to establish the optimal strategy in both open and laparoscopic surgery, but laparoscopy could be a valuable tool in the decision-making process for patients affected by gastric malignancy.

Technical and instrumental developments in laparoscopic surgery, conversely, allowed to perform a more aggressive surgery for gastric cancer and improved its diffusion. Several single institutional studies demonstrated that laparoscopy-assisted distal gastrectomy (LADG) caused less pain and enabled faster recovery and shorter hospital stay, which are parameters of early-phase quality of life (QOL). [5].

Most of the Korean and Japanese surgeons preferred the "laparoscopy-assisted" gastrectomy.

The number of laparoscopic gastrectomies is increasing in Japan and it is estimated that a laparoscopic approach is employed in about 20% of gastric cancer surgeries, according to the survey carried out by the Japan Society for Endoscopic Surgery and the statistical database of the Ministry of Health, Labor and Welfare of Japan. [6].

For these reasons, in Japan, a total of 5,271 laparoscopic gastrectomies were performed between 1991 and 2003, and more than 1,500 gastrectomies were carried out laparoscopically in 2003 [7].

Indications and Type of Gastrectomy

Currently, indications for gastrectomy vary from East to West. This aspect may reflect the higher incidence of early lesion found during the accurate screening program for gastric cancer performed in Eastern countries.

Early Gastric Cancer (EGC)

Laparoscopic gastrectomies in Japan were initially indicated only in presence of early gastric cancer without risk of lymphatic metastasis. The common resection types were laparoscopic wedge resections (LWR) and intra-gastric mucosal resection (IGMR). These procedures have declined in their use in favor of more advanced and less invasive endoscopic procedures: the endoscopic mucosal resection (EMR) and, recently, the endoscopic submucosal dissection (ESD).

Accordingly to the current indications [6] laparoscopy-assisted distal gastrectomy (LADG) is performed in EGC with risk of lymphnode metastasis, detected preoperatively (endoscopic US). The incidence of lymph node metastasis is about 2%–5% in EGC patients with mucosal cancer and 11%–20% in those with submucosal cancer, the latter being treated with resective surgery and adequate lymphadenectomy. [8-10]

Three types of laparoscopic lymph node dissection are performed in LADG: perigastric lymph node dissection (D1 + α), additional lymph node dissection along the common hepatic artery (D1 + β), and extended lymph node dissection (D2). The Japanese Gastric Cancer Association guidelines prescribe optimal lymph node dissectionin EGC as follows: D1 + αin mucosal cancer not suitable for EMR and in differentiated submucosal cancer less than 1.5 cm in diameter; D1 + βin other submucosal cancers without lymph node metastasis (N0) and in small EGC with perigastric lymph node metastasis (N1); D2 for larger EGC (> 2.0 cm in diameter) with N1 metastasis.

Advanced Gastric Cancer

Various types of gastrectomies have been described as feasible by laparoscopic approach for the treatment of AGC. They ranged from function preserving procedures (pilorus preserving -polar gastrectomies) to more radical ones (distal, subtotal and total gastrectomies). The most used approaches can be conventionally divided into three types: Totally laparoscopic gastrectomy (TLG), Laparoscopic Assisted Gastrectomy (LAG) and Hand Assisted Gastrectomy (HAG). During "totally laparoscopic" procedures, a minilaparotomy is necessary only for specimen extraction, but anastomoses are fashioned intracorporeally. A $\leq$10 cm minilaparotomy is necessary to carry out the reconstructive step and for the specimen extraction in the "laparoscopy-assisted gastrectomy" [11-12.]. In this case minilaparotomy is usually a median epigastric incision for extracorporeal reconstruction.

Two major issues arise when adopting a laparoscopic approach to treat AGC.The first is the extent and the adequacy of lymph node dissection and the second is the technical problems of reconstruction.

D2 lymph node dissection is routinely carried out for AGC in Asia, and even if criticized in Western countries, it represents the current standard of treatment. A laparoscopic D2 lymph node dissection technique was developed and is being performed in several Asian institutions. Nevertheless a national survey conducted by the Japan Society for Endoscopic Surgery (JSES) showed that D2 lymph node dissection was performed in 10% of patients treated by LADGs in Japan in 2003 [13].

Several debates arose on the oncological adequacy of laparoscopic D2 lymphadenectomy and issues related to the cell-dissemination and port site metastases. [7]

Another important issue of the laparoscopic gastric procedures is reconstruction, in particular the gastro-jejunostomy or the esophago-jejunostomy. Ifwe exclude hand-sewnanastomosis, which ispracticed invery fewcenters,the most commonly applied ones are: the linear "side - to - side" anastomosis [14,15] and, recently,the circular "end- to –side" anastomosis with transoral introduction of the anvil of a dedicated stapler (OrVil™).

Evidence Based Results of Laparoscopic D2 Gastrectomy

Seven randomized trials of laparoscopic versus open gastrectomies are, currently, published [17-23].

Quality of the randomized trials is rather heterogeneous, as the KLASS trial is the only multicenter trial with a large sample size (179 vs 161). Another limitation is the fact that in all the trials, LADG was compared with ODG and six of the trials enrolled only patients with clinically diagnosed EGC. Only one of the trials reported a 5-year follow-up of 59 patients with EGC or AGC.

Other retrospective studies have some biases such as the comparison to historical controls or patients who underwent open surgery during the same period.

Short Term Outcomes

Data extrapolated from the analysis of several retrospective case series [24-29] shows that laparoscopic D2 gastrectomy can be accomplished with less blood loss, although operative time is higher than open surgery.

Recent meta-analyses and reviews [30-32] clearly confirm these results and add some new issues. Probably thanks to the known technical advantages (magnification, less trauma), laparoscopy showed less morbidity than open surgery (9.3% vs 17.6%; OR 0.48 95%CI 0.30-0.79 $p<0.003$). Concerning thirty-day mortality, very few adverse events were registered and they were equally distributed between open and laparoscopic surgery (0.9% vs 0.6% OR 1.21 95%CI 0.13-11.21 p 0.86).

Another important issue is health-related quality of life. A small randomized trial from Korea observed considerable differences in the functioning scales and symptom scales of the European Organization for Research and Treatment of Cancer (QLQ-C30 and STO22) at 3 months after surgery, although outcomes in the long-term have not been analyzed [22].

Oncological Outcomes

Interesting and somewhat disappointing are the results on lymph nodes harvesting in the laparoscopic specimen. Lymph node retrieving was higher in open surgery than that in laparoscopy (mean difference -4.79 nodes 95%CI -6.79 - -2.79, p< 0.00001). This observation is very important as the number of retrieved nodes for laparoscopy was inferior to that in open surgery but above the minimum (15) recommended by current guidelines [33-35]. Mean number of harvested nodes in the trials, indeed, ranged between 20.2 and 39.

Cancer stages in most of these studies were early gastric cancers, which usually need D1+ α and D1+ β dissection and D2 lymphadenectomy only when tumor is more than 2 cm in diameter and nodal involvement is preoperatively diagnosed. An adequate D2 dissection is a challenging procedure and it can be achieved with low morbidity rates only in experienced centers (at least 50 procedures) [36]. The small number of retrieved nodes in specimens of stage I tumors raises the question whether laparoscopy can be adequate to treat more advanced stages in which nodes harvesting appears to be the major determinant of long term survival.

This issue is still under investigation by ongoing trials (KLASS trial and JCOG0912) and the results are pending. D1+ α and D1+ β, according to the Japanese Treatment Guidelines, may be performed in a limited population of patients (i.e. in presence of mucosal or smaller submucosal cancers). This category, characterized by an excellent prognosis, was the target of the vast majority of laparoscopic gastrectomies in the late 1990s and early 2000s. An extensive retrospective analysis of patients treated between 1994 and 2003 by expert laparoscopic surgeons revealed also excellent outcomes. [37] This analysis included 1,185 cases of laparoscopy-assisted distal gastrectomy (429 D1+ α, 549 D1+ β and 207 D2). At a median follow-up time of 36 months, estimated 5-year disease-free survival rates were 99.8% for stage IA, 98.7% for stage IB, and 85.7% for stage II.

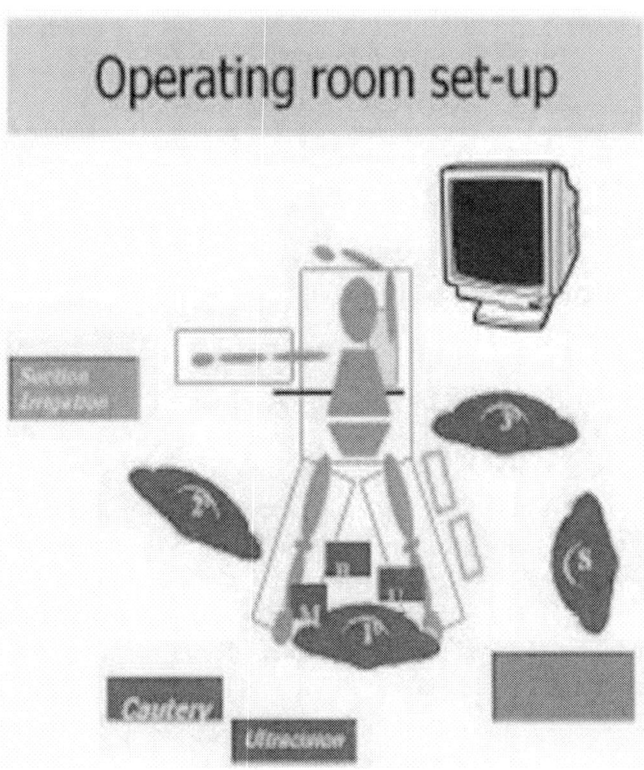

Figure 1. Operating room set-up.

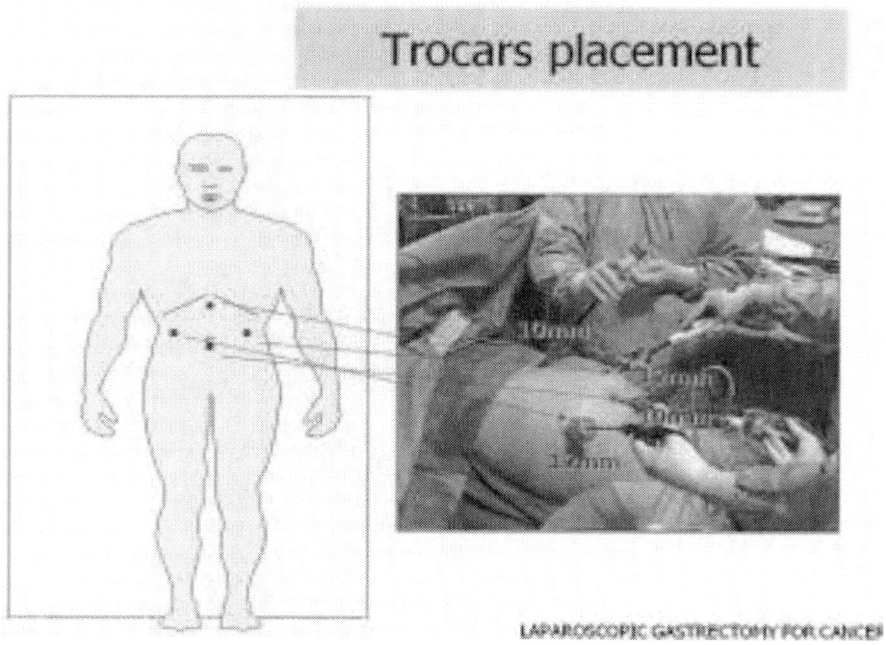

Figure 2. Trocars placement.

Similarly excellent retrospective data suggesting non inferiority of the laparoscopic approach to treat early-stage cancer have been reported from the KLASS group.[38] In addition, one randomized trial [17] with gastric cancer of varying clinical stages reported on the lack of difference in 5-year survival rates between the two approaches.

Our Technique

Totally Subtotal

The patient is placed in supine position with a 20 degree head up tilt, with his legs apart, and the left arm abducted with the intravenous line. The surgeon is positioned between patient's legs, the assistant stands at surgeon's left side and the scrub nurse on the right (Figure 1). Four ports are used. The pneumoperitoneum is established by Veress technique in left hypochondrium and the pressure is set at 14mmHg.

Four 10-12 mm ports are then inserted in the upper abdomen (Figure 2). The procedure starts with peritoneal washing. The first operative step is coloepiploic detachment with omentectomy (Figure 3). In case of a tumor of the posterior gastric wall, the supramesocolicsuprapancreatic fascia is removed, hence performing a "bursectomy"(Figure 4). All these maneuvers are performed with an ultrasonic scalpel. After the dissection of the lesser sac, the right gastroepiploic vesselsareisolated and sectioned (Figure 5) with right lymph nodes station No. 4 (Figure 6):the dissection is carried out to the pylorus, and the right gastro-epiploic vein is divided between absorbable clips (Figure 7). The right gastro-epiploic artery is sectioned between non-absorbable clips at its origin from the gastroduodenal artery just above the pancreatic head (Figure 8).

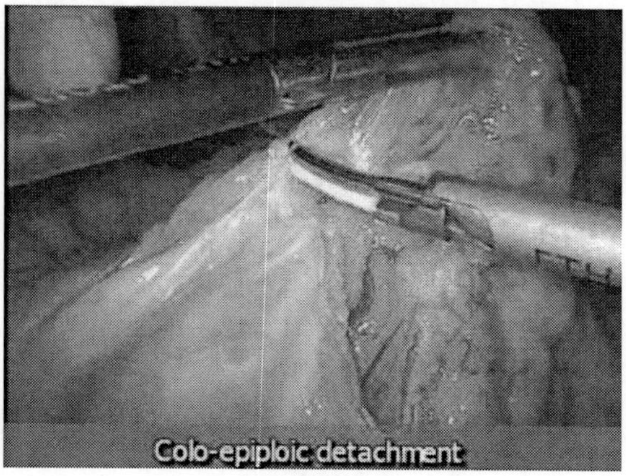

Figure 3. Colo-epiploic detachment.

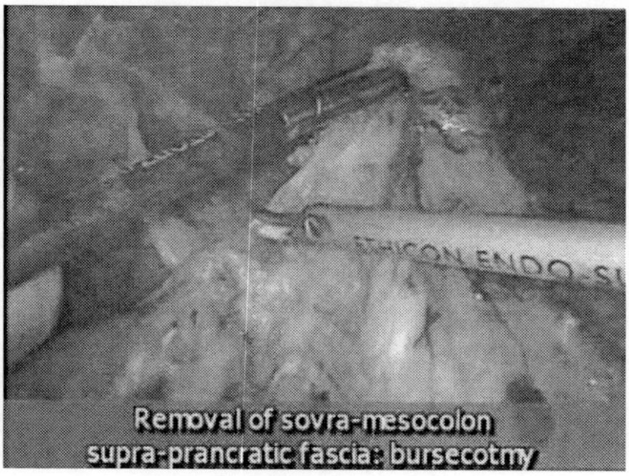

Figure 4. Bursectomy.

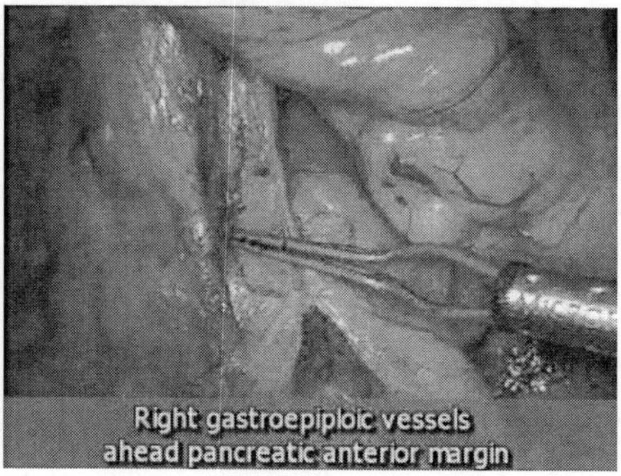

Figure 5. Isolation of right gastroepiploic vessels.

The pyloric vessels are divided. The pylorus and the duodenal stump are freed from the surrounding tissue. The inferior part of the lesser omentum (pars flaccida) is opened before starting with lymphadenectomy (Figure 9).

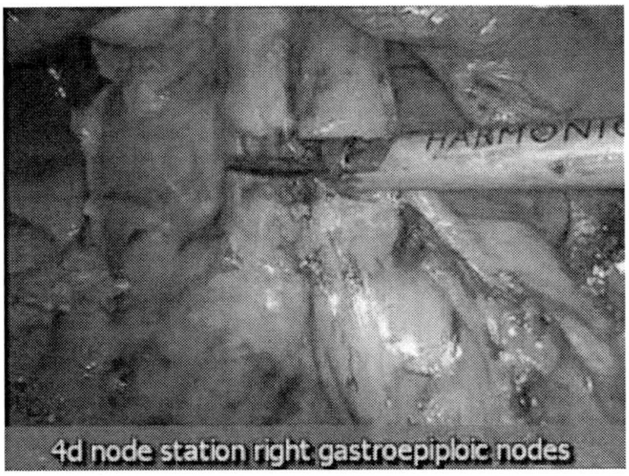

Figure 6. Isolation of node station 4.

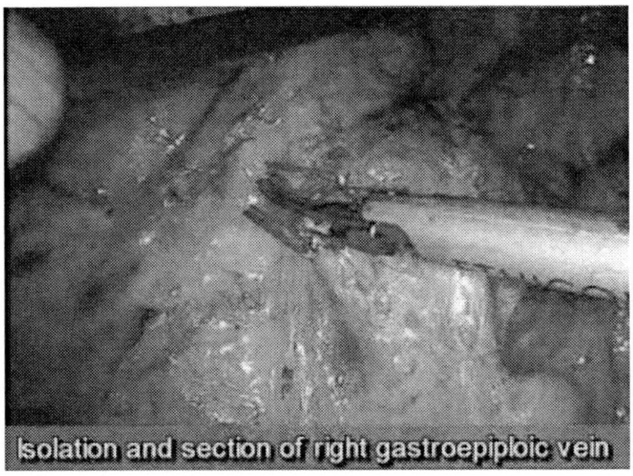

Figure 7. Isolation and section of right gastroepiploic vein.

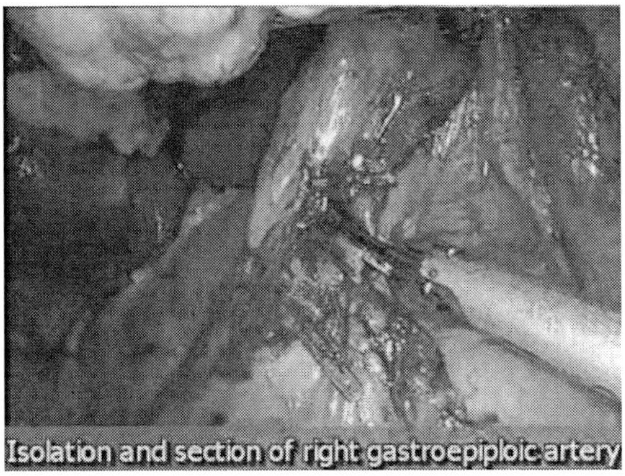

Figure 8. Isolation and section of right gastroepiploic artery.

D2 dissection involves removal of lymph node stations from No.7 to No.12. Lymph nodes of the hepatoduodenal ligament (No.12) are dissected and removed ‘en bloc’ (Figure 10). To complete the dissection, a cholecystectomy is performed and the elements of the hepatic pedicle are carefully isolated and encircled with vessel loops to facilitate the lymphadenectomy (Figure 11).

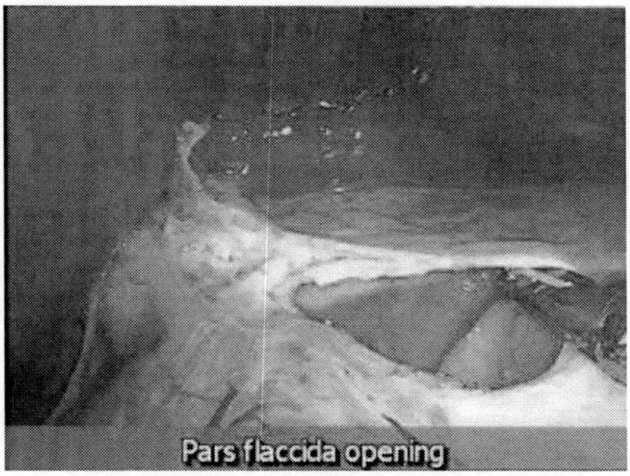

Figure 9. Pars flaccida opening.

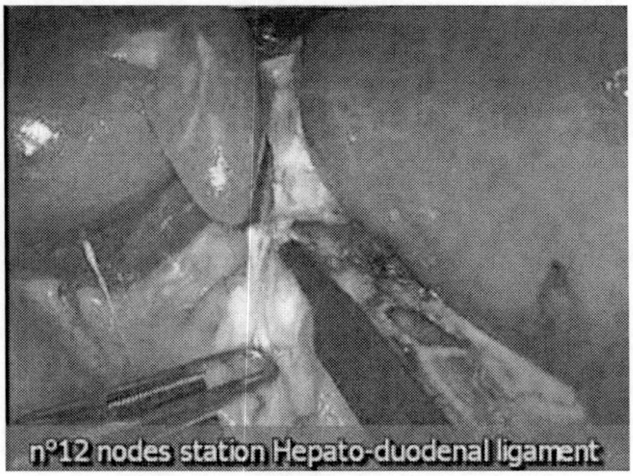

Figure 10. Isolation of node station 12.

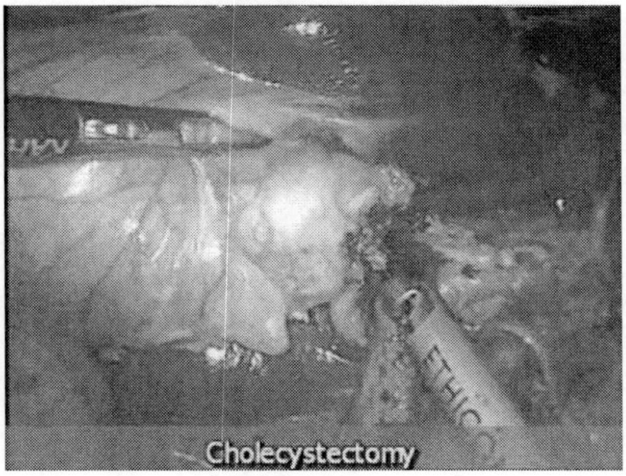

Figure 11. Cholecystectomy.

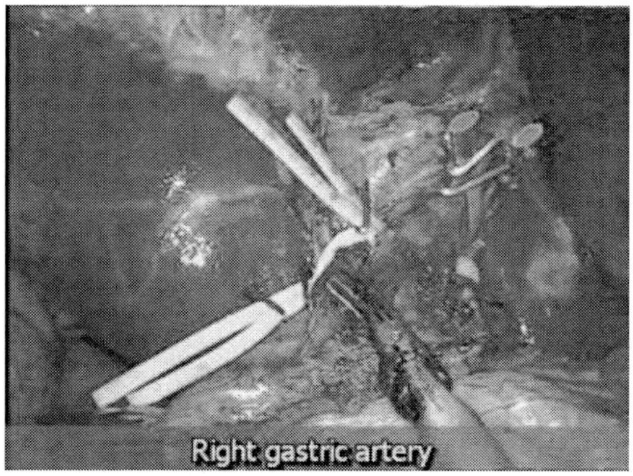

Figure 12. Section of right gastric artery.

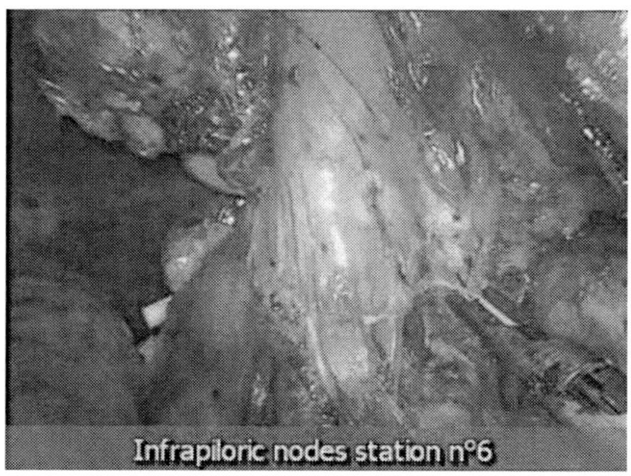

Figure 13. Isolation of infrapiloric node station 6.

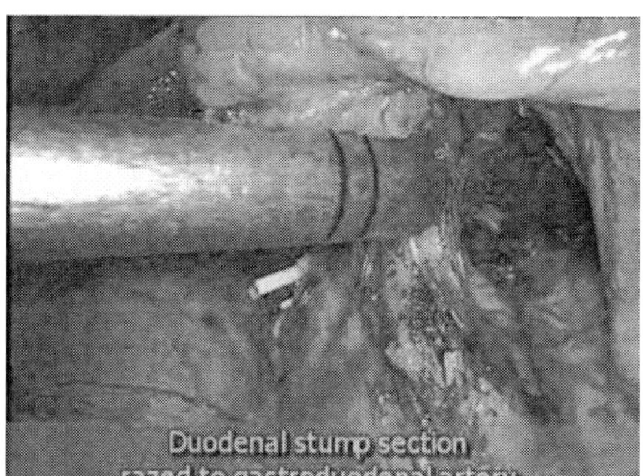

Figure 14. Duodenal stump section.

Infrapyloric nodes (No.6) and the right gastric artery are divided (Figure 12; 13).The duodenum is transected and closed with a 45mm linear stapler, blue cartridge, with triple staggered rows of staples (Figure 14). Starting from the common hepatic artery isolation, we removed all the nodes station No.8 on its anterior part (Figure 15).

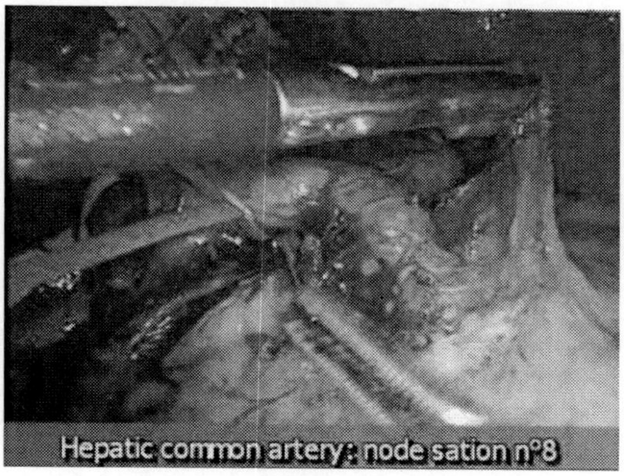

Figure 15. Isolation of hepatic common artery and node station 8.

Hence, he left gastric vein is closed and divided and the posterior part of the common hepatic artery, lymph nodes station No.8p, is removed (Figure 16; 17). The left gastric artery is isolated (nodes station No.7) (Figure 18); the splenic artery and celiac trunk origin are encircled by vessel loops (nodes station respectively No.11p and No.9) (Figure 19). The left gastric artery is divided between non-absorbable clips with removal of nodes station 7 (Figure 20). By lifting the remnant stomach up the excision of the posterior right paracardial nodes at the gastroesophageal region (station 1) is gained (Figure 21). The left gastro-epiploic artery is then isolated and divided with ultrasonic scalpel, and lymph node group 4s is resected (Figure 22). The stomach is always resected with two 60mm and one 45mm linear staplers, green cartridge, with triple staggered rows of staples (Figure 23). Two access openings are created, and the mechanical device, 45mm linear stapler, blue cartridge, with triple staggered rows of staples, is inserted to create a side-to-side aniso-peristaltic gastrojejunal anastomosis (Figure 24). The openings are joint with intra-corporeal continuous suture by3/0 PDS® material after nasogastric tube positioning. The transmesocolic jejunal loop is prepared by linear stapler (Figure 25). The jejuno-jejunal side-to-side stapled anastomosis of the Roux-en-Y loop restores the digestive tract continuity (Figure 26).

Totally Total

The first steps of Laparoscopic Total gastrectomy are the same as subtotal gastrectomy until left gastric artery dissection. The short vessels are then divided with the ultrasonic scalpel. The dissection is continued to the diaphragmatic crus, dividing the phrenoesophageal membrane and vagal nerves. Group 2 (left paracardial) is resected. The stomach is totally mobilized but not yet divided from the esophagus (Figure 27). The transmesocolicjejunal loop is prepared with linear stapler (Figure 28; 29).

The side-to-side stapled jejuno-jejunal anastomosis of the Roux-en-Y loop restores the digestive tract continuity. In our experience, it is easier to perform the jejuno-jejunal anastomosis before the esophagojejunal anastomosis (Figure 30).

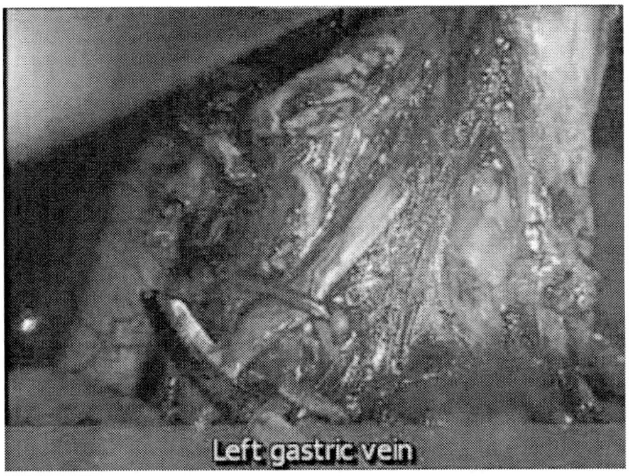

Figure 16. Section between clip of left gastric vein.

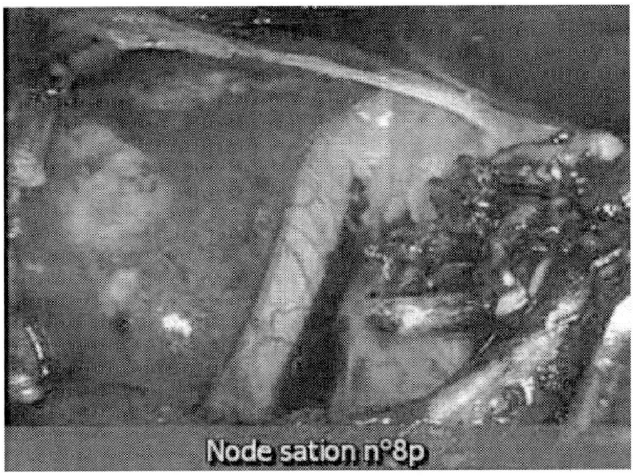

Figure 17. Node station 8.

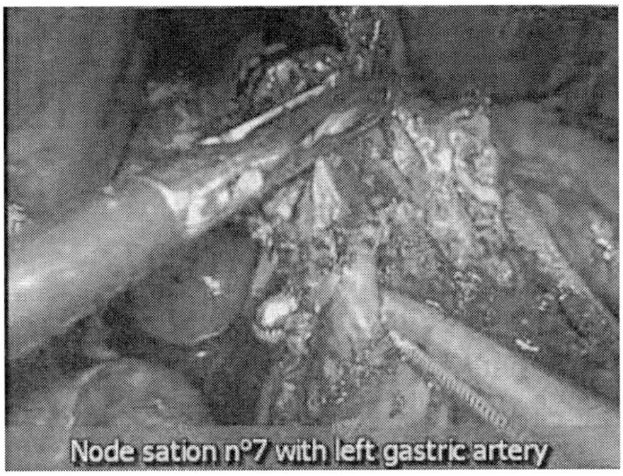

Figure 18. Isolation and resection of Node station 7 and left gastric artery.

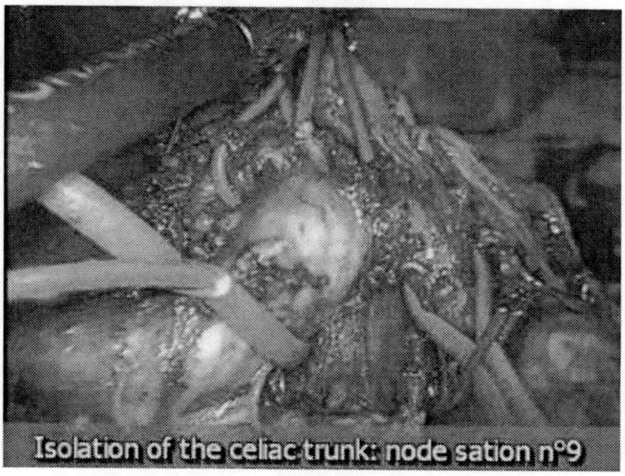

Figure 19. Isolation of the celiac trunk and node station 9.

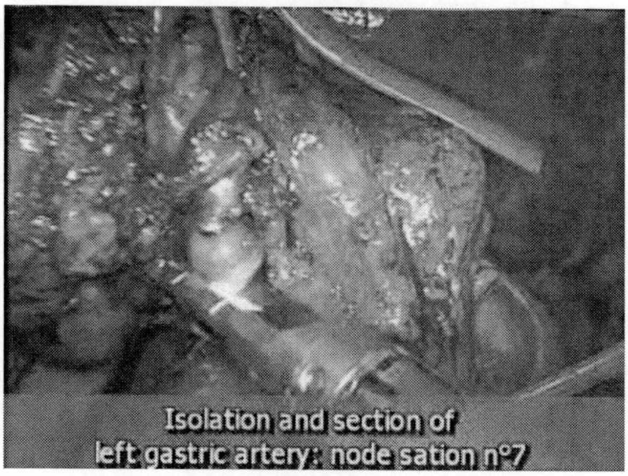

Figure 20. Section of left gastric artery and node station 7.

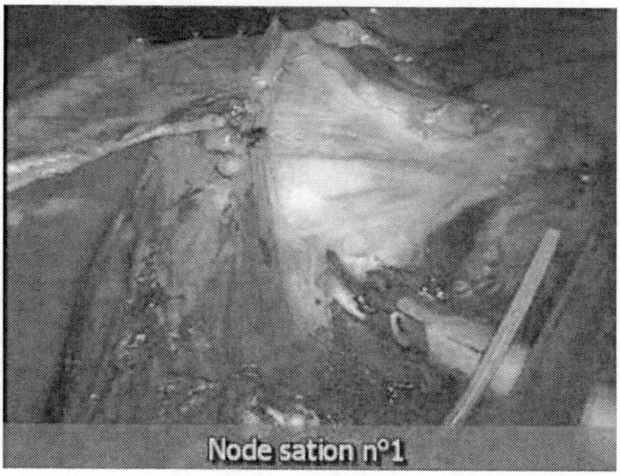

Figure 21. Node statiion 1 dissection.

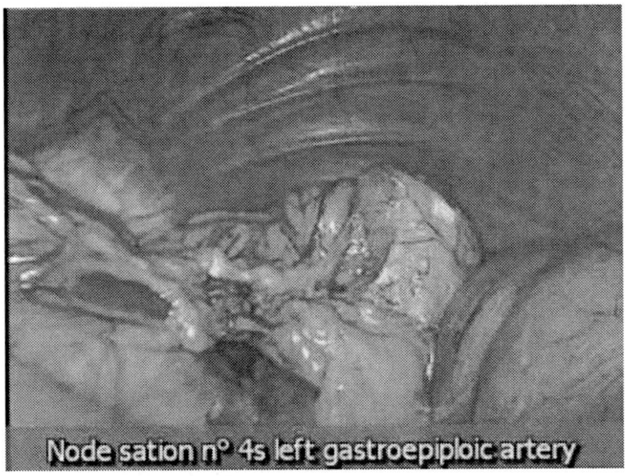

Figure 22. Node station 4 and left gastroepiploic artery dissection.

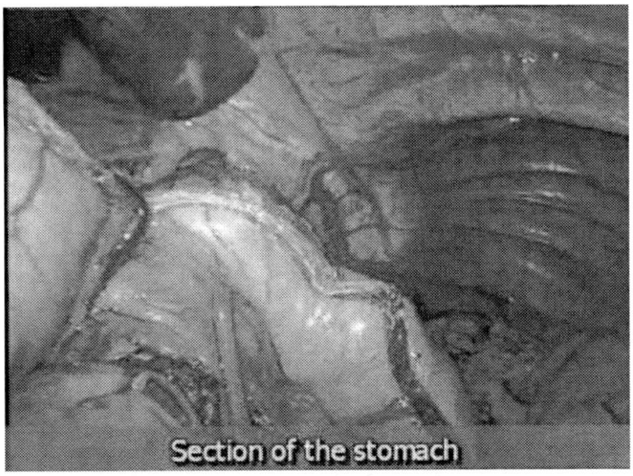

Figure 23. Section of the stomach.

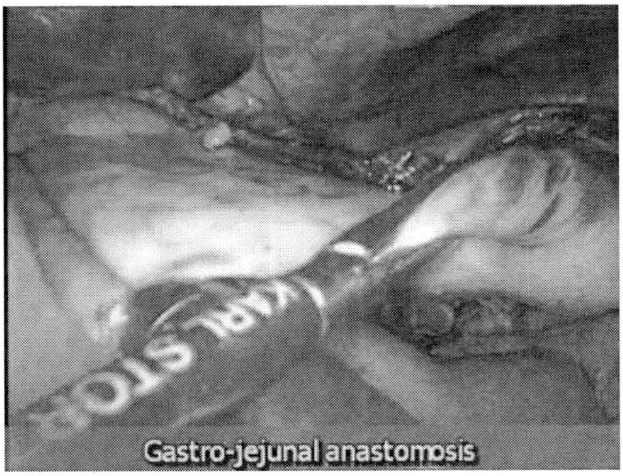

Figure 24. Gatro-jejunalanastomosis.

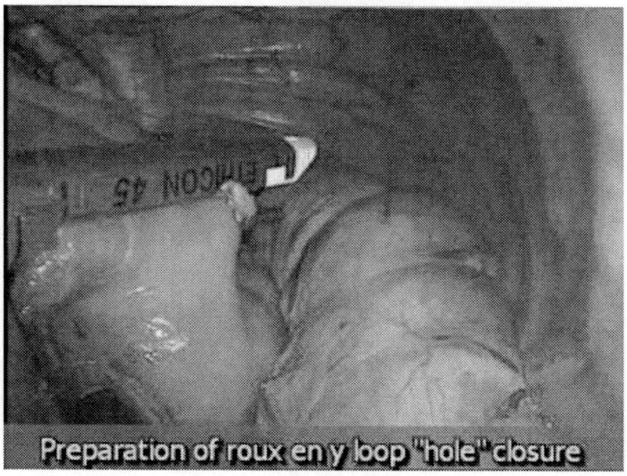

Figure 25. Preparation of Roux en y loop.

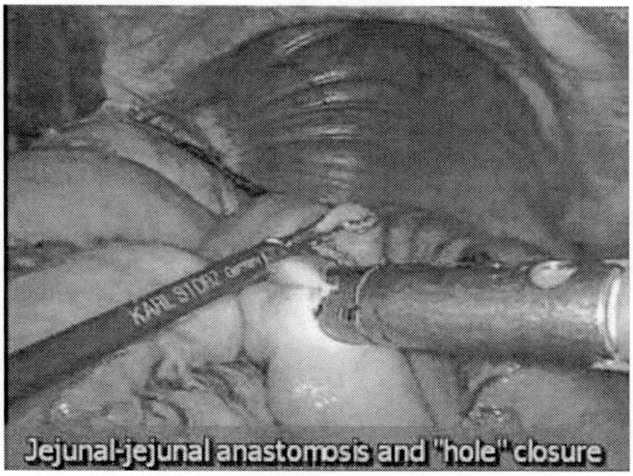

Figure 26. Jejunal-jejunal anastomosis.

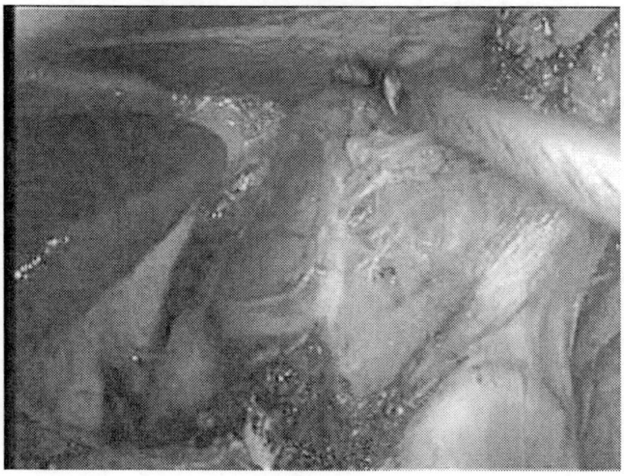

Figure 27. Completion of gastric mobilization.

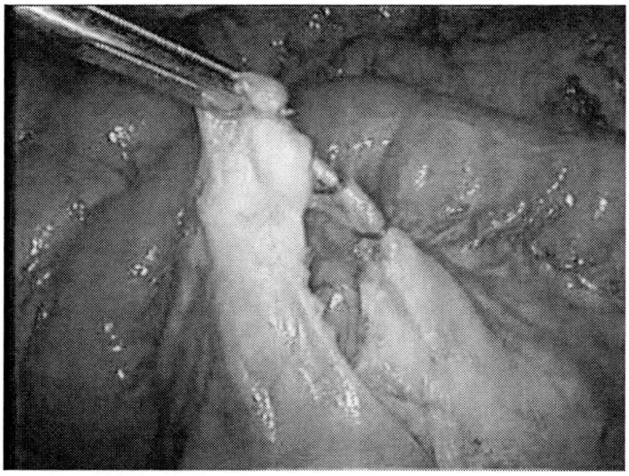

Figure 28. Transmesocolic loop Preparation.

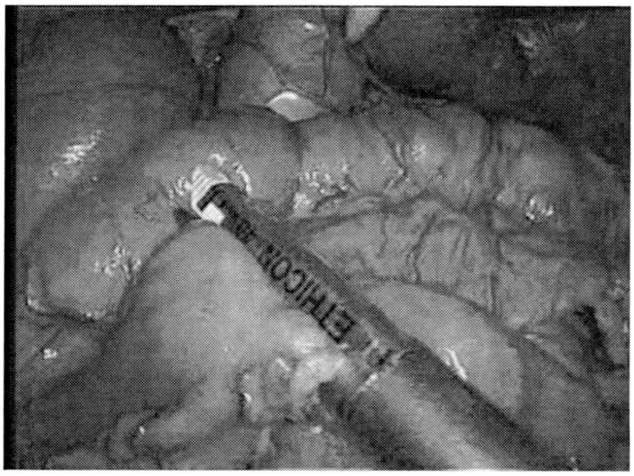

Figure 29. Transmesocolic loop preparation with stapler.

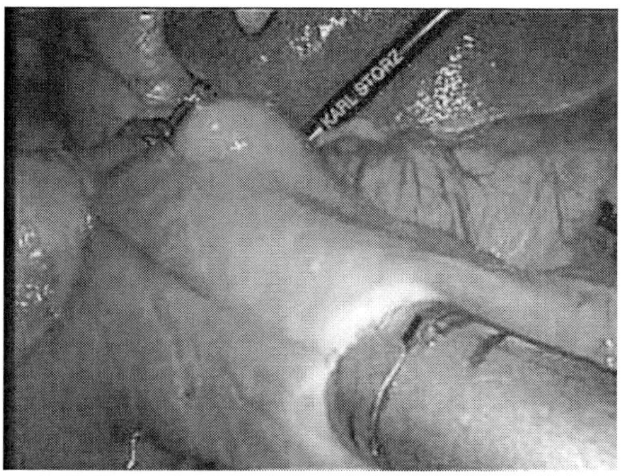

Figure 30. Side-to-side stapled jejuno-jejunal anastomosis at the foot of the Roux-en-Y loop.

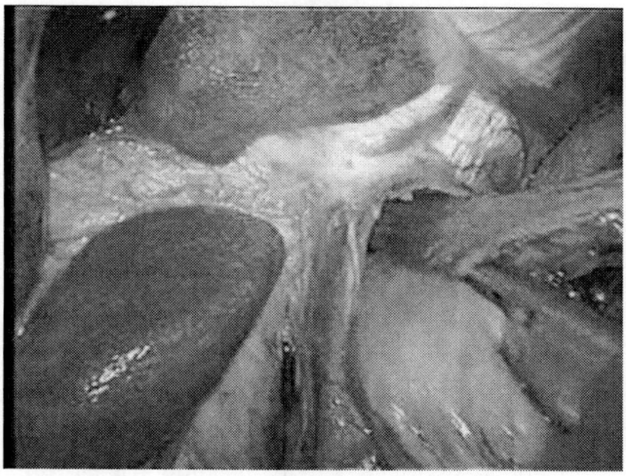

Figure 31. Esophago-jejunal anastomosis.

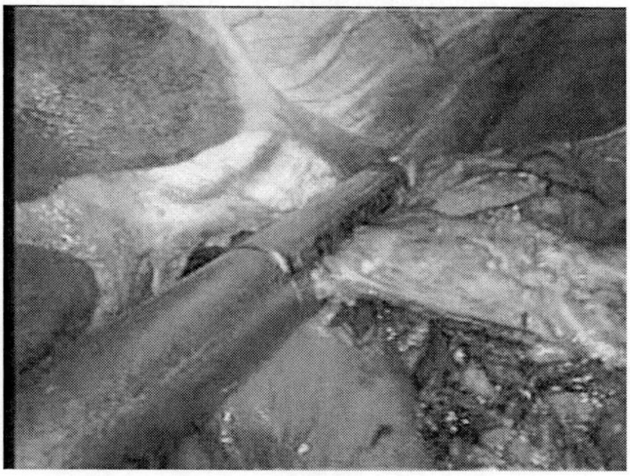

Figure 32. Gatric resection.

Two access openings are created, and the mechanical device, 45mm cartridge linear stapler (blue reloads, with triple staggered rows of staples), is inserted to create a side-to-side isoperistaltic esophagojejunal anastomosis according to Orringer's model [15] (Figure 31). The openings are closed with intracorporeal continuous sutures by 3/0 PDS® material after nasogastric tube positioning. The stomach is always resected with a 45mm cartridge linear stapler (Figure 32).

In female patients, the specimen is pulled out in an Endobag through a posterior vaginal incision, while in males a 5 cm Pfannesteil incision is made in order to remove the specimen. Drains are placed into the abdominal cavity. Closure of the last two port incisions with a subcuticular suture marks the end of the procedure.

Tips and Tricks

1. Use diagnostic laparoscopy in each patient, in order to confirm resective chance.

2. Use only 12mm trocars, due to use staples by both sides.
3. Duodenal resection should be performed with a stapler charged with triple staggered rows of staples, preserving an adequate blood supply to the duodenal stump.
4. It is useful to mobilize the first portion of the duodenum, by isolation of the right gastro-epiploic vessels and then of the gastro-duodenal artery. Placing a swab in this position as an anatomic landmark in order to dissect the pars flaccida.
5. Lymphadenectomy can be performed safely with bipolar devices, harmonic scalpel and monopolar hook. Placing vessel loops with a right-angle dissector around the vessels makes the vascular traction easier. In order to perform a good lymphadenectomy, it is necessary to proceed slowly, performing a correct hemostasis with bipolar device. We suggest to perform lymphadenectomy in a clockwise direction.
6. Celiac tripod and nodes station n 13 can be hidden by the pancreas. It is useful to change camera position in order to achieve a better v of the operative field.
7. Bursectomy in posterior wall gastric cancer can be also performed by exposing the retro-pancreatic peritoneum, without any injuries to the pancreas and using thermal devicesonly when necessary. High laparoscopic suture skills are needed in order to repair iatrogenic injuries.
8. Gastro-jejunal anastomosis must be performed with 45 or 60mm staples. The latter are preferred.Anastomosis has to be performed with intracorporeal continuous sutures. In Roux-en-Y reconstruction, it is better to perform thejejuno-jejunal anastomosis before gastrojejunostomy.
9. To avoid erroneous fashioning of the anastomoses, it is better to identify jejunal loops with conventional colored sutures.
10. Intracorporeal anastomosisis preferable in order to avoid stretching or twisting of the jejunal loop.
11. Conversion is mandatory in the early experience.
12. At the end of total gastrectomy, test intraoperatively the esophago-jejunal anastomosis with methylene blue.

Table 1. EGC treatment according to characteristics.The Japanese Gastric Cancer Association

Early Gastric Cancer		
FEATURES	TREATMENT	LYMPHADENECTOMY
differentiated mucosal non ulceration diameter>2cxm	EMR	-
mucosal cancer not amenable to EMR differentiated submucosal <1,5 cm	(LA)DG	D1+α
submucosal N0 EGC < 2.cm N1	(LA)DG	D1+β
EGC > 2cm N1	(LA)DG	D2

EGC = early gastric cancer.

EMR= endoscopic mucosal resection.

(LA)DG= laparoscopy-assisted distal gastrectomy.

DG= distal gastrectomy.

Conclusion

Laparoscopic Gastrectomy for gastric cancer, despite a longer operative time, overcomesOpen Gastrectomy in short-term results. No differences were assessed in morbidity and mortality rates and the extent of the lymphadenectomy is adequate.

In order to establish Laparoscopic Gastrectomy as the standard treatment for gastric cancer, RCTs with long-term follow-up should be conducted. We suggest that future studies should analyze data regarding surgical team's learning curve.

Gastrectomy is, however, one of the most difficult procedures to perform by a laparoscopic approach and we believe that it could be done only by high-skilled laparoscopic surgeon in high case-volume hospitals.

References

[1] Bai H. L., Chen B., Zhou Y., Wu X. T.Five-year long-term outcomes of laparoscopic surgery for colon cancer.*World J. Gastroenterol.* 2010 Oct. 21;16(39):4992-7.

[2] Abraham N. S., Byrne C. M., Young J. M. and Solomon M. J. Metaanalysis of non-randomized comparative studies of the short-term outcomes of laparoscopic resection for colorectal cancer. *ANZ J. Surg.* 2007;77:508–16.

[3] Kitano S., Iso Y., Moriyama M., Sugimachi K. Laparoscopy assisted Billroth I gastrectomy. *Surg. Laparosc. Endosc.* 1994; 4:146–8.

[4] Azagra J. S., Georgen M., De Simone P., Ibanez-Aguire J. L. Minimally invasive surgery for gastric cancer. *Surg. Endosc.* 1999;13:351–7.

[5] Kitagawa Y., Kitano S., Kubota T., Kumai K., Otani Y., Saikawa Y., Yoshida M., Kitajima M. Minimallyinvasivesurgery for gastriccancer -toward a confluence of two major streams: a review. *Gastric Cancer.* 2005;8(2):103-10.

[6] Japanese Gastric Cancer Association. Japanese gastric cancer treatment guidelines 2010 (ver. 3). *Gastric Cancer.* 2011 Jun.;14(2):113-23.

[7] Shiraishi N., Yasuda K., Kitano S. Laparoscopic gastrectomy with lymph node dissection for gastric cancer. *Gastric Cancer* 2006;9:167–76.

[8] Namieno T., Koito K., Higashi T., Takahashi M., Yamashita K., Kondo Y., et al. Assessing the suitability of gastric carcinoma for limited resection: endoscopic prediction of lymph node metastasis. *World J. Surg.* 1998;22:859–64.

[9] Nakamura K., Morisaki T., Sugitani A., Ogawa T., Uchiyama A., Kinukawa N., et al. An early gastric carcinoma treatment strategy based on analysis of lymph node metastasis. *Cancer* 1999;85:1500–5.

[10] Kurihara N., Kubota T., Otani Y., Ohgami M., Kumai K., Sugiura H., et al. Lymph node metastasis of early gastric cancer with submucosal invasion. *Br. J. Surg.* 1998;85:835–9.

[11] Tonouchi H., Mohri Y., Kobayashi M., Tanaka K., Ohi M., Kusunoki M. Laparoscopy-assisted distal gastrectomy with laparoscopic sentinel lymph node biopsy after endoscopic mucosal resection for early gastriccancer. *Surg. Endosc.* 2007 Aug.;21(8):1289-93.

[12] Kunisaki C., Makino H., Kosaka T., Oshima T., Fujii S., Takagawa R., Kimura J., Ono H. A., Akiyama H., Taguri M., Morita S., Endo I. Surgical outcomes of laparoscopy-assistedgastrectomy versus open gastrectomy for gastric cancer: a case-control study. *Surg. Endosc.* 2011 Oct. 15. [Epub ahead of print].

[13] Japan Society for Endoscopic Surgery. Nationwide survey on endoscopic surgery in Japan (in Japanese) *J. Jpn. Soc. Endosc. Surg.* 2004;9:475–563.

[14] Huscher C. G., Mingoli A., Sgarzini G., Sansonetti A., Di Paola M., Recher A., Ponzano C.Laparoscopic versus open subtotal gastrectomy for distal gastric cancer: five-year results of a randomized prospective trial. *Ann. Surg.* 2005 Feb.;241(2):232-7.

[15] Bracale U., Marzano E., Nastro P., Barone M., Cuccurullo D., Cutini G., Corcione F., Pignata G. Side-to-side oesophagojejunostomy during totally laparoscopic total gastrectomy for malignant disease: a multicenter study. *Surg. Endosc.* 2010 Oct.;24(10):2475-9. Epub 2010 Apr. 16.

[16] Sakuramoto S., Kikuchi S., Futawatari N., et al. Technique of esophagojejunostomy using transoral placement of the pretilted anvil head after laparoscopic gastrectomy for gastric cancer. *Surgery* 2010;147:742–747. [12;13].

[17] Huscher C. G., Mingoli A., Sgarzini G. et al (2005) Laparoscopic versus open subtotal gastrectomy for distal gastric cancer. Fiveyear results of a randomized prospective trial. *Ann. Surg.* 241:232–237.

[18] Kitano S., Shiraishi N., Fujii K. et al (2002) A randomized controlled trial comparing open vs laparoscopy-assisted distal gastrectomy for the treatment of early gastric cancer: an interim report. *Surgery* 131:s306–s311.

[19] Fujii K., Sonoda K., Izumi K. et al (2003) T lymphocyte subsets and Th1/Th2 balance after laparoscopy-assisted distal gastrectomy. *Surg. Endosc.* 17:1440–1444 Term Outcomes.

[20] Hayashi H., Ochiai T., Shimada H. et al (2005) Prospective randomized study of open vs laparoscopy-assisted distal gastrectomy with extraperigastric lymph node dissection for early gastric cancer. *Surg. Endosc.* 19:1172–1176.

[21] Lee J. H., Han H. S., Lee J. H. (2005) A prospective randomized study comparing open vs laparoscopy-assisted distal gastrectomy in early gastric cancer. *Surg. Endosc* 19:168–173.

[22] Kim Y. W., Baik Y. H., Yun Y. H. et al (2008) Improved quality of life outcomes after laparoscopy-assisted distal gastrectomy for early gastric cancer: results of a prospective randomized clinical trial. *Ann. Surg.* 248:721–727.

[23] Kim H. H., Hyung W. J., Cho G. S. et al (2010) Morbidity and mortality of laparoscopic gastrectomy versus open gastrectomy for gastric cancer. An interim report—a phase III multicenter, prospective, randomized trial (KLASS Trial). *Ann. Surg.* 251:417–420.

[24] Uyama I., Sugioka A., Matsui H., et al. Laparoscopic D2 lymph node dissection for advanced gastric cancer located in the middle or lower third portion of the stomach. *Gastric Cancer* 2000; 3:50–55.

[25] Tanimura S., Higashino M., Fukunaga Y., et al. Laparoscopic gastrectomy for gastric cancer: experience with more than 600 cases. *Surg. Endosc.* 2008;22:1161–1164.

[26] Kawamura H., Homma S., Yokota R., et al. Inspection of safety and accuracy of D2 lymph node dissection in laparoscopy assisted distal gastrectomy. *World J. Surg.* 2008;32:2366–2370.

[27] Song K., Kim S., Park C. Laparoscopy-assisted distal gastrectomy with D2 lymph node dissection for gastric cancer: technical and oncologic aspects. *Surg.Endosc.* 2008;22:655–659.

[28] Lee J., Ryu K., Park S., et al. Learning curve for total gastrectomy with D2 lymph node dissection: cumulative sum analysis for qualified surgery. *Ann. Surg. Oncol.* 2006;13:1175–1181.

[29] Lee J., Kim Y., Ryu K., et al. A phase-II clinical trial of laparoscopy-assisted distal gastrectomy with D2 lymph node dissection for gastric cancer patients. *Ann. Surg. Oncol.* 2007;14:3148–3153.

[30] Kodera Y., Fujiwara M., Ohashi N., Nakayama G., Koike M., Morita S., Nakao A. Laparoscopic Surgery for gastric cancer: a collective review with meta-analysis of randomized trials. *J. Am. Coll. Surg*. 2010; 211: 677-86.

[31] Koeda K., Nishizuka S., Wakabayashi G. Minimally Invasive surgery for gastric cancer: the future standard of care. *World J. Surg.* 2011;35:1469-77.

[32] Chen X. Z., Hu J. K., Yang K. et al (2009) Short-term evaluation of laparoscopy-assisted distal gastrectomy for predictive early gastric cancer: a meta-analysis of randomized controlled trials. *Surg. Laparosc Endosc. Percutan. Tech.* 19:277–284.

[33] NCCN Guidelines in Clinical Oncology version 2.2011 available at *http://www.nccn.org/professionals/physician_gls/pdf/gastric.pdf.*

[34] Hartgrink H. H., van de Velde C. J., Putter H., Bonenkamp J. J., Klein Kranenbarg E., Songun I., Welvaart K., van Krieken J. H., Meijer S., Plukker J. T., van Elk P. J., Obertop H., Gouma D. J., van Lanschot J. J., Taat C. W., de Graaf P. W., von Meyenfeldt M. F., Tilanus H., Sasako M. Extended lymph node dissection for gastric cancer: who may benefit? Final results of the randomized Dutch gastric cancer group trial. J. *Clin. Oncol.* 2004 Jun. 1;22(11):2069-77. Epub 2004 Apr. 13.

[35] Schwarz R. E., Smith D. D. Clinical impact of lymphadenectomy extent in resectable gastric cancer of advanced stage. *Ann. Surg. Oncol.* 2007 Feb.;14(2):317-28. Epub 2006 Nov. 9.

[36] Kim M., Kim W., Kim H., et al. Risk factors associated with complication following laparoscopy-assisted gastrectomy for gastric cancer: a large-scale Korean multicenter study. *Ann. Surg. Oncol.* 2008;15:2692–2700.

[37] Kitano S., Shiraishi N., Uyama I., et al. A multicenter study on oncologic outcome of laparoscopic gastrectomy for early cancer in Japan. *Ann. Surg.* 2007;245:68–72.

[38] Song J., Lee H., Cho G., et al. Recurrence following laparoscopy-assisted gastrectomy for gastric cancer: a multicenter retrospective analysis of 1,417 patients. *Ann. Surg.Oncol.* 2010;17:1777–1786.

In: Gastric Cancer
Editors: A. D'Annibale, V. Pende and I. Monsellato
ISBN: 978-1-62081-294-5

Chapter VII

Complications and Short - Term Results of Laparoscopic Gastrectomy for Cancer

Domenico D'Ugo**[*]**, Roberto Persiani, Ferdinando Cananzi and Francesco Santullo
General Surgery Unit, Department of Surgery,
Catholic University of Rome, Rome, Italy

Abstract

In recent years, due to the development of newly designed operative techniques and the introduction of better technological devices for laparoscopic surgery , together with the undoubted improvement of surgical skills, several surgeons have started applying laparoscopic assisted gastrectomy (LAG) for gastric cancer.

To date, in literature there are several studies which demonstrate both the feasibility of laparoscopic lymphadenectomy in terms of oncological radicality as well as the absence of differences in the complication rate and short-term results between laparoscopic and open surgery for Early Gastric Cancer (EGC). Laparoscopic-assisted distal gastrectomy (LADG) has been therefore increasingly used for EGC and T1-T2 tumors, but to date it has not reached a sufficient grade of recommendation as regards advanced gastric cancer (AGC), even if it is to be considered as a promising oncological procedure with adequate lymph node harvesting.

With the purpose of reaching a solid evidence-based validation, different prospective studies comparing the short- and long-term outcome are currently in progress to endorse the appropriateness and safety of laparoscopic assisted gastrectomy for patients with advanced gastric cancer.

---

[*] E-mail address: *ddugo@rm.unicatt.it.*

Introduction

In recent years, due to the development of minimally invasive techniques and improvement of the devices for laparoscopic surgery, several surgeons have started applying laparoscopic assisted gastrectomy (LAG) for gastric cancer. Up to date, the increase of laparoscopic procedures in gastric cancer has not followed the same chronological development observed in colorectal surgery whereas several prospective randomized studies have already shown that short-term outcomes and complications after laparoscopic surgery for colorectal cancer are clearly comparable to those observed for open surgery.

In spite of the many potential benefits of LAG compared to conventional open procedure -such as less post-operative pain, faster recovery, and shorter hospital stay- laparoscopic surgery for gastric cancer still lacks a solid evidence-based validation; up to 2010, the Japanese Gastric Cancer Treatment Guidelines did not recommend LAG in a curative cancer resection setting, but indicated laparoscopic gastrectomy just as an investigational procedure eligible for clinical trials [1].

To date, in literature, there are several retrospective studies together with two prospective trials (KLASS, JCOG 0703) [10, 11] which stand in favor of the safety and oncological feasibility of laparoscopic surgery for the treatment of Early Gastric Cancer (EGC). The results of these studies demonstrate both the reliability of laparoscopic lymphadenectomy in terms of oncological radicality as well as the absence of differences in the complication rate and short-term results between laparoscopic and open surgery. Therefore, along with the demonstration that the number of harvested lymph nodes by LAG to date has increased up to reach that observed during open gastrectomy, laparoscopic gastric surgery has now to be considered at least as "feasible".

Hereafter, if laparoscopy assisted distal gastrectomy (LADG) has been increasingly used for EGC and T1-T2 tumors, still it has been less investigated as regards advanced gastric cancer (AGC); it is currently matter for debate if LAG with D2 lymphadenectomy should represent an appropriate treatment for an advanced gastric cancer (AGC) as well [3, 4]. The worst general conditions of such patients due to the advanced status of the disease, indeed, imply an additional risk of complications. It would be therefore important to understand in which proportion the advantages of laparoscopic surgery are possibly counterbalanced by an increased incidence of complications in patients with AGC.

Complications

Complication following laparoscopic surgery for gastric cancer can be classified as intraoperative and postoperative.

Postoperative complications are essentially the same that may occur after open gastrectomy. On the other hand, intra-operative complications are often peculiar of the laparoscopic approach, such as laparoscopic organ or vascular injury caused by trocar placement or by the heat of energy devices which seldom occurs because of the restricted field of view and the reduction of the movement range.

Intraoperative bleeding due to vascular injury is the most frequent intraoperative complication and can occur during all phases of gastrectomy.

Colon injury can occur during total omentectomy (Figure 1), instead, spleen may be injured during isolation an exposure of the left gastroepiploic artery and the left gastroepiploic vein (Figure 2). During pancreatic lymph nodes dissection (Figure 3), when the splenic artery and vein are identified and exposed, the dorsal part of pancreatic parenchyma may be damaged. Such injury leads to the development of serious evolving complications, including anastomotic leakage and hemorrhage. Hepatic and bile duct injury can occur during the dissection of hepatic artery (Figure 4). Frequent postoperative complications after both LAG and open gastrectomy (OG) include: wound infection, pancreatic injury and fistula, abdominal abscess, abdominal bleeding, ileus, anastomotic stenosis, pulmonary complication, urinary tract infection, renal complication and anastomotic leakage. As regards patterns and incidence rate of anastomotic leakage there could be some differences between LAG and ODG due to the consistent development of newly designed operative techniques of mechanical suture and anastomosis for laparoscopic surgery which are sometimes consistently different from those used in open procedure. Kodera et al. [5] in a recent review compared the results of 6 different papers, showing that there is a decrease in the rate of complications for patients undergoing laparoscopic surgery compared to those undergoing conventional surgery. (Figure 5). According to published reports [6, 7, 8] the frequency of complications after laparoscopic surgery for gastric cancer ranges from 4.3% to 23.3%.

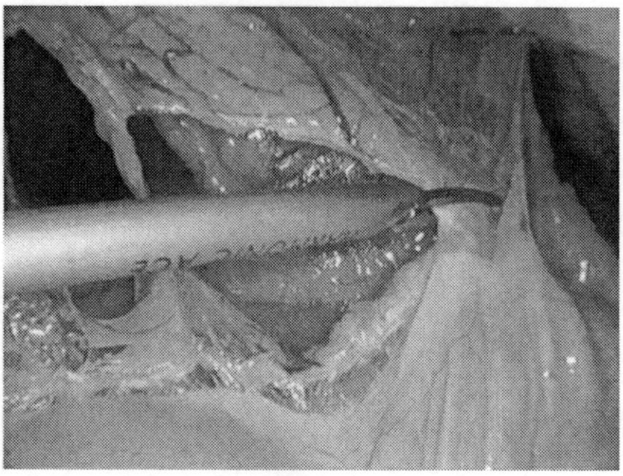

Figure 1. (sample) Original picture enclosed.

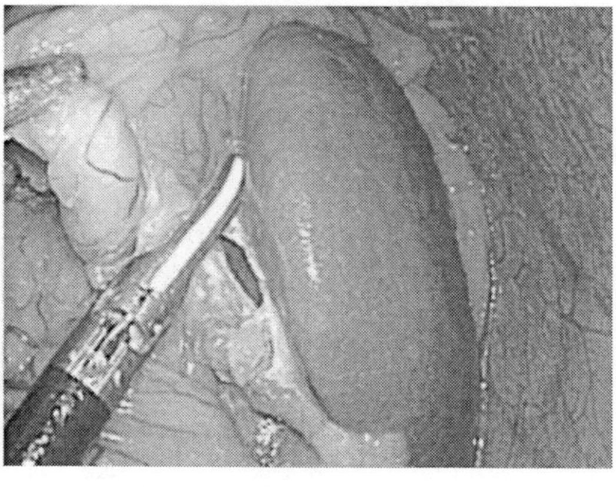

Figure 2. (sample) Original picture enclosed.

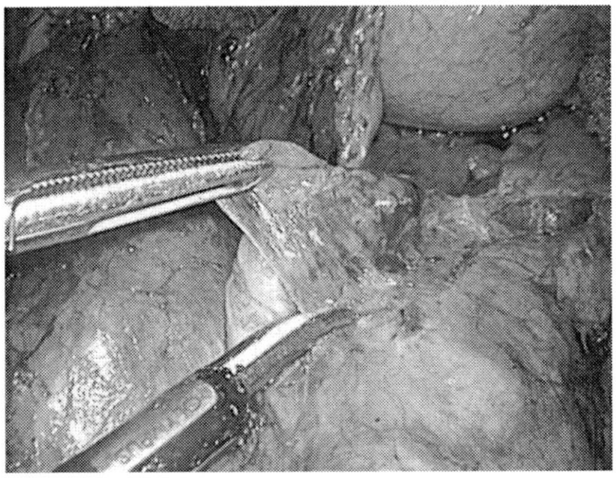

Figure 3. (sample) Original picture enclosed.

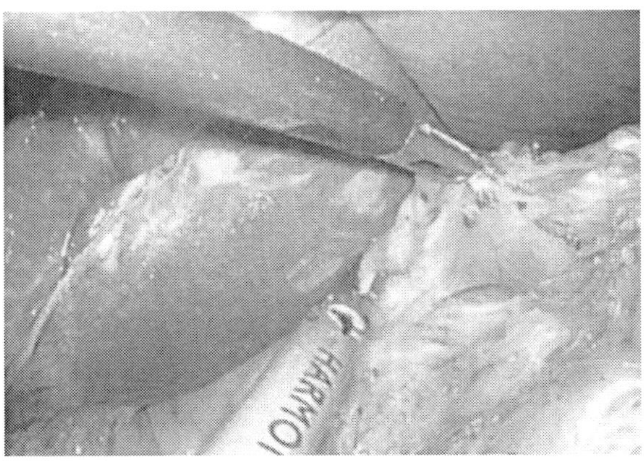

Figure 4. (sample) Original picture enclosed.

	LADG		ODG	
Reference	Events	Total	Events	Total
Huscher	8	30	9	29
Kitano	2	14	4	14
Hayashi	2	14	6	14
Lee	3	24	10	23
Kim YW	0	82	4	82
Kim HH	17	179	24	161

Figure 5.

In a multicenter retrospective study conducted by Kim HH et al. [9] the overall morbidity and mortality are 14.0% and 0.6%, respectively; these data are comparable to many other retrospective and some prospective randomized Japanese studies. The same authors in another multicenter prospective study (KLASS trial) [10] have shown for the LADG group a morbidity and mortality rates of 10.4% and 1.1%, and 14.7% and 0% for the open distal gastrectomy (ODG) group. Complications in this study were divided into two categories:

early postoperative complications (0-30 days) and late complications (>30 days). Early complications occurred in 20 patients (11.6%) in the LADG group and 27 patients (15.08%) in the ODG group (Figure 6), and late complications occurred in 3 patients for each group (1.74% and 1.67%) (Figure 7). However there were no statistical differences in terms of morbidity and mortality between the 2 groups.

Early PostoperativeComplications (0-30 days)			
Complications	LADG	ODG	p
Wound infection	1	6	
Fluid collection and abscess	1	3	
Intra abdominal bleeding	3	3	
Ileus	3	3	
Anastomotic stenosis	0	2	
Chyle leakage	0	1	
Anastomotic leakage	3	1	
Pulmunary complication	2	2	
Urinary tract infection	1	0	
Renal complication	2	0	
Hepatic	1	0	
Other	3	6	
Total (%)	20/172 (11.6%)	27/179 (15.08%)	0,137

Figure 6.

Reoperation was performed in 3 patients in the LADG group (intra-abdominal bleeding, intestinal obstruction, and anastomotic leakage), and in 3 patients in the ODG group (anastomotic leakage, adhesive ileus and wound dehiscence). Katai et al [11] showed in a phase II prospective trial comparing LADG and ODG that the proportion of patients who developed anastomotic leakage or pancreatic fistula after laparoscopic surgery is 1.7%, which is comparable to that observed in patients undergoing ODG (anastomotic leakage 0.6%–2.7%; pancreatic fistula 0.6%) [10, 12, 13]. In addition, the proportion of patients who developed these complications is lower than data reported in previous publications (anastomotic leakage 1.7%–14%; pancreatic fistula 1.0%) [2, 14]. Analysis of the pooled data revealed that the rate of pulmonary complication tend to be higher in the ODG group than in the LADG group.

Late Complications (>30 days)			
Complications	LADG	ODG	p
Incisional hernia	0	2	
Alkaline reflux	0	1	
Delayed emptyng	1	0	
Bronchiectasis	1	0	
Renal	1	0	
Total (%)	3/172 (1.74%)	3/179 (1.67%)	1

Figure 7.

	LADG			ODG			
Reference	n	Time (min)	SD	n	Time (min)	SD	Time difference (95%CI)
Huscher	30	196	21	29	168	29	28.00 (15.04-40.96)
Kitano	14	227	7	14	171	13	56.00 (48.27-63.73)
Hayashi	14	348	97	14	235	71	143.00 (80.03-205.97)
Lee	24	320	39	23	190	16	129.20 (112.21-146.19)
Kim YW	82	253	49	82	171	27	81.90 (69.85-93.95)
Total	164			162			81.83 (49.56-114.09)

Figure 8.

	LADG			ODG			
Reference	n	Blood loss(ml)	SD	n	Blood loss(ml)	SD	Time difference (95%CI)
Huscher	30	229	144	29	391	136	-162.00 (-233.45≈-90.55)
Kitano	14	117	30	14	258	53	-141.00 (-172.90≈-109.10)
Hayashi	14	327	245	14	489	301	-162.00 (-365.30≈-41.3)
Lee	24	336	180	23	294	156	42.00 (-54.35≈138.35)
Kim YW	14	112	30	14	258	53	-141.00 (-172.90≈-109.10)
Kim HH	179	109	133	161	200	166	-91.74 (-123.92≈-59.57)
Total	343			323			-115.60 (-159.18≈-72.03)

Figure 9.

Kitano et al. [15] and Lee et al. [8] reported that the lesser postoperative pain, which allow a faster mobilization of the patient due to laparoscopic surgery, results in a reduction of the incidence of pulmonary complications such as atelectasis.

Lee et al. [31] conducted an analysis on 601 patients, in which complications were reported according to the type of gastric resection performed (distal gastrectomy, proximal gastrectomy, pylorus-preserving gastrectomy, segmental gastrectomy, total gastrectomy). In this series bleeding was the most frequent intraoperative complication. However there were no statistical differences in the incidence of intraoperative complications between different types of resections. Postoperative complications occurred more frequently after total gastrectomy and in these patients there was a considerably higher incidence of pancreatic lesions (11.1%) and anastomotic leakage (11.1%).

Short Term Results

Most recent reports investigating the short-term results of laparoscopic gastric surgery refer to EGC; these data obviously cannot be directly transferred to what is expected for AGC and it is extremely important to differentiate the results related to early tumors from those related to advanced tumors.

Early Gastric Cancer (EGC)

Short-term outcome of LAG were analyzed by several studies and there are currently different parameters comparing laparoscopy-assisted distal gastrectomy with open distal gastrectomy: number of lymph nodes retrieved, operating time, estimated blood loss, duration, analgesic administration and length of hospital stay, recovery of gastrointestinal function.

Number of Harvested Lymph Nodes

It is well known that the number of lymph nodes removed during gastrectomy is to be correlated with the prognosis of gastric cancer. In past years the number of lymph nodes collected during laparoscopic lymphadenectomy was lower compared to open lymphadenectomy. Ohtani et al. showed in a meta-analysis conducted on four randomized control studies [8, 15, 16, 17] comparing LADG with ODG for EGC that the number of harvested lymph nodes was higher in the ODG group than in the LADG group, although this difference was not statistical significant except in one of the four studies.

In recent years, through the improvement of laparoscopic surgical techniques and skills of surgeons, the number of dissected lymph nodes has gradually increased, reaching that observed after open gastrectomy. A recent meta-analysis of eight case-control studies has revealed that there is no evident difference in the number of lymph nodes dissected, between LADG and ODG. [18]

Operative Time

The mean operative time for LADG is significantly higher than ODG. Kodera et al. [5] has shown that the mean operating time in the LADG group ranged from 196 to 348 minutes, a figure that appears to be certainly longer than the time needed to accomplish an open distal gastrectomy (ODG) in all studies. (Figure 8).

This finding could be due to the reduction of the field of view, lack of tactile sensation, and the steep learning curve needed for LADG. In the near future, with the advancements in surgical techniques and laparoscopic devices, the time required for laparoscopic-assisted gastrectomy is probably going to decrease.

Blood Loss

As observed in randomized control studies, intraoperative blood loss was significantly lower in the LADG group than in the ODG group. This difference may be due to the close vision of an enlarged surgical field obtained using a scope which allows a better detection of large and small vessels [19]. The expanded use of special equipment including ultrasonic dissectors and bipolar radiofrequency forceps also contributed to reduce blood loss.

Kodera et al. [5] showed, in a review that compared LADG with ODG for EGC, that an average blood loss of 200 ml in the LADG group and was significantly smaller than in the ODG group. (Figure 9) A reduction of bleeding in patients with gastric cancer decreases the chance or amount of transfusion. As noted by Pacelli et al. [33] the immunologic changes after blood transfusions such as decreased helper/suppressor T-cell ratios, decreased natural-killer cell activity, decreased macrophage antigen presentation, suppression of lymphocyte blastogenesis, and decreased delayed-type hypersensitivity may have somehow negative effect on the prognosis of gastric cancer patients.

Analgesic Administration and Length of Hospital Stay

The frequency of analgesic administration after LADG is lower than after ODG because of lower tissue injury. Laparoscopic surgery induces smaller wounds than those created during ODG, requiring less analgesic administration. Furthermore, a less painful surgery reduces the perioperative stress so that patients experience a faster recovery with a shorter hospital stay and an early resume of their daily activities. With the exception of complicated cases, most patients after LADG are discharged 7/8 days after surgery. [20].

Recovery of Gastrointestinal Function

Different studies show that the less surgical trauma of laparoscopic surgery allows a faster recovery of gastrointestinal function, a shorter time to first flatus and assumption of a normal diet. In addition, Braga et al. [21] found that the less-traumatic abdominal incision and the less traction on the mesentery due to laparoscopic surgery result in a higher oxygen tension inside the intestinal wall during the entire surgical procedure. This may improve the systemic response allowing early recovery of gut function.

Advanced Gastric Cancer (AGC)

To date, short-term results and complication rate of laparoscopy gastrectomy with D2 lymph nodes dissection for advanced gastric cancer are still controversial. A recent prospective randomized trial, comparing ODG versus LADG in advanced gastric cancer, has shown that, despite a prolonged operative time, there is no significant difference in most aspects including the number of harvested lymph nodes, time to first flatus, postoperative morbidity, days to first sips of water, blood loss, amount of transfusions and length hospital stay. (Figure 10)

Many authors have reported no difference between laparoscopic and open procedures in terms of number of harvested lymph nodes [23, 24, 25]. Shuang et al [26] reported a median number of 35 lymph nodes dissected in the laparoscopic group versus 38 in the open group, which is comparable to the number reported by other authors who performed laparoscopic surgery for AGC. [6, 24, 27]

	LAG group (n=49)	OG group (n=47)
Operative time	270± 55.26	187.66 ± 40.18
Amount of trasfusion (ml)	89.80 ± 168.62	74.47 ± 146.65
Estimatedbloodloss (ml)	293.67 ± 164.49	344.47 ± 219.65
Number of Linpho nodes dissected	22.98 ± 2.7	22.87 ± 2.42
Time to first Flautus	3.89 ± 1.64	4.21 ± 1.24
Number of day to get out of bed	4.77 ± 2.09	4.89 ± 1.53
Hospital stay (days)	11.63 ± 2.94	11.42 ± 1.17

Figure 10.

Analyzing the data in literature the postoperative morbidity rates of LAG for advanced gastric cancer ranges from 7.7% to 31.5% [10, 28, 29, 30]. Cai et al [22] reported that the overall morbidity rates were 12.24% in the LAG and 19.15% in the OG groups, with no significant difference. However, respiratory complications were more frequent in the OG group.

Conclusion

The achievement of reliability of laparoscopic lymphadenectomy in terms of oncological appropriateness and the absence of differences as regards the incidence of complications and short-term results between laparoscopic and open approach, have allowed the transferral of the many advantages of mini-invasiveness to the treatment of early gastric cancer. This has been made possible through the development of newly designed operative techniques and the introduction of better technological devices for laparoscopic surgery together with the undoubted improvement of surgical skills.

A phase III multicenter prospective randomized trial (KLASS Trial) [10] has concluded that there is no significance difference in morbidity and mortality between laparoscopy assisted distal gastrectomy and open distal gastrectomy as concerns early gastric cancer. Possible disadvantages are the longer operative time and the steep learning curve for laparoscopic surgery.

Because of these difficulties, an extensive case-load is required to individual surgeons in order to safely perform laparoscopy assisted gastrectomy; a precise standardization of laparoscopic procedures together with a considerable number of cases are needed for an efficient educational system. Therefore, clinical application and teaching of laparoscopic techniques for gastric cancer should be reserved only to high-volume certified centers [32].

Up to date laparoscopy assisted gastrectomy with D2 lymph node dissection for the treatment of advanced gastric cancer is a promising oncological procedure with adequate lymph node harvesting. The advantages of minimal invasion, including the reduced risks of surgical related trauma, the containment of blood loss, less postoperative pain and earlier recovery could lead to a reduction in complications for difficult patients such as those with advanced gastric cancer. Confirmation of the appropriateness and safety of laparoscopic assisted gastrectomy for patients with advanced gastric cancer are expected from the results of different prospective studies comparing the short- and long-term outcomes, such as the KLASS 2 trial, which are currently in progress.

References

[1] Japanese Gastric Cancer Association. Japanese gastric cancer treatment guidelines 2010 (ver. 3). *Gastric Cancer* 2011 Jun.;14(2):113-23.

[2] Kitano S., Shiraishi N., Uyama I., Sugihara K., Tanigawa N. Japanese Laparoscopic Surgery Study Group. A multicenter study on oncologic outcome of laparoscopic gastrectomy for early cancer in Japan. *Ann. Surg.* 2007;245:68–72.

[3] Goh P. M., Khan A. Z., So J. B., et al.: Early experience with laparoscopic radical gastrectomy for advanced gastric cancer. *Surg. Laparosc. Endosc. Percutan. Technol.* 2001;11:83–87.

[4] Ziqiang W., Feng Q., Zhimin C., et al.: Comparison of laparoscopically assisted and open radical distal gastrectomy with extended lymphadenectomy for gastric cancer management. *Surg. Endosc.* 2006;20:1738–1743.

[5] Kodera Y., Fujiwara M., Ohashi N., Nakayama G., Koike M., Morita S., Nakao A. Laparoscopic Surgery for Gastric Cancer: A Collective Review with Meta-Analysis of Randomized Trials. *J. Am. Coll. Surg.* 2010 2010 Nov.;211(5):677-86.

[6] Huscher C. G. S., Mingoli A., Sgarzini G., et al. Laparoscopic versus open subtotal gastrectomy for distal gastric cancer: five-year results of a randomized prospective trial. *Ann. Surg.* 2005;241:232–237.

[7] Hosono S., Arimoto Y., Ohtani H., et al. Meta-analysis of short term outcomes after laparoscopic-assisted distal gastrectomy. *World J. Gastroenterol.* 2006;12:7677–7683.

[8] Lee J. H., Han H. S., Lee J. H. A prospective randomized study comparing open vs laparoscopy assisted distal gastrectomy in early gastric cancer. Early results. *Surg. Endosc.* 2005;19:168 –173.

[9] Kim M. C., Kim W., Kim H. H., et al. Risk factors associated with complication following laparoscopy assisted gastrectomy for gastric cancer: a large-scale Korean multicenter study. *Ann. Surg. Oncol.* 2008;15:2692–2700.

[10] Kim H., Hyung W., Cho G., et al. Morbidity and mortality of laparoscopic gastrectomy versus open gastrectomy for gastric cancer: an interim report—a phase III multicenter, prospective, randomized trial (KLASS Trial). *Ann. Surg.* 2010;251:417–420.

[11] Katai H., Sasako M., Fukuda H., Nakamura K., Hiki N., Saka M., Yamaue H., Yoshikawa T., Kojima K.; JCOG Gastric Cancer Surgical Study Group. Safety and feasibility of laparoscopy-assisted distal gastrectomy with suprapancreatic nodal dissection for clinical stage I gastric cancer: a multicenter phase II trial (JCOG 0703). *Gastric Cancer.* 2010;13:238-244.

[12] Hori S., Ochiai T., Gunji Y., Hayashi H., Suzuki T. A prospective randomized trial of hand-sutured versus mechanically stapled anastomoses for gastroduodenostomy after distal gastrectomy. *Gastric Cancer* 2004;7:24–30.

[13] Sasako M., Katai H., Sano T., Maruyama K. Management of complications after gastrectomy with extended lymphadenectomy. *Surg. Oncol.* 2000;9:31–4.

[14] Fujiwara M., Kodera Y., Kasai Y., Kanyama Y., Hibi K., Ito K., et al. Laparoscopy-assisted distal gastrectomy with systemic lymph node dissection for early gastric carcinoma: a review of 43 cases. *J. Am. Coll. Surg.* 2003;196:75–81.

[15] Kitano S., Shiraishi N., Fujii K., et al. A randomized controlled trial comparing open vs laparoscopy-assisted distal gastrectomy for the treatment of early gastric cancer: an interim report. *Surgery* 2002;131:306–311.

[16] Hayashi H., Ochiai T., Shimada H., et al. (2005) Prospective randomized study of open versus laparoscopy-assisted distal gastrectomy with extraperigastric lymph node dissection for early gastric cancer. *Surg. Endosc.* 19:1172–1176.

[17] Kim Y. W., Baik Y. H., Yun Y. H., Nam B. H., Kim D. H., Choi I. J., Bae J. M.. Improved quality of life outcomes after laparoscopy-assisted distal gastrectomy for early gastric cancer: results of a prospective randomized clinical trial. *Ann. Surg.* 2008;248:721–727.

[18] Ding J., Liao G. Q., Liu L., Liu S., Tang J. Meta-Analysis of Laparoscopy-Assisted Distal Gastrectomy With D2 Lymph Node Dissection for Gastric Cancer. *J. Surg. Oncol.* 2011.

[19] Vamvakas E. C. Perioperative blood transfusion and cancer recurrence: meta-analysis for explanation. *Transfusion* 1995;35:760–768.

[20] Yoo C. H., Kim H. O., Hwang S., Son B. H., Shin J. H., Kim H. Short-term outcomes of laparoscopic-assisted distal gastrectomy for gastric cancer during a surgeon's learning curve period. *Surg. Endosc.* (2009) 23:2250–2257.

[21] Braga M., Vignali A., Gianotti L., et al.: Laparoscopic versus open colorectal surgery: A randomized trial on short-term outcome. *Ann. Surg.* 2002;236:759–766.

[22] Cai J., Wei D., Gao C. F., Zhang C. S., Zhang H., Zhao T. A. Prospective Randomized Study Comparing Open versus Laparoscopy-Assisted D2 Radical Gastrectomy in Advanced Gastric Cancer. D*ig. Surg.* 2011;28:331–337.

[23] Kawamura H., Homma S., Yokota R., Yokota K., Watarai H., Hagiwara M., Sato M., Noguchi K., Ueki S., Kondo Y. Inspection of safety and accuracy of D2 lymph node dissection in laparoscopyassisted distal gastrectomy. *World. J. Surg.* 2008;32:2366–2370.

[24] Hwang S. I., Kim H. O., Yoo C. H., Shin J. H., Son B. H. Laparoscopicassisted distal gastrectomy versus open distal gastrectomy for advanced gastric cancer. *Surg. Endosc.* 2009;23:1252–1258.

[25] Strong V. E., Devaud N., Allen P. J., Gonen M., Brennan M. F., Coit D. Laparoscopic versus open subtotal gastrectomy for adenocarcinoma: a case-control study. *Ann. Surg. Oncol.* 2009;16:1507–1513.

[26] Shuang J., Qi S., Zheng J., Zhao Q., Li J., Kang Z., Hua J., Du J. A Case–Control Study of Laparoscopy-Assisted and Open Distal Gastrectomy for Advanced Gastric Cancer. *J. Gastrointest Surg.* (2011) 15:57–62.

[27] Noshiro H., Nagai E., Shimizu S., Uchiyama A., Tanaka M. Laparoscopically assisted distal gastrectomy with standard radical lymph node dissection for gastric cancer. *Surg. Endosc.* 2005;19:1592–1596.

[28] Lee J., Kim W.: Long-term outcomes after laparoscopy-assisted gastrectomy for advanced gastric cancer: analysis of consecutive 106 experiences. *J. Surg. Oncol.* 2009; 100: 693–698.

[29] Huang J. L., Wei H. B., Zheng Z. H., Wei B., Chen T. F., Huang Y., Guo W. P., Hu B.: Laparoscopyassisted D2 radical distal gastrectomy for advanced gastric cancer. *Dig. Surg.* 2010; 27: 291–296.

[30] Shuang J., Qi S., Zheng J., Zhao Q., Li J., Kang Z., Hua J., Du J.: A case-control study of laparoscopy-assisted and open distal gastrectomy for advanced gastric cancer. *J. Gastrointest. Surg*. 2011; 15: 57–62.

[31] Lee S., Nomura E., Bouras G., Tokuhara T., Tsunemi S., Tanigawa N. Long-Term Oncologic Outcomes from Laparoscopic Gastrectomy for Gastric Cancer: A Single-Center Experience of 601 Consecutive Resections. *J. Am. Coll. Surg*. 2010 Jul;211(1):33-40.

[32] Tokunaga M., Hiki N., Fukunaga T., Miki A., Nunobe S., Ohyama S., Seto Y., Yamag T. Quality control and educational value of laparoscopy-assisted gastrectomy in a high-volume center. *Surg. Endosc*. (2009) 23:289–295.

[33] Pacelli F., Rosa F., Marrelli D., Pedrazzani C., Bossola M., Zoccali M., Marchet A., Di Cosmo M., Roata C., Graziosi L., Cavazzoni E., Covino M., D'Ugo D., Roviello F., Nitti D., Doglietto G. B. Do Perioperative Blood Transfusions Influence Prognosis of Gastric Cancer Patients? Analysis of 927 Patients and Interactions with Splenectomy. *Ann. Surg. Oncol*. (2011) 18:1615–1623.

In: Gastric Cancer
Editors: A. D'Annibale, V. Pende and I. Monsellato

ISBN: 978-1-62081-294-5

Chapter VIII

Robotic Gastrectomy: Technique, Complications and Short Term Results

Annibale D'Annibale, Vito Pende, Graziano Pernazza, Paolo Mazzocchi, Giorgio Lucandri, Giovanni Alfano and Igor Monsellato*

San Giovanni-Addolorata Hospital, Minimally-Invasive and Robotic Surgery Unit, Rome, Italy

Abstract

Laparoscopic surgery has become widely accepted and used as a minimally invasive approach for a number of procedures because it offers a number of patient benefits compared to open surgery such as milder morbidity, earlier time to walking, flatus, and oral intake, and quicker recovery with a shorter hospital stay.

The current standard of care for resectable locally advanced gastric cancer, in Japan and Europe, is R0- gastrectomy with extensive D2 lymph node dissection. Although laparoscopic D2-lymphadenectomy has been described and found to be feasible by several authors, widespread use of this technique was limited by the pitfalls of this complex procedure.

The anatomic complexity of the vascular structures, the technical limits of the conventional laparoscopic instrumentation, and the lack of a steady image, can consequently add to surgeons' stress, making this procedure quite complex even for minimally-invasive well-trained surgeons. In an effort to minimize the difficulty of laparoscopy, a robotic surgery system was introduced.

* E-mail address: *imonsellato@libero.it.*

Introduction

Since its introduction in the 1980s, laparoscopic surgery has become widely accepted and used as a minimally invasive approach for a number of procedures [1-6] because it offers a number of patient benefits compared to open surgery such as milder morbidity, earlier time to walking, flatus, and oral intake, and quicker recovery with a shorter hospital stay [7-10].

In the field of gastric cancer, laparoscopic gastrectomy was rapidly adopted in Eastern countries, initially on early stage diseases where a limited lymphadenectomy (D1) is accepted.

The current standard of care for resectable locally advanced gastric cancer, in Japan and Europe, is R0- gastrectomy with extensive D2 lymph node dissection [11-13]. D1 dissection involves group 1 lymph nodes: s1–s6 for lower middle and upper third localizations; s3, s4d, s5, s6 for lower third and duodenal localizations; s1, s3, s4sb, s4d, s5, s6 for middle third-lower localizations; s1–s6 for upper third-middle localizations; s1–s3, s4sa, s4sb for upper third localizations.

D2-lymphadenectomy involves group 1 plus group 2 stations: s1, s3, s4d, s4sb, s5–s7, s8a, s9, s11p, s12a for middle third localizations and s1, s3, s4d, s5–s7, s8a, s9, s11p, s12a, s14v for lower third-duodenal localizations. Although laparoscopic D2-lymphadenectomy has been described and found to be feasible by several authors [14–19], widespread use of this technique was limited by the pitfalls of this complex procedure. The anatomic complexity of the vascular structures, the technical limits of the conventional laparoscopic instrumentation, and the lack of a steady image, can consequently add to surgeons' stress, making this procedure quite complex even for minimally-invasive well-trained surgeons.

In an effort to minimize the difficulty of laparoscopy, a robotic surgery system was introduced [20-23]. The da Vinci Surgical System (Intuitive Surgical Inc., Sunnyvale, CA, US) aimed to relieve the shortcomings of laparoscopic surgery by maximizing the comfort of the surgeon, while providing instruments that enable technically demanding operations, three-dimensional views, and improved dexterity with an internal articulated EndoWrist that allows seven degrees of freedom.

Robotic surgery is spreading all over the world for many surgical procedures ranging from cardiac to general and urologic surgery thanks to its potential advantages overcoming the negative aspects of laparoscopic approach [5,23]. To date, the most successful application of robotic surgery is robot-assisted radical prostatectomy, which was rapidly adopted worldwide [24].

The first robot-assisted gastrectomy was reported by Hashizume et al [25]. in 2003. In 2009, Song et al. [26] presented their initial 100 cases of robot-assisted gastrectomy with lymph node dissection; it is the largest series for robotic surgery with gastric cancer in the literature. Then, Hur et al [27] reported total robotic gastrectomy using robot-sewn anastomosis and Ryu et al [28] reported a robot-assisted gastric wedge resection for gastric GIST.

The first report on intermediate survival after robot-assisted gastrectomy was recently presented by Pugliese et a l[29]. In April 2011, we published our research article on the first 24 total and subtotal gastrectomies for gastric cancer, showing acceptable short-term outcome [30].

Criteria in Selecting Patient for Minimally Invasive Surgery

Patient's selection is based on pathophysiological and pathological conditions. Absolute contraindications in colorectal cancer robotic surgery reflect those for whole minimally invasive surgery. Nevertheless, indications to minimally invasive approach are expanding rapidly suggesting the establishment of international guidelines in patient's selection.

There are several physiological parameters, which have been analyzed for patient's selection:

- *Age.* Age does not influence intraoperative or postoperative outcome as shown by several studies in which postoperative morbidity was lower than that in open surgery. Moreover, conversion rates were not statistically significant if different ages were considered (younger, middle-aged, elderly). Age is not a contraindication.
- *Cardiopulmonary condition.* Generally, altered cardiopulmonary functions are not considered a contraindication to minimally invasive approach. Nevertheless, minimally invasive approach needs continuous monitoring of patient's physiological parameters. The effect of the pneumoperitoneum on hemodynamics in patients ASA (American society of anesthesiologists score) I-II are not clinically relevant, while an invasive monitoring system of the blood pressure or circulating volume is advocated in patient ASA III-IV. In addition, gasless or low-pressure regimen should be maintained during the whole intervention in patients with limited cardiac function. Monitoring of end-tidal carbon-dioxide levels is mandatory, since pneumoperitoneum may causes a CO2-retention and head position and intrabdominal hypertension lead to ventilation-perfusion mismatch.
- *Obesity.* Obese patients' ventilation is often problematic because of pulmonary compliance reduced about 30% than in normal-weight patients. Although obesity is not considered an absolute contraindication, complications and conversion rate are higher at BMI (body mass index) greater than 30. Recently, similar postoperative short term outcomes have been demonstrated between obese and non-obese patients. Complication rates are comparable with those expected after open surgery.
- *Pathological criteria:* Characteristics of tumor may influence the surgical approach. A tumor invading adjacent structures (T4) is considered an "absolute" contraindication to minimally invasive approach, as the principles of atraumatic manipulation and wide resection margins could be not matched. Adhesions, localization and peritoneal carcinomatosis are not considered a contraindication by the majority of experts.

Operating Theater Setup

Patient Preparation

The patient undergoes bowel preparation with Polyethylene glycol one day before the procedure and a slag-free diet three days before the procedure. The banding technique of the inferior arms associated to administration of a low-molecular-weight heparin 12 hours before the procedure is performed for thromboembolism prophylaxis.

Venous Access

Before procedure starts, a venous access is needed to maintain correct blood volume and hydration of the patient and to infuse anesthetic agents during the whole procedure. The preferred choices of venous access are: right superior arm (18G catheter) for right colectomy and left superior arm for left colectomy and rectal resection (16/18 gauge catheter). If peripheral venous access is unavailable, a central catheter should be inserted before the day of the procedure. A heating system for venous access is needed in order to maintain the thermal homeostasis. Keeping patients warm has been associated with a threefold decrease in the rate of wound infection, reduction in operative blood loss, decrease in untoward cardiac events and patient discomfort. Maintenance of a normal temperature during surgery is important to reduce the stress of the surgical procedure and organ dysfunction.

Types of Anesthesia

General anesthesia with orotracheal intubation and mechanical dynamic ventilation is the preferred technique among anesthesiologists. Currently, both intravenous and gas-intravenous (Desforane, Sevorane) techniques are used by anesthesiologists as there is no evidence of better results by the one or the other procedure. The usual scheme provides an association with epidural access in order to better control postoperative pain. N2O (nitrous oxide) is contraindicated as it may increase the risk of pulmonary embolism. An optimal anesthesia may provide an acceptable muscular relaxation, better ventilation, thus minimizing the risk of pulmonary embolism and hemodynamics alteration, granting a wider operating field thus reducing the operative time.

Intraoperative Monitoring

Intraoperative monitoring differs between ASA I-III or III+ patients:

In ASA I-III:

ECG+HR, O2 saturation, Airways Pressure (PAW – Pressure plateau), capnography (EtCO2)

In ASA III+ in addition to previous tests:

Neuromuscular function (TOF), Diuresis monitoring (bladder catheterization), Swan-Ganz catheter, PeakPressure Monitoring, arterial catheterization, haemo-gas analysis.

A peripheral arterial access is mandatory for monitoring blood pressure in high-risk patients.

Surgical Instrumentation

- Stereoscopic endoscope (da Vinci Surgical System).
- CO2 insufflator.
- Irrigation/suction system device.

- Video processor.
- 1 Hasson-type trocart.
- 1 10/12mm trocart.
- 3 8mm robotic trocart.
- 2 Robotic Cadiere's graspers.
- 2 Robotic needle-holders.
- 1 Laparoscopic needle-holder.
- 1 Laparoscopic dissector.
- 3 Laparoscopic forceps type Johann.
- 1 Laparoscopic clip applier.
- 1 45-mm laparoscopic stapler device with 2-3 cartridges (intestinal and vascular type).
- 1 Robotic ultrasound device.
- 1 Robotic electrocautery hook.
- 1 Robotic bipolar forceps.
- 1 Wound protector for specimen extraction.

Patient's Position

Patient's position is similar both in robotic total gastrectomy and sub-total gastrectomy. Patient is placed in supine 15 degrees - reverse Trendelenburg position with shoulder supports. The legs are abducted and secured at the thigh and calf with straps. The assistant-surgeon stands between the patient's legs. The operating room scheme is shown in Figure 1.

Trocarts Setup

A conventional 12-mm port is placed by open technique just above the umbilicus, and a pneumoperitoneum to 12 mmHg is established. Under direct vision three 8-mm robotic trocarts are placed, two in the upper abdomen at the midclavicular line on the left (robotic arm no. 1) and on the right (robotic arm no. 2), and one at the right anterior axillary line for liver retraction (robotic arm no. 3). In addition, a 12-mm port for the assistant surgeon (Ax) is placed between the left robotic port and the camera port (Figure 1).

Once the abdominal cavity has been found to be free from metastatic disease, the four-arm da Vinci Surgical System is docked to the operative table above the patient's head and the operative arms are connected to the ports. The 30°-robotic endoscope is inserted through the umbilical port. The surgeon at the console controls the robotic arm no. 1 with the right master and the two left arms (no. 2 and no. 3) switching between both these arms depending on the steps of the procedure. The arm no. 2 is used for Cadiere forceps and the arm no. 3 is used to lift the liver. The robotic arm no. 1 carries the cautery hook or the harmonic scalpel (HS). The 12-mm Ax port is used to assist the surgeon in several steps of the procedure and for the introduction of aspiration/irrigation device, clip applier, linear stapler, sponges, and sutures.

Surgical Technique

Lymphadenectomy

According to JGCA guidelines, an extended (D2) lymphadenectomy is routinely performed both in total and in subtotal gastrectomy. The choice of the type of procedure is based on the location of the tumor. In total gastrectomy, involved lymph node stations are: 1, 2, 3, 4sa, 4sb, 4d, 5, 6, 7, 8a, 9, 10 (in middle-upper tumor location), 11 (p, d in middle-upper tumor location) and 12a.

In subtotal gastrectomy lymphadenectomy involves stations: 1, 3, 4 (sb in middle-lower location or d only in duodenal-lower location), 5, 6, 7, 8a, 9, 11p, 12a, 14v (in duodenal lower location).

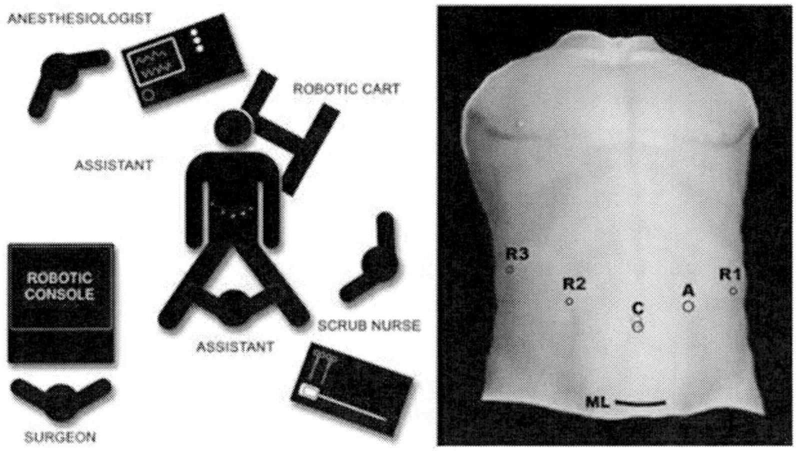

Figure 1. Operating room setup and trocarts position.

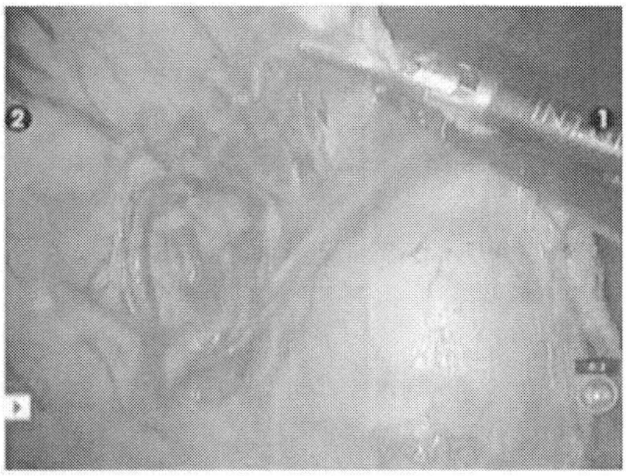

Figure 2. Coloepiploic detachment.

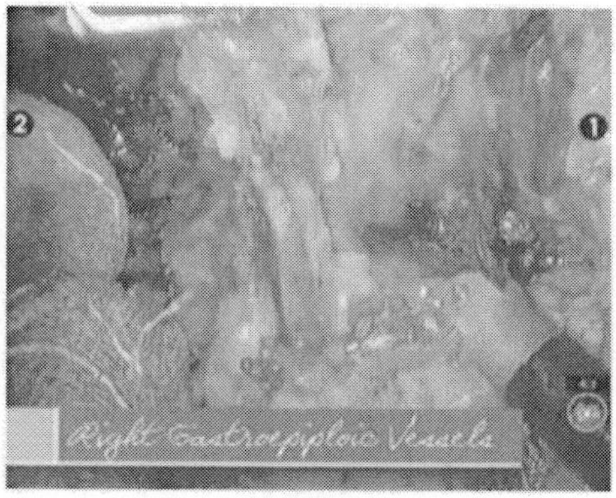

Figure 3. Right gastroepiploic vessels.

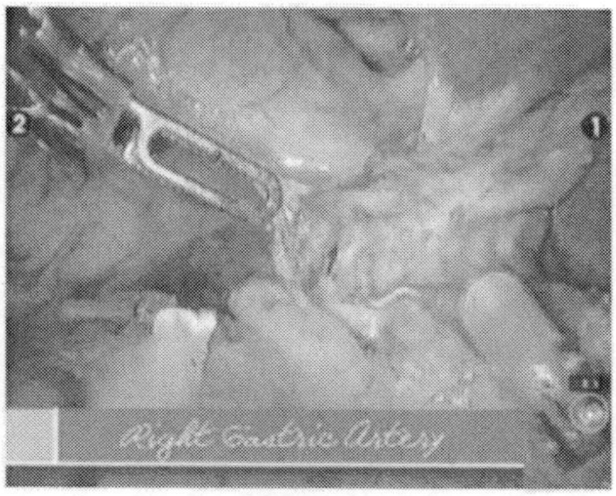

Figure 4. Right gastric artery.

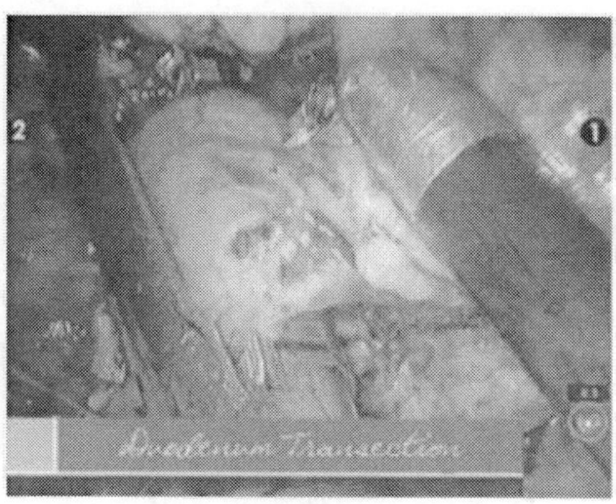

Figure 5. The duodenum has being transected.

Robotic Total Gastrectomy (RATG)

A complete colo-epiploic detachment is performed using the HS toward the lower pole of the spleen and the hepatic flexure (Figure 2). After the access to the bursa omentalis recess is gained, the surgeon lifts up cranially the posterior gastric wall by switching the arm no. 3 in order to expose the supramesocolic area.

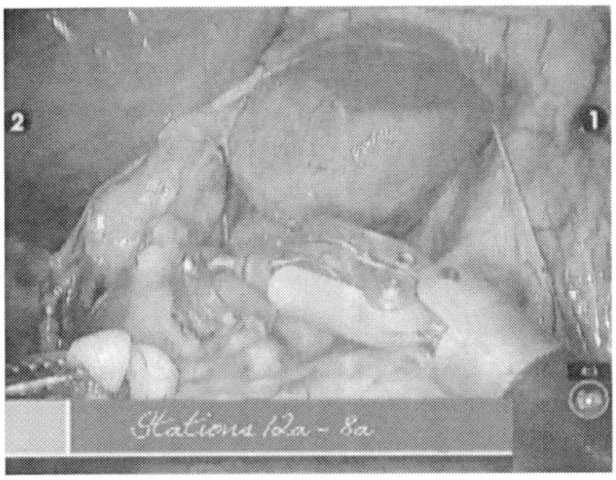

Figure 6. Hepatic pedicle (station 12a).

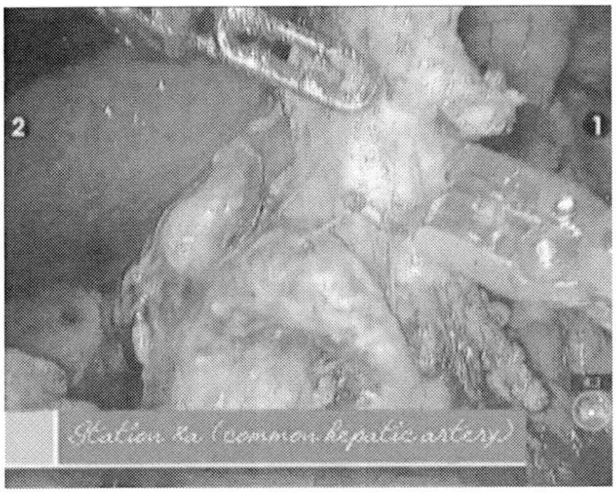

Figure 7. Lymphadenectomy of common hepatic artery.

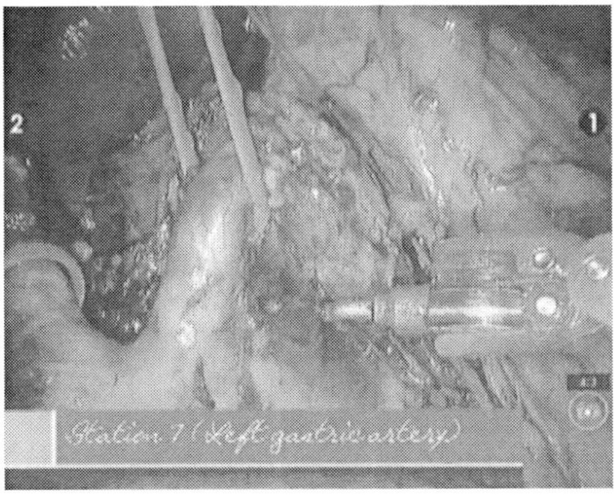

Figure 8. Lymphadenectomy of left gastric artery.

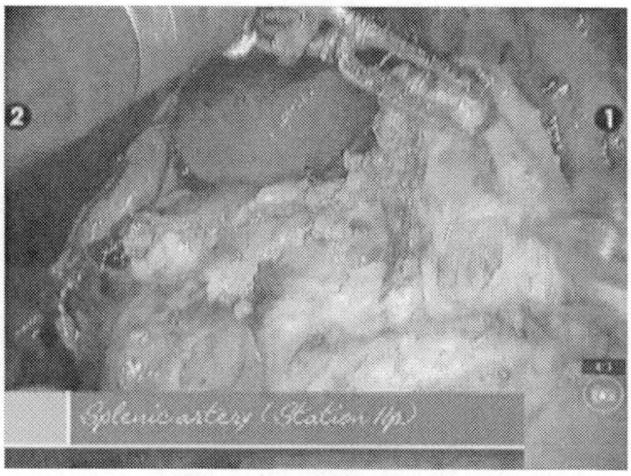

Figure 9. Proximal splenic artery (station 11p).

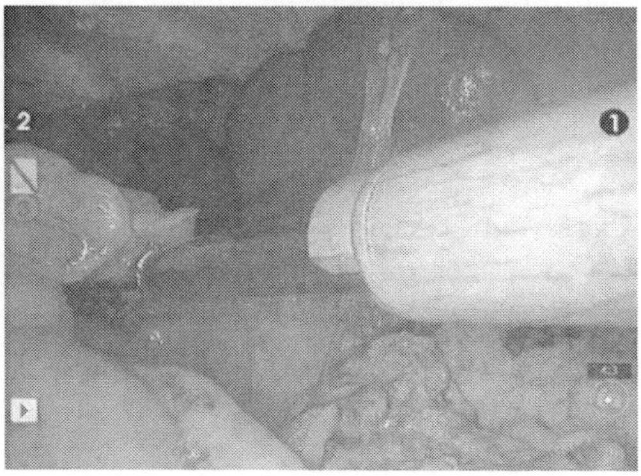

Figure 10. Dissection of gastrosplenic ligament.

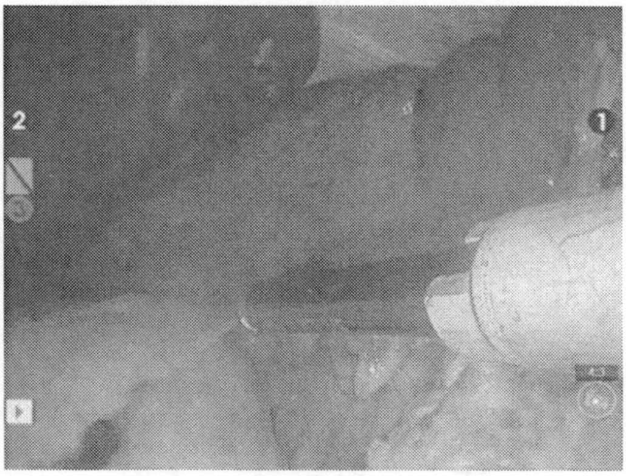

Figure 11. Dissection of gastrosplenic ligament.

The assistant-surgeon pulls caudally the transverse colon by using an atraumatic fenestrated forceps. The right gastroepiploic vessels are identified at the level of prepancreatic fascia and sectioned at their root between clips, including lymph node station 6 (infrapylorics) attached to the pyloric wall (Figure 3). The lesser sac is dissected and the right gastric artery is identified and sectioned close to the duodenal wall between clips, removing the lymphatic tissue of station 5 (suprapylorics) (Figure 4).

The duodenum is circumferentially dissected and transected 2 cm distal to the pylorus, using a 45 mm endoscopic linear stapler (LS–intestinal cartridge) (Figure 5). The assistant-surgeon pulls up the stomach and the surgeon switches the arm no. 3 for the liver retraction.

Extended lymphadenectomy begins at the station 12 (hepatic pedicle): the first assistant provides a gentle pressure on the pancreatic head to obtain an optimal tension of the hepato-duodenal ligament and to allow a complete dissection of the lymphatic tissue of the proper hepatic artery (station 12a). The dissection is prolonged above the pancreas along the common hepatic artery (station 8a) and lymph nodes are removed "en bloc" until reaching the origin of the celiac trunk (station 9) and the left gastric artery (station 7), which is divided at its origin between clips or by vascular stapler (Figures. 6 - 8).

When a functional accessory-left hepatic artery arising from the left gastric artery is identified, it should be preserved. In this case we use to section the left gastric artery distally to the emergence of the accessory-left hepatic artery, dissecting the lymphatic tissue encircling the main trunk. The origin of the splenic artery is then identified and freed from the surrounding lymphatic tissue (station 11p) (Figure 9). A careful dissection of the gastro-splenic ligament is performed by using either the US-device or clips. All the short gastric vessels are ligated and sectioned along the greater curvature of the stomach, thus removing station 4sa and mobilizing the gastric fundus (figures. 10 - 11).

A spleen-preserving dissection of the lymphatic tissue of the distal splenic artery (11d) and the splenic hilum (station 10) is performed. The phreno-esophageal ligament is sectioned superiorly and left crus of the diaphragm is exposed. The lymphatic tissue of left cardial station (2) is removed.

Subtotal Gastrectomy (RADG)

Subtotal gastrectomy starts as in total gastrectomy. A complete coloepiploic detachment is performed until the lower pole of the spleen. The bursa omentalis is accessed and the supramesocolic area is gained.

The Henle's trunk is identified and the soft tissue of station 14v (superior mesenteric vein) is dissected (Figure 13). D2-lymphadenectomy is completed by the dissection of lesser curvature (station 3) and right paracardial nodes (station 1) (Figure 14).

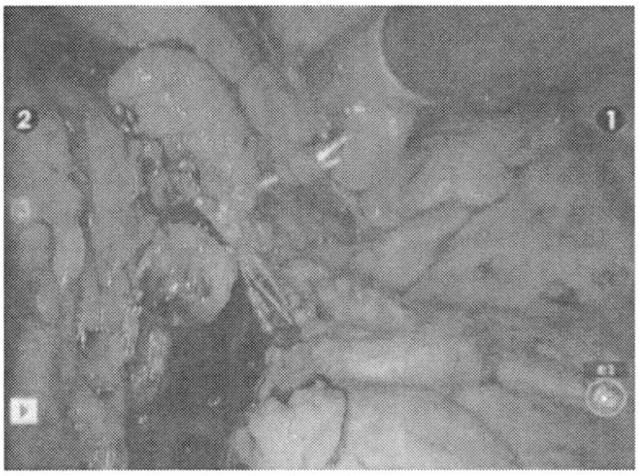

Figure 12. Distal splenic artery (station 11d).

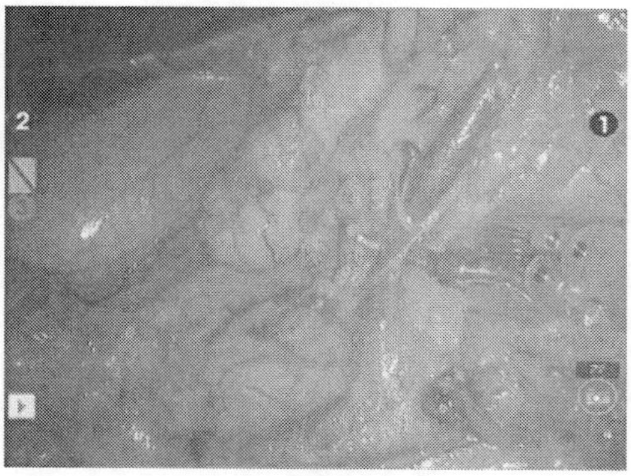

Figure 13. Henle's Trunk.

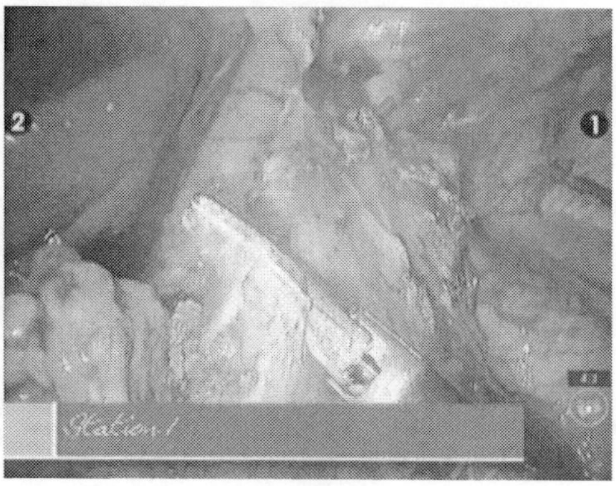

Figure 14. Right paracardial nodes (Station 1).

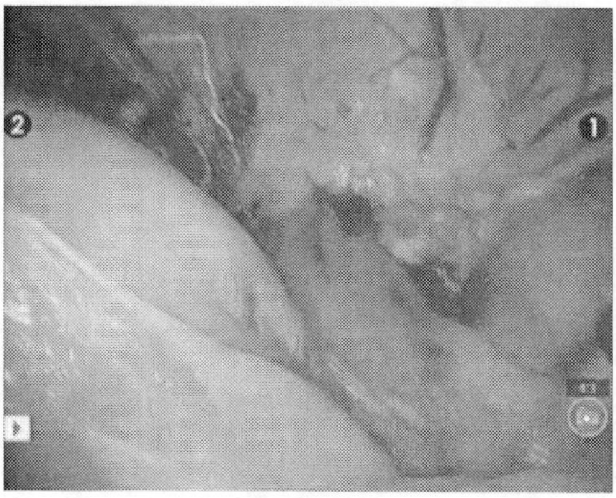

Figure 15. Transmesocolic retrieving of first jejunal loop.

Reconstruction

In total and subtotal gastrectomies, a Roux-en-Y reconstruction is routinely performed. An incision in the avascular area of the transverse mesocolon allowed us to gain access to the supramesocolic space and to identify the first jejunal loop (Figure 15). A robot-assisted mechanical side-to-side jejuno-jejunal anastomosis is performed (Figure 16).

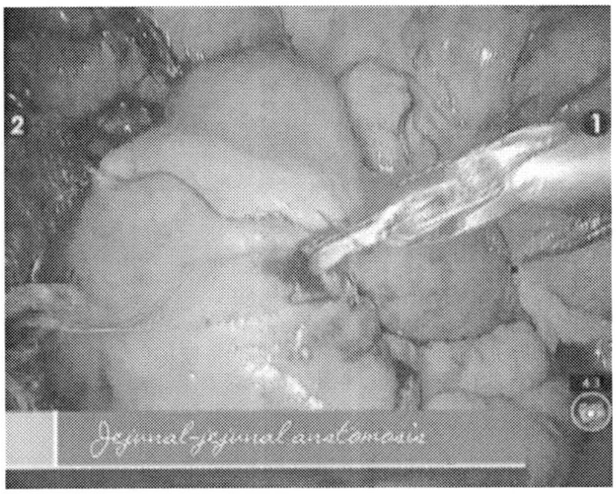

Figure 16. Robot-assisted side-to-side jejuno-jenunal anastomosis.

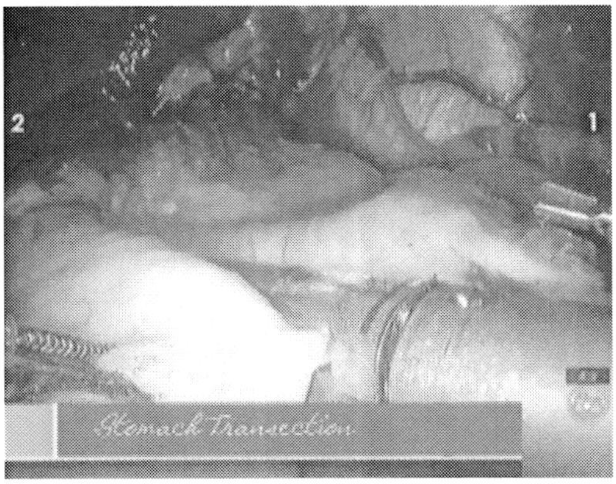

Figure 17. Transection of the stomach by laparoscopic stapler.

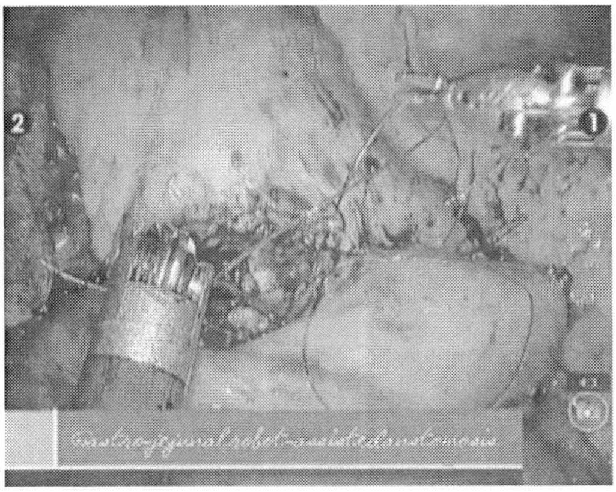

Figure 18. Robot-assisted end-to-side gastro-jejunal anstomosis.

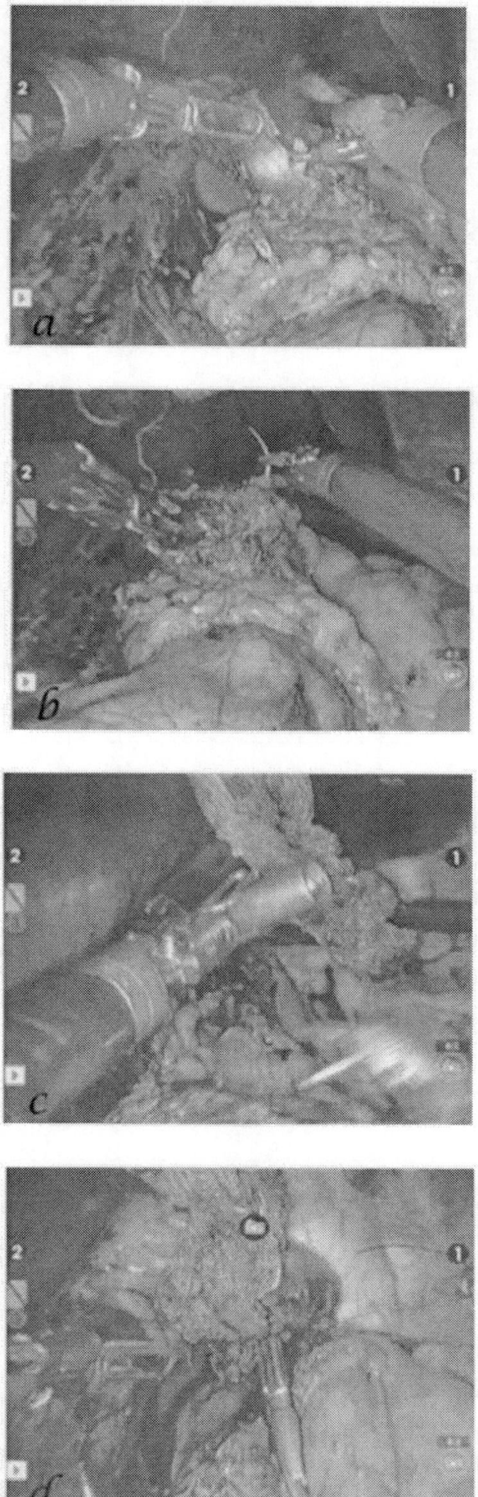

Figure19. a, anterior esophageal dissection; b, anterior esophageal half pursestring; c, anvil insertion into the esophagus; d, posterior half-pursestring.

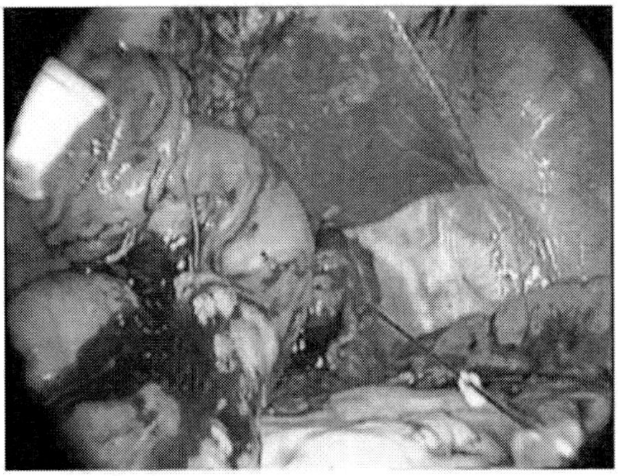

Figure 20. Intracorporeal end-to-side esophago-jejunal anastomosis.

Table 1. Intraoperative Data and Early Outcomes. RATG, robot-assisted total gastrectomy; RADG, robot-assisted distal gastrectomy; IBL, intraoperative blood loss; E-J, esophagojejunostomy; LOS, length of stay. *All values are median with interquartile range (IQR)

TYPE OF GASTRECTOMY	
RATG	19
RADG	21
OPERATIVE TIME (mins) Docking time	267,5 (255 – 305) 6 (5 – 13)
IBL (mL)	30 (0 – 100)
COMPLICATIONS	
Leakage	1 (E-J)
Pleural effusion	1
LIQUID DIET START (days)	5 (2 – 5)
LOS (days)	6 (5 – 8)

In subtotal gastrectomy, once lymphadenectomy is completed, the stomach is transected by the assistant from the left side port, using the laparoscopic stapler (Figure 17). The specimen, including stomach, omentum, and lymphatic tissue, is enclosed in an endoscopic bag and placed on the right hepatic lobe. A robot-assisted handsewn trans-mesocolic side-to-side doublelayer gastro-jejunal anastomosis is performed as in open surgery (Figure 18). In total gastrectomy, before sectioning the specimen and after a complete mobilization of the abdominal esophagus, the anterior wall of the esophagus is sectioned and a robot-assisted handsewn half pursestring suture is performed (Figure 19a-b). The assistant-port incision is enlarged and a lap disc is used in order to preserve the pneumoperitoneum. The anvil of a 25 mm circular stapler is inserted into the esophagus and the posterior purse string suture is completed (Figure 19b-c). The jejunum is transected at about 40 cm from the Treitz. The efferent jejunal loop is retrieved extracorporeally, and the circular stapler is then inserted into the jejunal loop and introduced into the abdomen in order to perform an intracorporeal end-to-side esophagojejunal anastomosis (Figure 20). The jejunal cul-de-sac is sectioned using LS. The stomach is removed ''en bloc'' with the omentum and the lymphatic tissue, then inserted into a large endobag lying in the right lower quadrant. The specimen is usually removed through a small muscle-splitting suprapubic protected incision.

Postoperative Patients' Care, Outcome and Technical Results

This chapter shows our results on 40 consecutive gastrectomies with extended (D2) lymphadenectomy performed with the da Vinci Surgical System for gastric adenocarcinoma. Nineteen robot-assisted total gastrectomies (RATG) and 21 robot-assisted distal gastrectomies (RADG) were performed. Intraoperative results and early outcomes are shown in table 1. Median overall operative time was 267.5 (255–305) min. Median docking time was 6 (5–13) min. Intraoperative blood loss (IBL) was 30 mL (IQR, 0–100). Liquid diet was resumed on postoperative d 5 (IQR, 2–5) after a routine postoperative contrast swallow. Length of stay was 6 d (IQR, 5–8). Surgery-related morbidity was 2/40 (5%): a left pleural collection and an asymptomatic leakage of the esophago-jejunostomy, both in RATG, diagnosed during a routinely postoperative contrast swallow and conservatively treated. Thirty-day mortality was 0%. Pathologic findings are shown in table 2.

Table 2. Pathologic findings

p-STAGE	
IA	12
IB	6
II	10
IIIA	5
IIIB	2
IIIC	5
HISTOLOGY	
Intestinal type	16
Diffuse type	24
SITE OF TUMOR	
Fundus	2
Body	18
Antrum	20
R0 (%)	100
RETRIEVED LYMPH NODESa	28 (23 – 34)

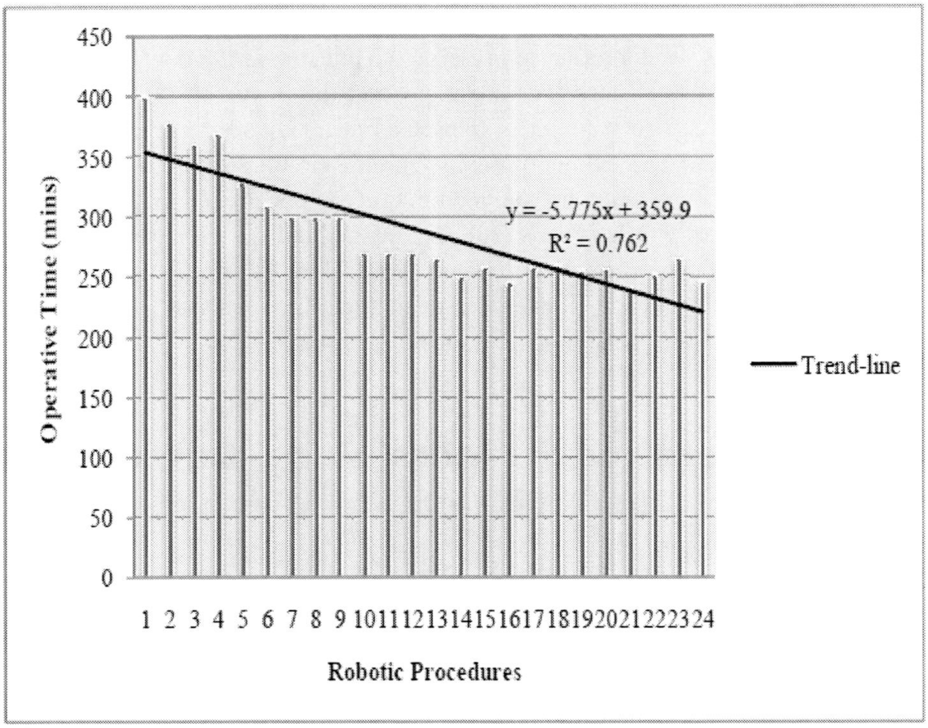

Figure 21. Analysis of operative time on the first 24 procedures.

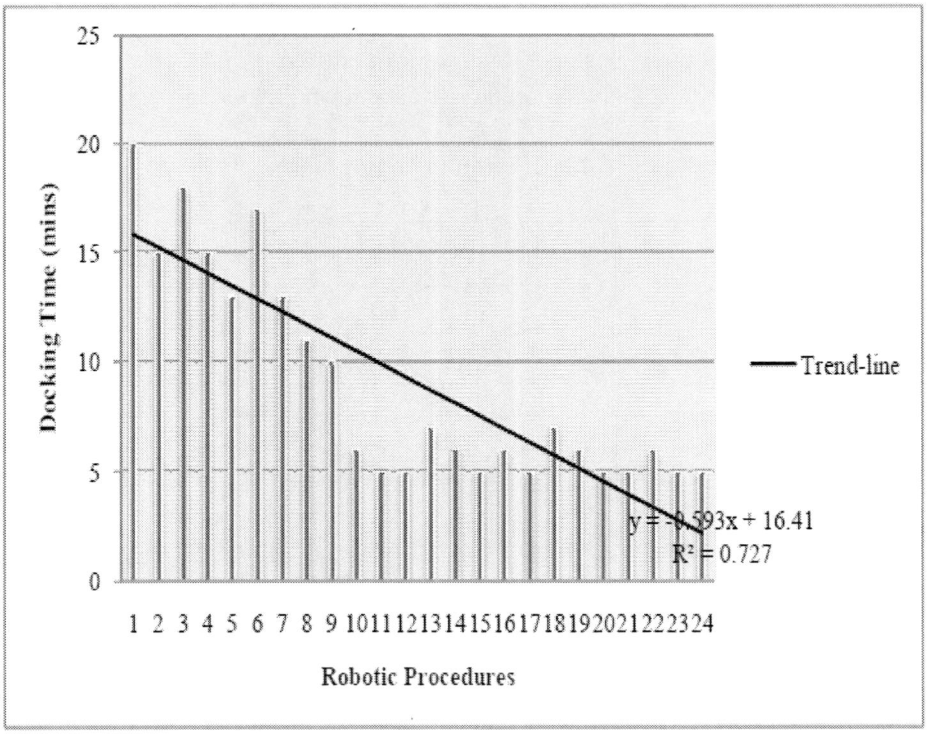

Figure 22. Analysis of the docking time on the first 24 procedures.

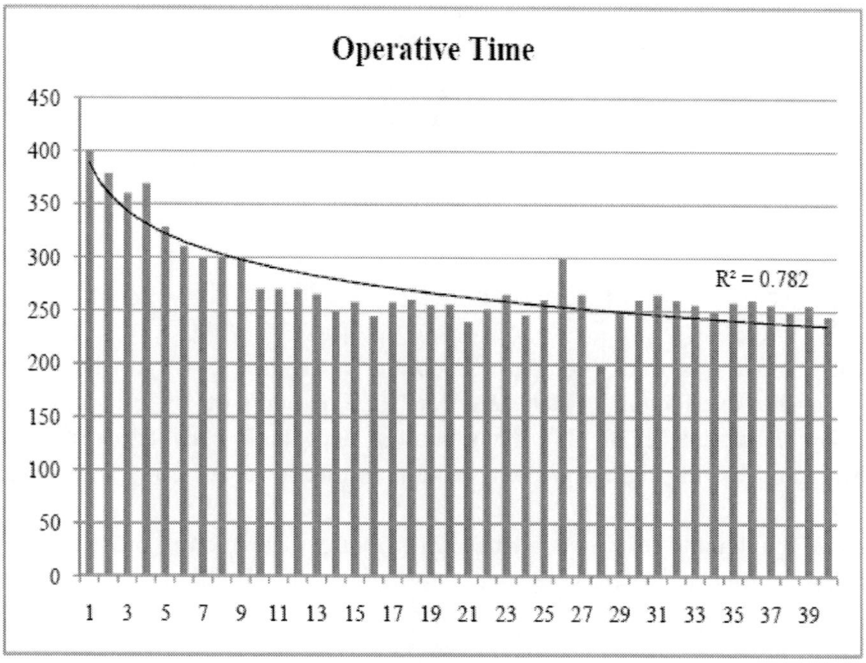

Figure 23. Analysis of the operative time of the whole experience of robotic gastrectomy.

Number of harvested lymph nodes was 28 (IQR, 23–34). Resection margins were negative in all cases. At a median follow up of 48 mo (IQR, 24–72), disease-free survival was 77,5%: 31 patients were alive with no evidence of disease, 1 patient had lymph nodal recurrence after 24 months from surgery and 1 after 10 months. Cancer-related mortality was 5/40 (12,5%). Two other patients died for other causes. We studied the trend of the operative time in the first 24 procedures. The analysis of the learning curve (LC) showed a decreasing trend of the operative time from 400 to 250 min (Figure 21) and a decreasing trend of the docking time from 20 to 5 min (Figure 22). The log-regression of the whole procedures is shown in Figure 23. The difference in operative time and docking time between the first five cases and the last five cases was statistically significant ($P < 0.05$).

Discussion

R0 surgery with extended (D2) lymphadenectomy is widely considered the optimal therapeutic option for resectable gastric cancer. Numerous studies comparing laparoscopic vs open procedures have demonstrated the benefits of laparoscopy to include better perioperative outcomes compared with the traditional open approach. Encouraging evidence from several randomized control trials and retrospective reviews suggests no difference in the oncologic outcomes such as tumor recurrence and long-term survival between patients undergoing laparoscopic vs open surgery in patients with gastric cancer. Although this technique is feasible and safe, with similar results to the open technique in terms of average number of harvested lymph nodes and postoperative outcome, the diffusion of this procedure has been limited to few advanced minimally invasive surgery centers [14,15,31,32].

The anatomic complexity of the vascular structures, the technical limits of the conventional laparoscopic instrumentation, and the lack of a steady image, can consequently add to surgeons' stress, making this procedure quite complex even for minimally-invasive well-trained surgeons. The analysis of bleeding during laparoscopic gastric surgery, indeed, showed that most of the surgeons experienced technical difficulties during laparoscopic lymph node dissection [33].

Robotic Gastric Surgery Experiences

Recently, several studies, comparing robotic vs laparoscopic gastric resections, are spreading in the international Literature. The first experience of gastric resection was published by Hashizume et al [25]. They showed acceptable short-term outcomes in two distal gastrectomies with higher operative time than that of laparoscopy and a long hospital stay.

In 2003, Giulianotti et al. described 21 robotic gastrectomy procedures (10 Total gastrectomies, 10 distal gastrectomies and 1 wedge resection) with acceptable postoperative morbidity and mortality (1 patient)[23]. The widest experience has been published by Song et al. in 2009 [26]. They showed acceptable results on 33 total gastrectomies and 67 subtotal gastrectomies. Complication rate was 13% (9 wound infections, 2 intraluminal bleedings, and 2 anastomotic leakages) with one intraoperative death. In 2011, D'Annibale et al published their experience on 24 robotic procedures showing acceptable short-term outcomes with low postoperative morbidity and no mortality [30].

Other studies, also, suggested that robot assistance facilitates laparoscopic surgery and has great impact on improving minimally invasive surgical techniques (table 3) [26,34-38]. Early evidence demonstrates that robot assistance may allow a surgeon to perform complicated minimally invasive procedures more accurately than with laparoscopy (table 4). There are several studies, indeed, comparing robotic vs laparoscopic technique. In 2009 Song et al. published their first 20 robotic procedures compared to early laparoscopic experience showing a reduced training time in robotic arm than laparoscopic one [39]. Moreover, the difference between operative time of both early robotic and laparoscopic procedures was not statistically significant.

In 2011 Eom et al. compared 62 laparoscopic gastric procedures vs 30 robotic ones showing with the exception of operating time and cost, that the numbers of retrieved lymph nodes and the short-term clinical outcomes of robotic procedures were comparable to those of laparoscopic ones, despite the surgeon's familiarity with laparoscopy and lack of robotic experience [40].

Woo et al. showed robotic gastrectomy to have better short-term and comparable oncologic outcomes compared with laparoscopic gastrectomy in early gastric cancer asserting that robotic approach is a promising alternative to laparoscopic surgery [41]. Kim et al. published the first comparative study between robotic, laparoscopic and open gastric resection techniques [42].

They concluded that robotic gastrectomy for the treatment of gastric cancer is a feasible and safe procedure in the hands of experienced laparoscopic surgeons. Moreover, they asserted that robotic gastrectomy offers better short-term surgical outcomes than the open and laparoscopic methods.

The Role of Robotic Gastric Surgery

Robotic surgery has recently emerged as a newer minimally invasive technique that may offer surgeons technical solution to the limitations of conventional laparoscopy surgery [43,44].

The intrinsic advantages of the da Vinci Surgical System, such as the elimination of physiologic tremor, the 3-D view, the steady image, and the articulation of the tip of the instruments (EndoWrist), may be helpful in making lymph node dissection easier by allowing more precise movements of the instruments circumferentially around the vessels [30]. The infrapyloric area and the inferior mesenteric vein, including stations 6 and 14, are valued as the most frequent sources of intraoperative bleeding, while the suprapancreatic area including stations 7, 8, and 9 is the second most frequent source [33]. Robotics can improve surgeon's dexterity and may be especially helpful during maneuvers in restricted fields such as during the extended lymphadenectomy [30,45].

Table 3. Robotic published experiences. Technical outcomes

Author Year	N	Procedures	Op. time (mins)	Conversions	Complications
Hashizume 2002 [25]	2	2 D2 RADG	320	0	0
Giulianotti 2003 [23]	21	10 D2 RATG 10 D2 RADG (2 BEN) 1 WEDGE	350 (TG) 365(DG)	1 (TG)	4
Kakeji 2006 [34]	5	2 D2 RADG (Da Vinci) 3 D2 RADG (Zeus)	445 656	0	0
Anderson 2007 [35]	7	7 D2 RADG	420 (390–480)	0	1 colonic ischemia 1 Pulmonary edema 3 Blood transfusion
Patriti 2008 [36]	13	4 D2 RATG 8 D2 RATG 1 D2 RAPG	286 ± 32,6	0	1 Duodenal stump leakage 1 Trocar bleeding 1 Prolonged ileus 1 Hyperamylasemia 1 Pulmonary edema 1 Pleural effusion
Pugliese 2009 [37]	11	9 D2 STG	350 ± 71 (240 - 460)	2	1 pancreatic leak 1 mortality (heamorragic stroke)
Song 2009 [26]	10 0	33 TG (D1 + β or D2) 67 STG (D1 + β or D2)	231,3 ± 43,2 (155 – 330)	0	9 Wound 2 Intraluminal bleeding 2 leakage 1 operative mortality
Lee 2011 [38]	12	RADG (EGC)	253 (170-365)	0	1 acute pancreatitis
D'Annibale 2011 [30]	24	11 RATG 13 RADG	267,5 (255-305)	0	1 Leak 1 Pleural effusion

Table 4. Robotic published experiences. Technical outcome

Author Year	N	LN	R0	Hospital Stay	Soft Diet Start	EBL	Mortality
Hashizume 2002 [25]	2	NR	2	32	-	65	0
Giulianotti 2003 [23]	21	NR	-	11 (TG) 9 (DG) 1 (WEDGE)	-	-	1 (30 DAYS)
Kakeji 2006 [34]	5	24,4	-	32	-	65	0
Anderson 2007 [35]	7	24 (17-30)	7	4 (3-9)	1 (1-6)	300 (100-900)	0 (30 days)
Patriti 2008 [36]	13	28.1 ± 8.3	13	11.2 ± 4.3	5	103 ± 87.5	0
Pugliese 2009 [37]	11	27.5 ± 5 (18-40)	11	11 ± 1 (10-13)	5 ± 1.1	92 ± 58	1 (haemorragic stroke)
Song 2009 [26]	100	36.7 ± 13.3	100	7.8	4.2	128	1
Lee 2011 [38]	12	46 ± 25.5 (21-115)	12	6.6 ± 1,6	4.6 ± 0.8	135.8 ± 133.9 (30-500)	0
D'Annibale 2011 [30]	24	28 (23-34)	24	6 (5-8)	5 (2-5)	30 (0-100)	0

Table 5. Robotic vs laparoscopic surgery comparative studies

Author Year	N	Proc	Op. time (mins) (mean ± SD)	Conv	Blood Loss	Retrieved LN	Hospital stay	Soft Diet Start
Song 2009 [39]	20	Rob ADG	230 ± 34,9	0	94,8 ± 121,5	35,3 ± 10,5	5,7 ± 1,0	4 ± 0
	20	INITIAL Lap ADG	289.5 ± 59.3	0	nd	31.5 ± 17.1	7.7 ± 3.5	4.95 ± 1.47
	20	RECENT Lap ADG	134,1 ± 40,0	0	39,5 ± 27,7	42,7 ± 14,9	6,2 ± 3,1	4,1 ± 0,45

Author Year	N	Proc	Op. time (mins) (mean ± SD)	Conv	Blood Loss	Retrieved LN	Hospital stay	Soft Diet Start
Eom 2011 [40]	30	RADG (20 D2 21 D1 + β)	229.1	0	152.8	30.2	7.9	3.4
	62	LADG (34 D2 28 D1 + β)	189.4	0	88.3	33.4	7.8	3.4
Woo 2011 [41]	236	172 RADG 62 RATG 2 DEGASTRO	219.5	0	91.6	39	7.7	-
	591	481 LADG 108 LATG 2 DEGASTRO	170.7	0	147.9	37.4	7	-

Table 6. Robotic vs laparoscopic vs open surgery comparative study

Author Year	N	Proc	Op. time (mins)	Conv	EBL	LN	Hospital stay	Compl	Soft Diet Start
Kim 2010 [42]	16	Rob ADG	259.2 ± 38,1	0	30.3 ± 15.1	41.1 ± 10.9	5.1 ± 0.3	O	-
	11	Lap ADG	203.9 ± 36.4	0	44.7 ± 37.1	37.4 ± 10.0	6.5 ± 0.8	1	-
	12	Open DG	126.7 ± 24.1	0	78.8 ± 74.1	43.3 ± 10.4	6.7 ± 1.4	2	-

All these aspects give the surgeon a significant technical advantage while performing the dissection of the lymphatic tissue around the portal vein, common hepatic artery, celiac trunk, and splenic artery. Moreover, the magnification and steadiness of the image and the tremor filtration allows the surgeon to drive the vascular dissection under the tunica adventitia, completely clearing the lymphatic tissue and identifying and preserving the vascular supply of the pancreas. Several comparatives studies showed that the estimated blood loss in the robot-assisted gastrectomy group was significantly less than in laparoscopic or open surgery[37-42]. In our previous published experience, the lymphadenectomy of the hepatic pedicle was much easier to perform, and we did not register any vascular injury or intraoperative bleeding. Moreover, we were able to perform a correct spleen-preserving dissection of stations 10, 11d in all RATG, without any related morbidity, and a precise dissection of the esophageal hiatus carrying out a correct extended lymphadenectomy in every case. The median number of retrieved lymph nodes was above the minimum recommended by the Japanese and Western guidelines in all published robotic experience and comparable to major open gastric surgical series reported in the literature. The analysis of the learning curve showed an early progressively decreasing trend in function of the number of performed procedures in the robotic experiences showing easy adaptability of robot-assisted surgery. Owing to its easier maneuverability, the robot surgical system can be said to enable the rapid acquisition of dexterity and accuracy in a short time.

Moreover, in our series, we observed that the operative time decreased gradually until case no. 10. After case no. 11, the variability between the operative times was not statistically significant, thus configuring the landmark of the optimization of the LC ($P = 0.051$)[30]. As clearly reported by several authors, operative time can be reduced, in addition, by the completion of the learning curve of the surgical and nursing team. In our experience, median docking-time decreased in the last procedures as well as previously reported in robotic colorectal surgery [46]. The trend of the LC of the docking time showed a plateau after case no. 10 ($P = 0.22$).

Most studies have reported that anastomosis after robot-assisted gastrectomy was performed by extracorporeal hand-sewing sutures or intracorporeal stapler. Hur et al [27] showed in a pilot study that both esophagojejunostomy and gastrojejunostomy may be successfully achieved by a robot-sewing technique showing the possibility of a "full" robotic approach to gastric cancer. This technique seems to maximize the advantage for patients with a high BMI, because of the complexity of performing a "minilaparotomy" in such patients [45].

Conclusion

Robot-assisted surgery can facilitate some surgical steps that are technically challenging in laparoscopic surgery. The learning curve appears to be shorter than in laparoscopic surgery, thus representing a useful tool for a wider diffusion of MIS for gastric cancer. Since the oncologic and survival outcomes are the mandatory conclusions in surgical oncology, at least one prospective study comparing open, laparoscopic and robotic gastrectomy and lymphadenectomy is required. Moreover, all these results seem to justify the setting of RCTs for the evaluation of quality of life, disease-free, and overall survival in gastric cancer patients.

References

[1] Memon M. A., Brow G. Laparoscopic closure of an acutely perforated duodenal ulcer an early experience. *Irish Med. J.* 1993;86:106–7.

[2] Hackett T. R., Memon M. A., Fitzgibbons Jr. R. J., Mixter C. G. Laparoscopic resection of heterotopic gastric pancreatic tissue. *J. Laparoendosc Adv. Surg. Tech*. 1997;7: 307–12.

[3] Memon M. A., Fitzgibbons Jr. R. J. Hand assisted laparoscopic surgery (HALS): a useful technique for complex laparoscopic abdominal procedures. *J. Laparoendosc. Adv. Surg. Tech*. 1998; 8:143–50.

[4] Koopmann M. C., Heise C. P. Laparoscopic and minimally invasive resection of malignant colorectal disease. *Surg. Clin. North Am.* 2008;88:1047–72.

[5] Piazza L., Caragliano P., Scardilli M., Sgroi A. V., Marino G., Giannone G. Laparoscopic robot-assisted right adrenalectomy and left ovariectomy (case reports). *Chir. Ital.* 1999;51(6):465–6.

[6] Reichenspurner H., Boehm D. H., Gulbins H., et al. Three-dimensional video and robot-assisted port-access mitral valve operation. *Ann. Thorac. Surg*. 2000;69(4): 1176–81.

[7] Law W. L., Lee Y. M., Choi H. K., et al. Impact of laparoscopic resection for colorectal cancer on operative outcomes and survival. *Ann. Surg*. 2007;245(1):1–7.

[8] Schwenk W., Bohm B., Muller J. M. Postoperative pain and fatigue after laparoscopic or conventional colorectal resections. A prospective randomized trial. *Surg. Endosc.* 1998; 12(9):1131–6.

[9] Soper N. J., Brunt L. M., Kerbl K. Laparoscopic general surgery. *N. Engl. J. Med.* 1994;330: 409-19.

[10] Trus T. L., Laycock W. S., Waring J. P., Branum G. D., Hunter J. G. Improvement in quality of life measures after laparoscopic antireflux surgery. *Ann. Surg.* 1999;229: 331-6.

[11] Nakajima T. Gastric cancer treatment guidelines in Japan. *Gastric Cancer* 2002;5:1.

[12] Allum W. H., Griffin S. M., Watson A., et al. Guidelines for the management of oesophageal and gastric cancer. *Gut*. 2002;50.(Suppl. 5):v1.

[13] Japanese Gastric Cancer Association. Guidelines for Diagnosis and Treatment of Carcinoma of the Stomach. *Gastric Cancer* 1998;1:10.

[14] Huscher C., Mingoli A., Sgarzini G., et al. Laparoscopic versus open subtotal gastectomy for distal gastric cancer: Five-year results of a randomized prospective trial. *Ann. Surg*. 2005;241:232.
[15] Pugliese R., Maggioni D., Sansonna F., et al. Total and subtotal laparoscopic gastrectomy foradenocarinoma. *Surg. Endosc*. 2007;21:21.
[16] Tanimura S., Higashino M., Fukunaga Y., et al. Laparoscopic distal gastrectomy with regional lymph node dissection for gastric cancer. *Surg. Endosc*. 2003;17:758.
[17] Tanimura S., Higashino M., Fukunaga Y., et al. Laparoscopic gastrectomy with regional lymph node dissection for upper gastric cancer. *Br. J. Surg*. 2007;94:204.
[18] Uyama I., Sugioika A., Fujita J., et al. Completely laparoscopic extraperigastric lymph node dissection for gastric malignancies located in the middle or lower third of the stomach. *Gastric Cancer* 1999;2:186.
[19] Uyama I., Sugioka A., Fujita J., et al. Laparoscopic total gastrectomy with distal pancreatosplenectomy D2 lymphadenectomy for advanced gastric cancer. *Gastric Cancer* 1999;2:230.
[20] Berguer R. Surgical technology and the ergonomics of laparoscopic instruments. *Surg. Endosc*. 1998; 12: 458-462.
[21] Dakin G. F., Gagner M. Comparison of laparoscopic skills performance between standard instruments and two surgical robotic systems. *Surg. Endosc*. 2003; 17: 574-579.
[22] Ballantyne G. H., Merola P., Weber A., Wasielewski A. Robotic solutions to the pitfalls of laparoscopic colectomy. *Osp. Ital. Chir*. 2001;7:405–12.
[23] Giulianotti P. C., Coratti A., Angelini M., Sbrana F., Cecconi S., Balestracci T., et al. Robotics in general surgery: personal experience in a large community hospital. *Arch. Surg*. 2003;138(7):777–84.
[24] Patel V. R., Chammas M. F., Shah S. Robotic assisted laparoscopic radical prostatectomy: a review of the current state of affairs. *Int. J. Clin. Pract*. 2007; 61: 309-314.
[25] Hashizume M., Sugimachi K. Robot-assisted gastric surgery. *Surg. Clin. North. Am*. 2003; 83: 1429-1444.
[26] Song J., Oh S. J., Kang W. H., Hyung W. J., Choi S. H., Noh S. H. Robot-assisted gastrectomy with lymph node dissection for gastric cancer: lessons learned from an initial 100 consecutive procedures. *Ann. Surg*. 2009; 249: 927-932.
[27] Hur H., Kim J. Y., Cho Y. K., Han S. U. Technical feasibility of robot-sewn anastomosis in robotic surgery for gastric cancer. *J. Laparoendosc. Adv. Surg. Tech. A*. 2010; 20: 693-697.
[28] Ryu K. J., Jung S. R., Choi J. S., Jang Y. J., Kim J. H., Park S. S., Park B. J., Park S. H., Kim S. J., Mok Y. J., Kim C. S. Laparoscopic resection of small gastric submucosal tumors. *Surg. Endosc*. 2011; 25:271-277.
[29] Pugliese R., Maggioni D., Sansonna F., Costanzi A., Ferrari G. C., Di Lernia S., Magistro C., De Martini P., Pugliese F. Subtotal gastrectomy with D2 dissection by minimally invasive surgery for distal adenocarcinoma of the stomach: results and 5-year survival. *Surg. Endosc*. 2010; 24: 2594-2602.

[30] D'Annibale A., Pende V., Pernazza G., Monsellato I., Mazzocchi P., Lucandri G., Morpurgo E., Contardo T., Sovernigo G. Full robotic gastrectomy with extended (D2) lymphadenectomy for gastric cancer: surgical technique and preliminary results. *J. Surg. Res.* 2011 Apr.; 166(2):e113-20. Epub 2010 Dec. 13.

[31] Lee J. H., Han H. S., Lee J. H. A prospective randomized study comparing open vs laparoscopy-assisted distal gastrectomy in early gastric cancer: Early results. *Surg. Endosc.* 2005;19:168.

[32] Hur H., Jeon H. M., Kim W. Laparoscopy-assisted distal gastrectomy with D2 lymphadenectomy for T2b advanced gastric cancers: Three years' experience. *J. Surg. Oncol.* 2008;98:515.

[33] Kim M. C., Choi H. J., Jung G. J., et al. Techniques and complications of laparoscopy-assisted distal gastrectomy (LADG) for gastric cancer. *Eur. J. Surg. Oncol.* 2007;33:700.

[34] Kakeji Y., Konishi K., Ieiri S., Yasunaga T., Nakamoto M., Tanoue K., Baba H., Maehara Y., Hashizume M. Robotic laparoscopic distal gastrectomy: a comparison of the da Vinci and Zeus systems. *Int. J. Med. Robot.* 2006 Dec.;2(4):299-304.

[35] Anderson C., Ellenhorn J., Hellan M., Pigazzi A. Pilot series of robot-assisted laparoscopic subtotal gastrectomy with extended lymphadenectomy for gastric cancer. *Surg. Endosc.* 2007 Sep.; 21(9): 1662-6. Epub 2007 Mar. 8.

[36] Patriti A., Ceccarelli G., Bellochi R., Bartoli A., Spaziani A., Di Zitti L., Casciola L. Robot-assisted laparoscopic total and partial gastric resection with D2 lymph node dissection for adenocarcinoma. *Surg. Endosc.* 2008 Dec.;22(12):2753-60. Epub 2008 Sep. 24.

[37] Pugliese R., Maggioni D., Sansonna F., Ferrari G. C., Forgione A., Costanzi A., Magistro C., Pauna J., Di Lernia S., Citterio D., Brambilla C. Outcomes and survival after laparoscopic gastrectomy for adenocarcinoma. Analysis on 65 patients operated on by conventional or robot-assisted minimal access procedures. *Eur. J. Surg. Oncol.* 2009 Mar.;35(3):281-8. Epub 2008 Mar. 14.

[38] Lee H. H., Hur H., Jung H., Jeon H. M., Park C. H., Song K. Y. Robot-assisted distal gastrectomy for gastric cancer: initial experience. *Am. J. Surg.* 2011 Jun.;201(6):841-5.

[39] Song J., Kang W. H., Oh S. J., Hyung W. J., Choi S. H., Noh S. H. Role of robotic gastrectomy using da Vinci system compared with laparoscopic gastrectomy: initial experience of 20 consecutive cases. *Surg. Endosc.* 2009 Jun.;23(6):1204-11. Epub 2009 Mar. 5.

[40] Eom B. W., Yoon H. M., Ryu K. W., Lee J. H., Cho S. J., Lee J. Y., Kim C. G., Choi I. J., Lee J. S., Kook M. C., Rhee J. Y., Park S. R., Kim Y. W. Comparison of surgical performance and short-term clinical outcomes between laparoscopic and robotic surgery in distal gastric cancer. *Eur. J. Surg. Oncol.* 2012 Jan.;38(1):57-63. Epub 2011 Sep. 25.

[41] Woo Y., Hyung W. J., Pak K. H., Inaba K., Obama K., Choi S. H., Noh S. H. Robotic gastrectomy as an oncologically sound alternative to laparoscopic resections for the treatment of early-stage gastric cancers. *Arch. Surg.* 2011 Sep.;146(9):1086-92. Epub 2011 May 16.

[42] Kim M. C., Heo G. U., Jung G. J. Robotic gastrectomy for gastric cancer: surgical techniques and clinical merits. *Surg Endosc.* 2010 Mar.;24(3):610-5. Epub 2009 Aug. 18.

[43] Lanfranco A. R., Castellanos A. E., Desai J. P., Meyers W. C. Robotic surgery: A current perspective. *Ann. Surg*. 2004; 239: 14-21.
[44] Ballantyne G. H., Moll F. The da Vinci telerobotic surgical system: The virtual operative field and telepresence surgery. *Surg. Clin. North. Am.* 2003;83:1293.
[45] Baek S. J., Lee D. W., Park S. S., Kim S. H. Current status of robot-assisted gastric surgery. *World. J. Gastrointest. Oncol*. 2011 Oct. 15; 3(10):137-43.
[46] D'Annibale A., Pernazza G.,Morpurgo E., et al. Robotic Right Colon Resection:Evaluation of First 50Consecutive Cases forMalignant Disease. *Ann. Surg. Oncol*. 2010;17:2856. Epub 2010 Jun. 22.

In: Gastric Cancer
Editors: A. D'Annibale, V. Pende and I. Monsellato
ISBN: 978-1-62081-294-5

Chapter IX

Pancreatic Lesions After Gastrectomy

Susumu Matsukuma*
Department of Pathology,
Japan Self Defense Forces Central Hospital, Japan

Abstract

Increased hyalinosis or atrophy of the pancreatic islets of Langerhans may occur in gastrectomized patients with an incidence of 55%. These changes would be partly associated with the alteration in glucose metabolism. Some authors suggested that the islets of Langerhans may show hyperplasia within 5 years from gastrectomy, and thereafter, B cells in the islets of Langerhans would become wasted, finally resulting in hyalinization. Recent articles have described unique neural changes of postmortem pancreas after gastrectomy. These changes consisted of prominently thickened and/or proliferated neural fascicles, focally or multifocally involving pancreatic parenchyma and/or interlobular septa, and were found in 11.8% (6/51) of pancreases after gastrectomy. These lesions closely mimicked those of rarely reported pancreatic neuroma, but the pathogenesis is different. In one case, antemortem ultrasonography detected pancreatic mass lesions suggesting neoplasm or recurrence of gastric cancer, but autopsy revealed pancreatic neuroma-like lesions with marked fibrosis. An increased risk of pancreatic cancer was also reported to be associated to a remote partial gastrectomy. The knowledge of the possible occurrence of pancreatic neuroma-like lesions after gastrectomy would be useful in the follow-up of patients undergoing gastric resections.

Introduction

Pancreatic alterations which may be expected after gastric resections are usually inflammatory lesions due to its operative procedure [1]. Gastrectomy can induce, however, changes in food transit or absorption, dissection or injuries of vagal or other nerves, or blood

* E-mail address: skuma@cocoa.plala.or.jp.

supply alterations, which would influence physiological processes of the pancreas. This chapter focuses on unusual pancreatic pathological features (endocrine lesions and neural alterations) following gastric resections.

Hyalinosis of the pancreatic islets of Langerhans is a characteristic of type 2 diabetes mellitus, although similar features may be found in 4% to 23% of elderly non-diabetic people [2]. Suda et al [3] examined postmortem pancreases removed from patients who underwent gastrectomy and identified similar islet's alterations in 9 of 15 cases (60%) of Billroth I anastomosis and in 8 of 16 cases (50%) of Billroth II anastomosis. Dumping syndrome, which is a well-known complication after gastrectomy, induces a rapid absorption of carbohydrates and causes an excessive stimulation of Langerhans' islets [4]. This prolonged excessive impulse induces islet cells hyalinization. Moreover, Suda et al. [3] suggested that gastrectomy-associated vagotomy may activate and induce the islets cells hyalinization too. Another study [3] demonstrated that pancreatic islets showed hyperplasia within 5 years from gastrectomy, and, thereafter, hyalinization of the islets gradually increased. These hyaline alterations of the pancreatic islets of Langerhans would be partly associated to impaired glucose tolerance in gastrectomized patients [3,5].

Our recent study [6] has detected unique neural alterations in postmortem pancreases after gastrectomy. All these alterations consisted in prominent thickened and/or proliferated neural fascicles (>300 micrometer in the longest dimension of neural fascicles), focally or multifocally involving pancreatic parenchyma and/or interlobular septa. Focal lesion represented a nodular and/or nested proliferation of neural fascicles in pancreatic lobule (Figure 1) or interlobular region (Figure 2). Diffuse proliferated lesions involved interlobular regions, partially retaining preexisting structures of interlobular neural fascicles (Figure 3). In our series, [6] these neural changes were found in 11.8% (6/51) of examined pancreases. Similar prominent thickened neural lesions were not identified in pancreases of 51 aged- and sex-matched group-control patients. These findings suggest that these neural lesions are unusual senescent features.

These prominent thickened neural alterations mimicked those of pancreatic neuroma. To date, only 2 cases of pancreatic neuroma [7,8] have been reported: one [7] case after splenectomy, and one [8] case after the excision of a pancreatic pseudocyst. The occurrence of pancreatic neuromas can be explained by reparative or proliferative reaction in surgically injured para- or intra-pancreatic neural tissues. Amputation or traumatic neuroma in the bile duct has been also reported after cholecystectomy [9,10]. Gastrectomy-related neural injuries would be, however, in a more proximal or central portion of the vagal and/or splanchnic nerves, rather than pancreatic sites. Vagotomy-related neuromas involving lower esophagus [11] and gastrectomy-associated neuroma around the celiac trunk [12] have been reported, but no similar pancreatic neuromas have been reported in the literature. Therefore, pathogenesis of pancreatic neuroma-like lesions following gastrectomy differs from those of previously reported pancreatic neuromas. Moreover, many researchers asserted that pancreatic nerves can become thicker in chronic pancreatitis [13-15]. Recent studies [14,15] described that enhanced neural density and hypertrophy are closely linked to the severity of perineural inflammatory infiltrates. These neural changes appear to generate and enhance pancreatic neural pain [14]. In our series, [6] three (50%) of six pancreases showing neuroma-like changes after gastrectomy were accompanied by moderate to severe chronic pancreatitis and/or pancreatic fibrosis (Figure 4), which may support the theory of pancreatitis-induced neural thickening. The other six pancreases containing neuroma-like lesions showed, however, a mild form of chronic pancreatitis and/or pancreatic fibrosis.

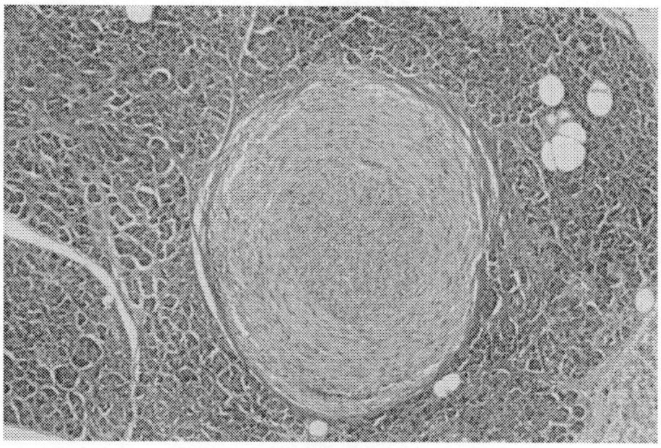

Figure 1. Nodular proliferation of neural fascicle involving the pancreatic lobule.

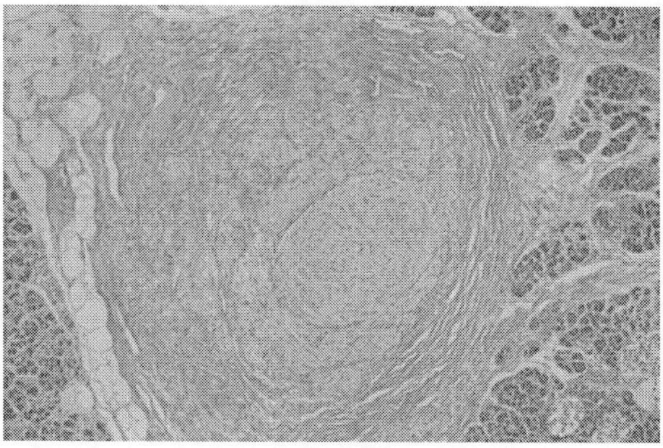

Figure 2. Nodular and nested proliferation of neural fascicles involving interlobular septum of pancreas after gastrectomy.

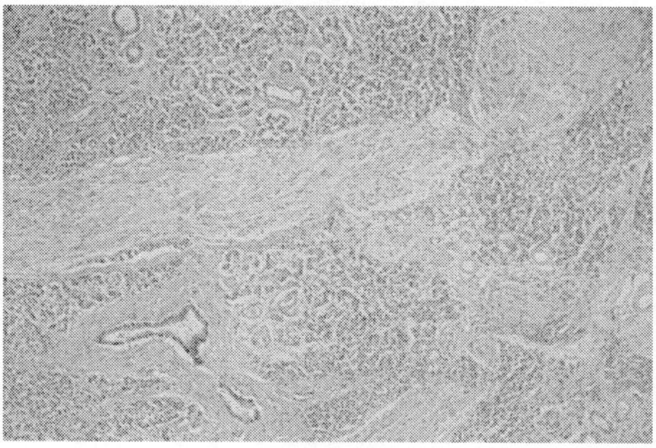

Figure 3. Prominently and diffusely thickened neural fascicles involving interlobular septa and pancreatic lobule.

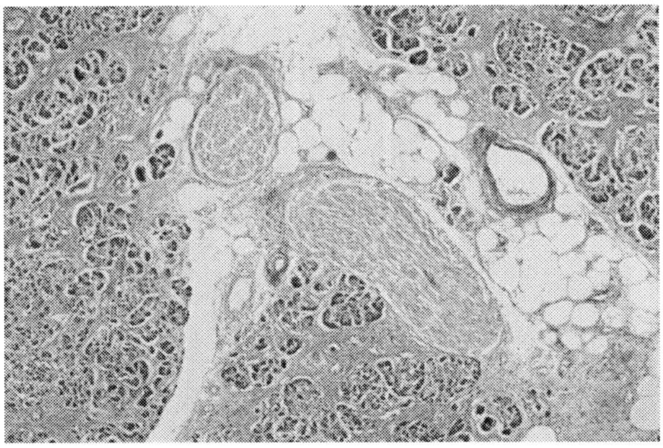

Figure 4. Neuroma-like lesion in pancreas after gastrectomy and pancreatic fibrosis.

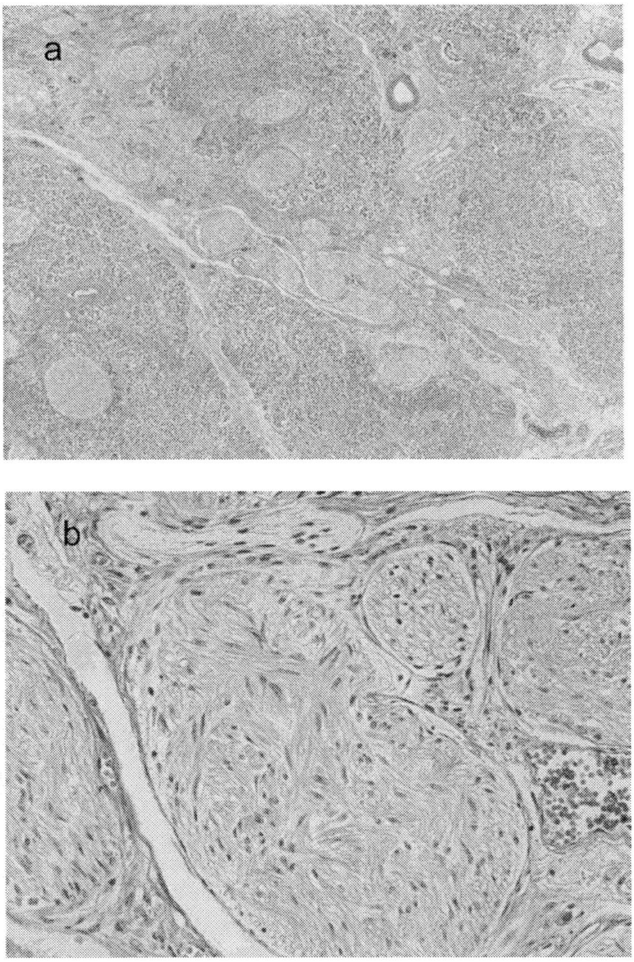

Figure 5. Pancreatic neuroma-like lesion detected by antemortem ultrasonography. (a) Low-power view showing diffusely thickened neural fascicles in the interlobular and intralobular regions with pancreatic fibrosis. (b) High-power view showing neuroma-like thickening and proliferation of neural fascicles.

Moreover, secondary pancreatitis and/or pancreatic fibrosis caused by neural changes cannot be excluded. None of the six patients with pancreatic neuroma-like lesions complained of abdominal pain. These findings suggest that the occurrence of neuroma-like changes after gastrectomy cannot be explained by chronic pancreatitis-related etiology alone. Furthermore, we speculate that neural irritation or activation due to gastrectomy or other upper abdominal surgery, similar to hyalinosis of pancreatic islets after gastrectomy, may promote neuroma-like changes. In our series, [6] the highest dimension of the neural fascicles in 57 pancreases after upper abdominal surgery including gastrectomy was significantly greater than that present in 57 aged- and sex-matched group-control patients. This evidence supports our hypothesis even though four of these control pancreases contained non-prominent but moderately swollen neural fascicles. These findings also showed the possibility that pancreatic neural changes might be influenced by additional unknown factors beyond gastrectomy-related injury and chronic pancreatitis.

Recent advances in imaging procedures have been able to detect relatively small neurogenic tumors [16]. Therefore, pancreatic neuroma-like lesions after gastrectomy may be found in imaging examination during follow-up of patients with malignancy requiring partial or total gastrectomy, such as gastric cancer, esophageal cancer, or pancreatic cancer. One case of pancreatic neuroma-like lesion in our series, indeed, was detected by antemortem ultrasonography as a low-echoic mass [6]. These clinical findings had suggested that pancreatic lesions are a recurrence or metastases of previously removed gastric cancer. Autopsy revealed, however, no malignant lesions and demonstrated pancreatic lesions composed of markedly thickened neural fascicles multifocally involving both the lobules and the interlobular septa in a tortuous fashion with prominent fibrosis (Figure 5).

Conclusion

An increase in pancreatic cancer risk after gastrectomy has been noted previously [17]. Therefore, we believe that consideration of the possible occurrence of pancreatic neuroma-like lesions after gastrectomy is important in differential diagnosis of true primary or secondary pancreatic neoplasms.

References

[1] Warren K. W. (1951). Acute pancreatitis and pancreatic injuries following subtotal gastrectomy. *Surgery*, 29, 643-657.

[2] Maitra A. (2010). The endocrine system. In Kumar V., Abbas A. K., Fausto N., and Aster J.C. (Ed.), *Robbins and Cotran Pathologic basis of disease* (8th edition, pp. 1097-1164). Philadelphia, P. A., US: Saunders/Elsevier.

[3] Suda K., Takei K., Suzuki F., Kamano T., and Yamane T. (1997). Histopathologic study of islets of Langerhans in patients after gastrectomy. *J. Clin. Gastroenterol.*, 25, 546-549.

[4] Roth D. A., and Meade R. C. (1965). Hyperinsulinism-hypoglycemia in the postgastrectomy patients. *Diabetes*, 14, 526-528.

[5] Itoh H., and Takei K. (2000). Immunohistochemical and statistical studies on the islets of Langerhans pancreas in autopsied patients after gastrectomy. *Hum. Pathol.*, 31, 1368-1376.

[6] Matsukuma S., and Sato K. (2010). Pancreatic neuroma-like lesions after upper abdominal surgery: a clinicopathological postmortem study. *Virchows Arch.*, 457, 651-657.

[7] Geddy P. M., and Venables C. W. (1991). Traumatic neuroma at the tail of the pancreas following splenectomy. *Postgrad. Med. J.*, 67, 90-91.

[8] Kim J. W., Choi G., Hwang J. E., Kang S. K., Han D. J., and Jang S. J. (2006). Traumatic neuroma in the pancreas head following excision of pseudocyst: a brief case report. *Korean J. Pathol.*, 40, 385-388.

[9] Fujino Y., and Satoh Y. (1991). A case report of amputation neuroma of the common bile duct occurred two months after cholecystectomy. *Jpn. J. Gastroenterol Surg.*, 24, 2437-2441.

[10] Nagata Y., Tomioka T., Chiba K., and Kanematsu T. (1995). Traumatic neuroma of the common hepatic duct after laparoscopic cholecystectomy. *Am. J. Gastroenterol*, 90, 1887-1888.

[11] Gillesby W. J., and Wu K. H. (1965). Amputation neuromas of vagus nerves. *Am. J. Surg.*, 110, 673-676.

[12] Kwon J. H., Ryu S. W., and Kang Y. N. (2007) Traumatic neuroma around the celiac trunk after gastrectomy mimicking a nodal metastasis: a case report. *Korean J. Radiol.*, 8, 242-245.

[13] Bockman D. E., Buchler M., Malfertheiner P., and Beger H. G.(1988). Analysis of nerves in chronic pancreatitis. *Gastroenterology*, 94, 1459-1469.

[14] Ceyhan G. O., Bergmann F., Kadihasanoglu M., Altintas B., Demir I.E., Hinz U., Müller M. W., Giese T., Büchler M. W., Giese N. A., and Friess H. (2009). Pancreatic neuropathy and neuropathic pain – a comprehensive pathomorphological study of 546 cases. *Gastroenterology*, 136, 177-186.

[15] Ceyhan G. O., Demir I. E., Rauch U., Bergmann F., Müller M. W., Büchler M. W., Friess H., and Schäfer K-H. (2009). Pancreatic neuropathy results in "neural remodeling" and altered pancreatic innervation in chronic pancreatitis and pancreatic cancer. *Am. J. Gastroenterol*, 104, 2555-2565.

[16] Murphey M. D., Smith W. S., Smith S. E., Kransdorf M. J., Temple H. T.(1999). From the archives of the AFIP. Imaging of musculoskeletal neurogenic tumors: radiologic-pathologic correlation. *Radiographics*, 19, 1523-1580.

[17] Tascilar M., van Rees B. P., Sturm P. D. J., Tytgat G. N. J., Hruban R. H., Goodman S. N., Giardiello F. M., Offerhaus G. J. A., and Tersmette A. C. (2001) Pancreatic cancer after remote ulcer surgery. *J. Clin. Pathol.*, 55, 340-345.

In: Gastric Cancer
Editors: A. D'Annibale, V. Pende and I. Monsellato
ISBN: 978-1-62081-294-5

Chapter X

Neoadjuvant and Adjuvant Chemotherapy in Gastric Cancer: Focus on Oncological Results After Minimally Invasive Surgery

Giuseppe Tonini[1], Loretta D'Onofrio, Bruno Vincenzi and Daniele Santini
Department of Medical Oncology, University Campus Bio-Medico, Italy

Abstract

Over the past two decades, surgical techniques, adjuvant chemotherapy, preoperative chemotherapy and radiation therapy for gastric cancer treatment improved. The choice of the optimal treatment, however, varies by regions. Minimally invasive surgery rapidly increased after the first report on laparoscopic wedge resection for early gastric cancer in 1992 [1]. Since then, many retrospective studies evaluating short and long-term advantages of laparoscopic surgery compared to open procedures were reported and prospective randomized trial are still ongoing. In this chapter, main international studies focusing on the role of adjuvant and neoadjuvant chemotherapy in the treatment of gastric cancer are reviewed. Oncological adequacy of minimally invasive surgery is also discussed.

Introduction

Gastric cancer is the second cause of death worldwide. In 2010, there were 21 000 new cases in US [2], even though its incidence has reduced. Nevertheless, the incidence of gastric cancer varies by regions: the highest rates are reported in East Asia, South America and

[1] Email address: *g.tonini@unicampus.it.*

Eastern Europe [3]. In the United States, migration of gastric cancer site from the antrum-body to the proximal part of the stomach was reported since 1970s and improvements in identification of important physiopathological factors involved in tumor genesis (i.e. Helicobacter Pylori infection) were carried out [4]. Genetic susceptibility, pathological profile, clinical presentation and prognosis of proximal and distal lesions are different. Oncologists, indeed, consider all gastric tumors as different entities [5]. Therefore, a standard treatment strategy cannot be carried out. Further studies on molecular mechanisms involved in the genesis of gastric cancer and on identification of predictive and prognostic biomarkers are needed in order to allow oncologists to perform a "tailored" treatment on each patient.

Radical surgery is the main treatment for resectable gastric cancer. Nevertheless, long-term survival and disease-free survival rates in Western countries are 20–30% and 60% respectively after surgery alone, since most patients present with advanced stage disease at diagnosis [6]. Multimodal treatment (a cooperation between oncologists, surgeons and radiotherapists) was suggested by experts in order to improve oncological outcome in gastric cancer patients. Several trials confirmed that multimodal treatment can improve survival than surgery alone but a standard multimodal treatment is not defined yet. In the United States adjuvant chemoradiation is routinely performed, while perioperative chemotherapy (before and after surgery) is the current standard of care in Europe. In Eastern countries, especially in Japan, gastric cancer is often diagnosed at an early stage and radical resection followed by oral adjuvant chemotherapy is usually performed.

The role of minimally invasive surgery in gastric cancer and its oncological adequacy are currently under evaluation. In Eastern countries, laparoscopic gastrectomy with limited lymphadenectomy (D1), which is easier to perform than extended node dissection, was rapidly adopted in the treatment of early stage diseases. Laparoscopic gastric resection with D1 lymph node dissection is considered an oncologically adequate procedure for the treatment of early gastric cancer. The current standard of care for resectable locally advanced gastric cancer, in Japan and Europe, is R0-gastrectomy with extended D2 lymphadenectomy [7]. Oncological adequacy of minimally invasive surgery for locally-advanced gastric cancer, however, is under evaluation.

Primary endpoint is to determine whether combination of minimally invasive techniques and systemic therapies might improve long-term efficacy and overall survival in gastric cancer patients. An accurate selection of patients who may benefit from multimodality approach is mandatory.

Multimodality Treatment for Resectable Gastric Cancer

Radical surgery (R0) is the only curative treatment for localized, non-metastatic gastric cancer. Nevertheless, less than 50% of gastric cancer patients undergo curative-intent surgery as about 65% of gastric cancer patients usually present with stage III–IV disease at first diagnosis, 85% have lymph node involvement and 30% have liver metastases [8].

Moreover, ten-years overall survival rate is less than 20% [9] and recurrence rate reported by Western studies is about 60%. There are few studies in the literature focused on chemotherapy for advanced gastric cancer and all of these studies reported a median overall survival of less than 1 year. Multimodality approach did not improve survival until the introduction of chemoradiation (chemotherapy plus radiotherapy) in the treatment of gastric cancer.

Table 1. Multi-chemotherapy Regimens in Adjuvant Treatment

References	Adjuvant Chemotherapy	OS (%)	DFS (%)
ACTS-GC trial [17]	*S-1* 40 mg/m^2	80.1% (3-years)	72.2% (3-years)
Popiela et al. [18]	*5-Fluorouracil* 600 mg/m^2 *Doxorubicin* 30 mg/m^2 *Mitomicyn C* 10 mg/m^2	47.1 % (10-years)	-
Bajetta et al. [19]	*Etoposide* 120 mg/m^2 *Doxorubicin* 20 mg/m^2 *Cisplatin* 40 mg/m^2 *Leucovorin* 100 mg/m^2 *5-Fluorouracil* 375 mg/m^2	52 % (5-years)	49% (5-years)
Bouché et al. [20]	*5-Fluorouracil* 800 mg/m^2 *Cisplatin* 100 mg/m^2	46.6 % (5-years)	47.6 % (5-years)
Nitti et al. [21]	*5-Fluorouracil* 1.5 g/m^2 *Doxorubicin* 30 mg/m^2 *Metotrexate + Leucovorin* (1.5 g/m^2 + 15 g/m^2)	43% (5-years)	41 % (5-years)

Recent findings on biological mechanisms involved in gastric tumor genesis and progression allowed selecting new standard cytotoxic combinations and targeted therapies. Median survival increased to about 14 months, thanks to the use of these innovative therapies.

Adjuvant Chemotherapy and Chemoradiation

Over the past two decades, several phase III trials comparing surgery alone to adjuvant chemotherapy combination were reported. In eastern countries, especially in Japan, adjuvant chemotherapy is the gold standard treatment for gastric cancer, supported by the results of the Adjuvant Chemotherapy Trial of S-1 for Gastric Cancer (*ACTS-GC trial*) reported in 2007 [10]. Five hundred twenty-nine patients with stage II-III gastric cancer were randomly assigned to gastrectomy with extended (D2) lymphadenectomy and adjuvant therapy with S-1 40 mg/m2 or to surgery alone. *S-1* is an oral active combination of tegafur with 5-chloro-2,4-dihydroxypyridine (CDHP) and potassium oxonate (Oxo). Tegafur is a prodrug which converts to 5-fluorouracil (5-FU) in the body. Three-year overall survival rate was higher in the S-1 group (80.1% versus 70.1%) than that in surgery group. Relapse-free survival rate also improved (p= 0.001). G3 or G4 toxicity in S-1 group included anorexia, nausea, diarrhea, leukopenia and anemia, elevated serum level of bilirubin, stomatitis, and skin rash. Nevertheless, overall toxicity was acceptable. Japanese oncologists recommend administration of S-1 adjuvant chemotherapy to patients with stage IIA, IIB, IIIA, IIIB, or IIIC, except T1, within 6 weeks after surgery, for one year. The American First-Line

Advanced Gastric Cancer Study (FLAGS trial) in advanced disease [11] compared cisplatin and S-1 vs cisplatin and fluoropyridines. FLAGS trial, however, failed to demonstrate any advantage of using S-1 to improve survival rates but confirmed its safety.

In 2010, a comprehensive meta-analysis on adjuvant chemotherapy for gastric cancer was performed by the GASTRIC (Global Advanced/Adjuvant Stomach Tumor Research International Collaboration) Group [12]. Data from 3838 patients were collected in a database and clinical outcomes, median overall survival (OS) and median disease free survival (DFS), were analyzed. Median follow-up was 7 years. Adjuvant chemotherapy after curative resection showed a reduced risk of death (HR 0.82, 95% CI: 0.76–0.90; p=0.001) and an increased overall survival by 18% and 6% respectively, after 5 years. Most of the studied included a fluorouracil-based treatment (table 1). Postoperative chemotherapy is not the only adjuvant treatment for gastric cancer. Chemoradiation, indeed, showed some encouraging results [13]. In 2001, a well-designed phase III randomized trial (INT0116 trial) analyzed adjuvant chemoradiation on 556 patients with resected adenocarcinoma of the stomach or gastroesophageal junction.

Patients were randomly assigned to surgery plus postoperative chemoradiation or to surgery alone. Adjuvant treatment consisted in 425 mg/m2/die of fluorouracil and 20 mg/m2/die of leucovorin, over 5 days, followed by RT in dose of 4500 cGy (180 cGy/die, 5 days a week) over 5 weeks, with modified doses of fluorouracil and leucovorin on the first four and the last three days of radiotherapy. Two five-day cycles of fluorouracil (425 mg/m2/die) plus leucovorin (20 mg/m2/die) were administered to patients, after one month from radiation treatment. [14].

Median overall survival and relapse-free survival significantly increased in the chemoradiation group (36 months versus 27 months, P=0.005 and 30 months versus 19 months, respectively). This trial was criticized by the experts because of its suboptimal surgery, high toxicity rates (54% of patients complained with grade 3/4 hematological and gastrointestinal toxicity), outdated chemotherapy regimen and suboptimal radiotherapy technique.

The role of postoperative chemoradiation in patients receiving neoadjuvant chemotherapy followed by curative-intent gastric surgery is still an unresolved issue. A prospective multicenter phase III study (the *CRITICS trial*) including 788 patients is ongoing. Patients undergo preoperative chemotherapy (three courses of *epirubicin, cisplatin and capecitabine - ECC*) and surgery followed by either postoperative chemotherapy (another three cycles of ECC) or chemoradiation [15].

Recent discoveries in carcinogenesis molecular biology promoted the adoption in cancer treatment of biological agents which inhibit cell growth (targeted therapy). Efficacy of targeted therapy in gastric cancer is still under evaluation. In Europe, a randomized phase III study (*MAGIC-2*) is currently recruiting patients affected by resectable gastric or gastroesophageal junction cancer in order to analyze the effect of combined therapy with *bevacizumab*, an anti-VEGF monoclonal antibody, and standard chemotherapy (*ECC*) administered to patients before and after surgery. The Radiation Therapy Oncology Group *(RTOG) 04026* trial is ongoing. Patients are randomly assigned to chemoradiation with or without *cetuximab,* an anti-EGFR antibody. A phase III study by Van Cutsem et al showed improved survival to about 14 months in her2/neu overexpressing metastatic diseases (*TOGA trial* [16]) by the use of *trastuzumab* (an anti-her2/neu antibody), thus promising better outcomes in resectable disease.

Neoadjuvant Chemotherapy

Potential advantages of neoadjuvant therapy are listed below:

- Early identification of patients who will benefit by adjuvant treatment;
- Early management of occult micrometastatic disease, with improved long-term outcomes;
- Tumor downstaging (higher R0 resection rates);
- "Sterilization" of the operating field, with reduced risk of seeding.

No phase III data are currently available to support the use of the sole neoadjuvant therapy for resectable gastric cancer and available results are disappointing.

The Dutch trial based on four courses of preoperative chemotherapy with 5-fluorouracil, doxorubicin and methotrexate (FAMTX) versus surgery alone, failed to show any benefit on patient outcomes [22]. In 2009, a phase III trial by Schuhmacher C et al. [23] analyzed the role of preoperative chemotherapy versus surgery alone in locally-advanced gastric cancer. One hundred and forty-four patients were randomly assigned either to neoadjuvant chemotherapy (a combination of *cisplatin* 50 mg/m^2 days 1-15-29, *folic acid* 500 mg/m^2 and continuous infusion of *5-FU* 2 g/m^2 over 24 hours on days 1-8-15-22-29-36, for two cycles before surgery) or to surgery alone. Results were considered not valid by several experts, but an increased rate of R0 resections (81.9% compared with 66.7% with surgery alone, $p = 0.036$) was reported in the chemotherapy group. No increase in survival rates (HR 0.84, 95% CI 0.52–1.35; $p = 0.466$), however, was reported. *Neoadjuvant radiotherapy* seems to be a promising treatment even though limited data are available in order to define its role.

In 2007, a meta-analysis on nine randomized controlled trials (1700 patients) comparing adjuvant radiotherapy and radiotherapy before and after surgery for resectable gastric carcinoma (with or without chemotherapy) was performed by Fiorica et al. Preoperative radiation reduced significantly 3-year (OR 0.57, 95% CI 0.43-0.76; $p = 0.0001$) and 5-year (OR 0.62 95% CI 0.46-0.84; $p = 0.002$) overall mortality versus surgery alone [24]. Since then, several studies analyzed neoadjuvant chemotherapy or chemoradiation for the treatment of lower esophageal and type I/II gastroesophageal junction resectable adenocarcinoma. Preoperative treatment showed significant and promising results, but it is not widely accepted as the standard treatment in Europe.

Prospective studies are needed to establish the role of preoperative systemic treatment. New therapeutic regimens based on promising combinations of taxanes, oxaliplatin or oral fluoropyrimidines, and recently, targeted therapies, are currently undergoing phase I/II analysis.

Perioperative Chemotherapy

The current standard treatment in Europe for resectable adenocarcinoma of the stomach, gastroesophageal junction, and lower esophagus is based on the results of the UK Medical Research Adjuvant Gastric Infusional Chemotherapy (*MAGIC*) study. It was the first randomized trial demonstrating effective benefits of perioperative chemotherapy on survival

[25]. Five hundred three patients were randomized either to three courses of perioperative chemotherapy (*ECF: epirubicin* 50 mg/m2 and *cisplatin* 60 mg/m2 on day 1, and continuous infusion of *5-fluorouracil* 200 mg/m2 for 21 days) or to surgery alone. *ECF regimen*, used since the late 80s [26], showed curative rates (between 49% and 56%) higher than those observed in other regimens (*FAMTX: 5-fluorouracil, doxorubicin and methotrexate*) and acceptable toxicity grades [27-28]. Five-year survival in the multimodality approach group and in the surgery alone group was 36% and 23%, respectively (HR 0.75; 95% CI 0.60–0.93; P = 0.009). Progression-free survival improved in the multimodality treatment group (HR 0.66; 95% CI 0.53–0.81; P < 0.001). Postoperative complication and mortality rates were similar in both two arms. Length of hospital stay and curative resections were not affected by chemotherapy. Only 55% of patients, who were assigned to perioperative chemotherapy, however, underwent postoperative therapy, and only 42% underwent all six cycles of chemotherapy. Others biases of MAGIC trial are: use of non-standardized surgery, inaccurate preoperative staging (no preoperative laparoscopy) and low rates of adjuvant therapy completion.

The French *ACCORD07-FFCD 9703 trial* presented in 2007, confirmed MAGIC results, assessing the need of a multimodality approach in patients with resectable cancer than surgery alone.

Twenty hundred twenty-four patients with histologically-proven adenocarcinoma (stage II or higher) of the lower third of the esophagus (11%), esophagogastric junction (64%), or stomach (25%), were randomly assigned either to surgery or to neoadjuvant chemotherapy. Preoperative chemotherapy-plus-surgery group received *cisplatin* 100 mg/m2 on days 1-2 in association to *5-FU* 800 mg/m2 in continuous infusion for 5 days for two-three cycles. Adjuvant chemotherapy was administered to downstaged patients (neoadjuvant therapy) and to patients with lymph node involvement and no signs of disease progression. Eighteen-nine percent of chemotherapy group patients underwent complete preoperative chemotherapy and 51% received one to four cycles of postoperative therapy. Five-year disease-free survival and overall survival improved in the chemotherapy arm (DFS: 34% vs. 19%; HR 0.65; 95% CI 0.48-0.89; p = 0.003; OS: 38% vs. 24%; HR 0.69; 95% CI 0.50- 0.95; p = 0.02) [29].

Table 2. Comparison of INT0116, MAGIC and CRITICS trial

	Intergroup 0116	MAGIC	CRITICS
Stage Location	Ib-IV (M0) GOJ/ Stomach	II-IV (M0) Lower 1/3 oesophagus/ GOJ/ Stomach	Ib-IV (M0) GOJ/ Stomach
N° of patients	556	503	788 (needed)
Preoperative Therapy	Not applicable	A: ECF (3 courses) B: none	A: ECC/EOC B: ECC/EOC
Postoperative Therapy	A:5-FU/LV/RT (45Gy) B: none	A: ECF (3 courses) B: none	A: CC/RT B: ECC/EOC
Main Endopoint (5-year OS)	A: 42% B: 25%	A: 36% B: 23%	ongoing

Abbreviations: A (experimental arm), B (control arm), ECF (epirubicin, cisplatin, 5 fluorouracil), RT (radiotherapy), ECC (epirubicin, cisplatin, capecitabine), OS (overall survival), GOJ (gastroesophageal junction).

Oral prodrug *capecitabine* has been demonstrated to have similar effects in tumor control than intravenous 5-FU but less toxicity. Moreover, use of oral drugs avoids implantation of central venous port connected to portable infusion pumps requested by continuous infusional 5-FU [30]. Combination of epirubicin with cisplatin and capecitabine (*ECX*) as perioperative chemotherapy regimen, therefore, seems to be appropriate for resectable gastric cancer.

Currently, two phase III studies are evaluating the role of bevacizumab + ECX (capecitabine for 5-FU) and adjuvant radiation, showing the same results than 5-FU in the treatment of advanced stage disease.

Oncological Outcomes After Minimally Invasive Surgery

Minimally invasive surgery (MIS) has been slowly introduced in the treatment of gastric cancer. Nevertheless, MIS has several advantages, including early postoperative recovery, reduced hospital stay, less pain and improved quality of life [31]. MIS has been extensively analyzed in colorectal cancer and, recently, several studies reported MIS experiences on gastric cancer treatment.

Randomized clinical trials in colorectal cancer (*Barcelona* [32], *COST* [33], *COLOR* [34] and *CLASICC* trials [35]) showed oncological adequacy of laparoscopic surgery for both colonic and rectal cancer, offering acceptable long-term oncological results than open surgery. Applications of MIS in gastric cancer may vary from preoperative staging to curative-intent surgery for early and locally-advanced disease.

Diagnostic Laparoscopy

Staging laparoscopy for gastric cancer is an essential tool for detecting potentially curable patients and avoiding nontherapeutic laparotomies [36]. Standard staging methods, such as computed tomography (CT) and positron emission tomography (PET) are accurate in detecting gross metastatic disease but may fail to diagnose small peritoneal metastases or lymph node involvement. A retrospective analysis by De Graaf et al. showed that preoperative laparoscopy can avoid inappropriate laparotomies in 28-44% of patients with potentially resectable disease [37].

Current guidelines suggest that laparoscopic staging is not indicated in T1 lesions, which have low risk of distant metastases and affected patients should undergo surgery. Conversely, staging laparoscopy is indicated in T3 and T4 tumors in which the risk of peritoneal metastasis is high. In Japan, where MIS is routinely performed, a classification of the types of peritoneal dissemination found at staging laparoscopy was proposed in order to manage clinical decisions [38].

Aggressive surgery (P1 disease) or neoadjuvant chemotherapy (P2-P3 diseases) may be performed on the basis of staging laparoscopy findings: locally metastatic seeding adjacent to the stomach (P1 disease), few scattered distant metastases (P2) or numerous distant peritoneal metastases (P3).

Table 3. Long-term oncologic outcomes of Laparoscopic Gastrectomy in EGC

Study	N of patients	Indication	Median Follow Up	SURVIVAL (%)						
				Ia	Ib	IIa	IIb	IIIa	IIIb	IV
Kitano et al. (2007)	1,294	EGC	36	99.8	98.7	85.7	-	-	-	-
Hwang et al. (2009)	197	EGC, cT2N0MO	45	100	96.4	87.7	-	-	100	100
Song et al. (2010)	1,485	EGC, AGC	41	98.6	-	86.0	-	44.7	-	50
Lee et al. (2010)	601	EGC, cT2N0-1M0	35.9	94.2	87.4	80.8	69.6	-	-	-

Minimally Invasive Surgery for Early Gastric Cancer

Since the first report in 1994, laparoscopic gastrectomy for early gastric cancer (EGC) has rapidly diffused in Japan. Although there are evidence supporting short-term efficacy of laparoscopic approach for EGC, long-term outcomes are still under evaluation. In 2010, Lee et al reported a single-center experience of 601 consecutive laparoscopic resections in patients with tumors confined to the muscularis propria not suitable for endoscopic mucosal resection with limited lymph node involvement (N1) [39]. Adjuvant chemotherapy with S-1, was administered for 1 year to patients with stage higher than IIA, in order to reduce local and distant recurrence.

Median follow-up was 35.9 months: 14 (2.3%) patients experienced distant relapses (8 peritoneal, 4 hepatic, 1 paraortic and 1 bone recurrences). Five-year overall and disease-free survival rates were 94.2% and 89.9% in stage IA, 87.4% and 82.7% in stage IB, 80.8% and 70.7% in IIA, 69.6% and 63.1% in stage IIB, respectively. Overall survival and disease-free survival rates were similar to those in open surgery.

Similar results were showed in other Japanese experiences, including a multicenter retrospective study on 1,294 laparoscopic gastrectomies, reported by Kitano et al [40]. A meta-analysis comparing MIS and open surgery for gastric cancer has been recently presented [41]. A multicenter retrospective study was carried out in South Korea and included 1.417 laparoscopic gastric procedures showing a recurrence rate of 3.5%, similar to that in open procedures.

Japanese Gastric Cancer Association clinical guidelines (*2004 edition*) [42] recommend laparoscopic gastrectomy alone in gastric cancer patients with clinical stages *IA (T1(SM)N0)* and *IB (cT1N1 – cT2N0)*, laparoscopic gastrectomy with adjuvant treatment in patients with clinical stages *II (T2N1)*, *IIIA (T2N2 – T3N1)* and *IIIB (T3N2)*, laparoscopic gastrectomy with neoadjuvant/adjuvant treatment in patients with clinical stages *II (cT3N0)* and *IIIB (T3N2 – T4N1)* and laparoscopic gastrectomy with neoadjuvant/adjuvant treatment plus radiation therapy in patients with stage *IIIA (T4N0)*. Patinets with clinical stage *IA (T1(M)N0)* are referred to endoscopic mucosal resection (EMR) or endoscopic submucosal dissection (ESD).

In conclusion, laparoscopic gastrectomy for EGC appears safe and feasible with acceptable short and long-term oncologic outcomes and decreased overall and postoperative morbidity.

Minimally Invasive Surgery for Advanced Gastric Cancer

Few studies analyzed laparoscopic approach for advanced gastric cancer (AGC). Baker et al reported 111 consecutive laparoscopic-assisted esophago-gastrectomies for local advanced cancer of distal esophagus (40.5%) and esophagogastric junction (55.9%). Sixty-eight percent of patients received neoadjuvant chemotherapy (*CF* 40.5%, *ECX* 21.65% and *ECF* 5.4%) [43]. Median number of retrieved lymph nodes increased from 5 in the first phase (1998 to 2001) to 28 in the last phase (2006 to 2009, $p < 0.001$). Complication rate was 38.7% and median survival was 38.5 ± 5.4 months, confirming laparoscopy as a safe procedure in advanced disease when combined to chemotherapy.

Huscher et al [44] reported the first experience on minimally-invasive surgical treatment for advanced gastric cancer in Europe. They reported better outcomes in minimally invasive technique (LG) than in open surgery (OG). Mortality rate was 3.3% versus 6.7%, 5-year recurrence rate was 58.9% versus 55.7% and disease-free survival rate was 57.3% versus 54.8% in LG and in OG group respectively.

In 2009, Zhou DL et al reported improved outcomes in advanced gastric cancer patients which underwent laparoscopic surgery plus neoadjuvant chemotherapy. Fifty patients with stage II, III, IV (M0) gastric adenocarcinoma were treated with *neoadjuvant FOLFOX 7* regimen (*oxaliplatin* 130 mg/m2 day 1, *folic acid* 400 mg/m2 day 1, followed by continuous infusion of *5-FU* 2400 mg/m2) every two weeks for 4 cycles. Conversely, thirty patients received laparoscopic gastrectomy alone (control group). Overall toxicity was acceptable (less than grade 3), 2 patients had complete remission, 10 experienced partial remission and 3 were non-responders. Ten patients, who received neoadjuvant therapy, underwent laparoscopic-assisted radical gastrectomy.

R0 resection rate (80.0%) and pN0 rate (60.0%) in patients receiving chemotherapy were significantly higher than those in the control group (46.7% R0 and 20.0% pN0), while positive lymph node rate (11.0%) was significantly lower than that in the control group (23.8%). Operative time and postoperative complications were not affected by preoperative chemotherapy. This trial suggests that chemotherapy delivered before MIS allows downstaging of the disease and increase R0 resection rates

Conclusion

Over the past few decades, gastric cancer incidence and mortality decreased in most areas of the world [45]. Surgery has been considered the sole curative strategy for a long time, but recent clinical data showed that multidisciplinary approach is mandatory to improve patients survival. Both *SWOG 9008/INT 0116* and *MAGIC* studies are large, well-designed, randomized trials which showed statistically and clinically significant improvements in survival in patients with resectable gastric cancer. Nevertheless, multidisciplinary treatment methods are not standardized: postoperative chemoradiation is performed in the United States, adjuvant chemotherapy in Japan and perioperative chemotherapy in Europe. There is no evidence, indeed, to prefer perioperative chemotherapy on postoperative chemoradiation and viceversa. Management of patients, therefore, needs to be discussed by a qualified multidisciplinary team, consisting in oncologists, surgeons, gastroenterologists, radiologists, and pathologists.

Since failure rates after current multimodality strategies are still high, clinical research on targeted agents and translational biology is needed. Biomarkers predictive of good/worse response to chemotherapy and radiotherapy are also needed.

References

[1] Goh P., Tekant Y., Isaac J., Kum C. K., Ngoi S. S. The technique of laparoscopic Billroth II gastrectomy. *Surg. Laparosc. Endosc.* 1992;2(3):258-260.

[2] Jemal A., Siegel R., Xu J., Ward E. Cancer statistics, 2010. *CA Cancer. J. Clin.* 2010 Sep.-Oct.;60(5):277-300.

[3] Forman D., Burley V. J. Gastric cancer: global pattern of the disease and an overview of environmental risk factors. *Best Pract. Res. Clin. Gastroenterol* 2006; 20: 633–649.

[4] González C. A., Megraud F., et al. Helicobacter pylori infection assessed by ELISA and by immunoblot and noncardia gastric cancer risk in a prospective study: the Eurgast-EPIC project. *Ann. Oncol.* 2011 Sep. 14. [Epub ahead of print].

[5] Rohde H., Bauer P., et al. Proximal compared with distal adenocarcinoma of the stomach: differences and consequences. German Gastric Cancer TNM Study Group. *Br. J. Surg.* 1991 Oct.;78(10): 1242-8.

[6] Hartgrink H. H., Jansen E. P., van Grieken N. C., van de Velde C. J. Gastric cancer. *Lancet.* 2009;374(9688): 477-490.

[7] Allum W. H., Griffin S. M., Watson A., et al. Guidelines for the management of oesophageal and gastric cancer. *Gut.* 2002;50(Suppl. 5):v1.

[8] Adachi Y., Kitano S., Sugimachi K. Surgery for gastric cancer: 10-year experience worldwide. *Gastric. Cancer.* 2001;4(4):166–174.

[9] Hundahl S. A., Phillips J. L., Menck H. R. The National Cancer Data Base Report on poor survival of U.S. gastric carcinoma patients treated with gastrectomy: fifth edition American Joint Committee on Cancer staging, proximal disease, and the 'different disease' hypothesis. *Cancer* 2000; 88:921–932.

[10] Sakuramoto S., Sasako M., Yamaguchi T., et al; ACTS-GC Group. Adjuvant chemotherapy for gastric cancer with S-1, an oral fluoropyrimidine. *N. Engl. J. Med.* 2007;357(18):1810-1820.

[11] Ajani J. A., Rodriguez W., Bodoky G., et al. Multicenter phase III comparison of cisplatin/S-1 with cisplatin/ infusional fluorouracil in advanced gastric or gastroesophageal adenocarcinoma study: the FLAGS trial. *J. Clin. Oncol.* 2010;28(9):1547-1553.

[12] Oba K., Burzykowski T., Michiels S., Ohashi Y., Pignon J. P., et al. Benefit of adjuvant chemotherapy for resectable gastric cancer: a meta-analysis. GASTRIC (Global Advanced/Adjuvant Stomach Tumor Research International Collaboration) Group. *JAMA.* 2010 May 5;303(17):1729-37.

[13] Zhang Z. X., Gu X. Z., Yin W. B., et al. Randomized clinical trial on the combination of preoperative irradiation and surgery in the treatment of adenocarcinoma of gastric

cardia (AGC): report on 370 patients. *Int. J. Radiat. Oncol. Biol. Phys.* 1998; 42: 929–934.

[14] Macdonald J. S., Smalley S. R., Benedetti J., et al. Chemoradiotherapy after surgery compared with surgery alone for adenocarcinoma of the stomach or gastroesophageal junction. *N. Engl. J. Med.* 2001; 345(10): 725–730.

[15] Dikken J. L., van Sandick J. W., et al. Neo-adjuvant chemotherapy followed by surgery and chemotherapy or by surgery and chemoradiotherapy for patients with resectable gastric cancer (CRITICS). *BMC Cancer.* 2011 Aug. 2;11:329.

[16] Van Cutsem E., Kang Y., Chung H., et al. Efficacy results from the ToGA trial: A phase III study of trastuzumab added to standard chemotherapy (CT) in firstline human epidermal growth factor receptor 2 (HER2)-positive advanced gastric cancer (GC) [abstract #LBA4509]. *J. Clin. Oncol.* 2009; 27:18s.

[17] Sakuramoto S., Sasako M., Yamaguchi T., et al; ACTS-GC Group. Adjuvant chemotherapy for gastric cancer with S-1, an oral fluoropyrimidine. *N. Engl. J. Med.* 2007;357(18):1810-1820.

[18] Popiela T., Kulig J., Czupryna A., Szczepanik A. M., Zembala M. Efficiency of adjuvant immunochemotherapy following curative resection in patients with locally advanced gastric cancer. *Gastric. Cancer.* 2004; 7(4):240-245.

[19] Bajetta E., Buzzoni R., Mariani L., et al. Adjuvant chemotherapy in gastric cancer: 5-year results of a randomized study by the Italian Trials in Medical Oncology (ITMO) Group. *Ann. Oncol.* 2002;13(2):299- 307.

[20] Bouche′ O., Ychou M., Burtin P., et al; Fe′ de′ ration Francophone de Cance′ rologie Digestive Group. Adjuvant chemotherapy with 5-fluorouracil and cisplatin compared with surgery alone for gastric cancer: 7-year result of the FFCD randomized phase III trial (8801). *Ann. Oncol.* 2005;16(9):1488-1497.

[21] Nitti D., Wils J., Dos Santos J. G., et al; EORTC GI Group; ICCG. Randomized phase III trial of adjuvant FAMTX or FEMTX compared with surgery alone in resected gastric cancer: a combined analysis of the EORTC GI group and the ICCG. *Ann. Oncol.* 2006; 17(2):262-269.

[22] Hartgrink H. H., van de Velde C. J. H., Putter H., et al.: Neoadjuvant chemotherapy for operable gastric cancer; long-term results of the Dutch randomised FAMTX trial. *Eur. J. Surg. Oncol.* 2004, 30:643–649.

[23] Schuhmacher C., Gretschel S., Lordick F., et al. Neoadjuvant chemotherapy compared with surgery alone for locally advanced cancer of the stomach and cardia: European Organisation for Research and Treatment of Cancer randomized trial 40954. *J. Clin. Oncol.* 2010; 28(35):5210–5218.

[24] Fiorica F., Cartei F., Enea M., et al.: The impact of radiotherapy on survival in resectable gastric carcinoma: a meta analysis of literature data. *Cancer Treat. Rev.* 2007, 33:729–740.

[25] Cunningham D., Allum W. H., Stenning S. P., et al. Perioperative chemotherapy versus surgery alone for resectable gastroesophageal cancer. *N. Engl. J. Med.* 2006; 355: 11–20.

[26] Findlay M., Cunningham D., Norman A.,et al. A phase II study in advanced gastroesophageal cancer using epirubicin and cisplatin in combination with continuous infusion 5-fluorouracil (ECF). *Ann. Oncol.* 1994;5:609-16.

[27] Webb A., Cunningham D., Scarffe J. H., et al. Randomized trial comparing epirubicin, cisplatin, and fluorouracil versus fluorouracil, doxorubicin, and methotrexate in advanced esophagogastric cancer. *J. Clin. Oncol.* 1997;15:261-7.

[28] Ross P., Nicolson M., Cunningham D., et al. Prospective randomized trial comparing mitomycin, cisplatin, and protracted venous-infusion fluorouracil (PVI 5-FU) with epirubicin, cisplatin, and PVI 5-FU in advance esophagogastric cancer. *J. Clin. Oncol.* 2002;20:1996-2004.

[29] Ychou M., Boige V., Pignon J. P., Conroy T., et al.: Perioperative chemotherapy compared with surgery alone for resectable gastroesophageal adenocarcinoma: an FNCLCC and FFCD multicenter phase III trial. *J. Clin. Oncol.* 2011; 13:1715-21.

[30] Evans T. R., Pentheroudakis G., Paul J. et al. A phase I and pharmacokinetic study of capecitabine in combination with epirubicin and cisplatin in patients with inoperable oesophago-gastric adenocarcinoma. *Ann. Oncol.* 2002; 13: 1469–1478.

[31] Weeks J. C., Nelson H., Gelber S. et al (2002) Short-term quality-of life outcomes following laparoscopic-assisted colectomy vs open colectomy for colon cancer: a randomized trial. *JAMA* 287:321–328.

[32] Lacy A. M., Garcia-Valdecasas J. C., Delgado S., et al: Laparoscopy-assisted colectomy versus open colectomy for treatment of non-metastatic colon cancer: A randomised trial. *Lancet* 359:2224-2229, 2002.

[33] The Clinical Outcomes of Surgical Therapy Study Group: A comparison of laparoscopically assisted and open colectomy for colon cancer. *N. Engl. J. Med.* 350:2050-2059, 2004.

[34] Veldkamp R., Kuhry E., Hop W. C., et al: Laparoscopic surgery versus open surgery for colon cancer: Short-term outcomes of a randomised trial. *Lancet Oncol.* 6:477-484, 2005.

[35] Guillou P. J., Quirke P., Thorpe H., et al: Short-term endpoints of conventional versus laparoscopic-assisted surgery in patients with colorectal cancer (MRC CLASICC trial): Multicentre, randomised controlled trial. *Lancet.* 365:1718-1726, 2010.

[36] Patel A. N., Buenaventura P. O., et al Current staging of esophageal carcinoma. *Surg. Clin. North. Am.* 200585:555-567.

[37] De Graaf G. W., Ayantunde A. A., Parsons S. L., et al.: The role of staging laparoscopy in oesophagogastric cancers. *EJSO* 2007, 33: 988–992.

[38] Song K. Y., Kim J. J., Kim S. N., et al.: Staging laparoscopy for advanced gastric cancer: is it also useful for the group which has an aggressive surgical strategy. *World. J. Surg.* 2007, 31:1228–1233.

[39] Lee S. W., Nomura E., et al. Long-term oncologic outcomes from laparoscopic gastrectomy for gastric cancer: a single-center experience of 601 consecutive resections. *J. Am. Coll. Surg.* 2010 Jul.;211(1):33-40.

[40] Kitano S., Shiraishi N., Uyama I., et al. A multicenter study on oncologic outcome of laparoscopic gastrectomy for early cancer in Japan. *Ann. Surg.* 2007;245:68–72.

[41] Zorcolo L., Rosman A. S., et al. A meta-analysis of prospective randomized trials comparing minimally invasive and open distal gastrectomy for cancer. *J. Surg. Oncol.* 2011 Oct;104(5):544-51.

[42] The Japanese Gastric Cancer Association (2004) Guidelines for the treatment of gastric cancer. Kanehara, Tokyo.

[43] Baker C. R., Bailey M. E., et al. Two-phase laparoscopic-assisted oesophago-gastrectomy: a single-unit experience of 111 consecutive cases and outcomes. *Surg. Endosc*. 2011 Jun. 8.

[44] Huscher C. G., Mingoli A., Sgarzini G., Sansonetti A., Di Paola M., Recher A., Ponzano C: Laparoscopic versus open subtotal gastrectomy for distal gastric cancer: five-year results of a randomized prospective trial. *Ann. Surg*., 241: 232-237, 2005.

[45] Jemal A., Thomas A., Murray T., Thun M. Cancer statistics, 2002. *CA Cancer. J. Clin*. 2002; 52: 23-47.

In: Gastric Cancer
Editors: A. D'Annibale, V. Pende and I. Monsellato
ISBN: 978-1-62081-294-5

Chapter XI

The Relevance of Nutrition Before and After Gastrectomy for Gastric Cancer

Esther Uña Cidón
Digestive Oncology Unit, Clinical University Hospital
and Faculty of Medicine of Valladolid, Spain

Abstract

Incidence of gastric cancer is reduced, but gastric cancer is still the second most common cause of death worldwide. Overall survival rates need to be improved by innovations in treatment methods, since higher rates of overall survival are needed (about 50%, currently about 20%). Surgical treatment of gastric cancer is a procedure which can cause mild to severe alterations of nutritional and metabolic processes. These alterations may affect prognosis and quality of life. The most commonly used technique for bowel reconstruction in total gastrectomy is the Roux-en-Y esophagojejunostomy. Roux technique, however, may cause a slow and incomplete recovery. Further research on food transit restoring techniques are still required to improve postoperative nutrition in gastrectomized patients. Most treated patients, indeed, suffer from rapid weight loss, low energy intake, and malnutrition, which is the most important postoperative complication causing high postoperative morbidity and mortality rates.

Introduction

Although incidence of gastric carcinoma is reduced, gastric cancer is still the second most common cause of cancer-related death. Incidence varies by regions: 26.9/100 000 per year in Asia and 7.4 in North America. Variability in incidence rates can be caused by different exposure to several risk factors. Non-cardiac tumors are related to a diet poor in fruits and vegetables, high consumption of salty and smoked foods, Helicobacter pylori and lower socio-economic status. Other risk factors are familiar clustering, genetic syndromes, and atrophic gastritis. Five-year overall survival rate in Western countries is still about 20%. Overall survival rate needs to be improved further (about 50%). Surgical treatment of gastric cancer is a procedure causing mild to severe alterations of nutritional and metabolic processes which can have a relevant impact on prognosis and quality of life (QoL). The most commonly used technique for Roux technique, however, may cause a slow and incomplete recovery. Further research on food transit restoring techniques are still required to improve postoperative nutrition in gastrectomized patients. Most treated patients, indeed, suffer from rapid weight loss and low energy intake. Malnutrition is the most important postoperative complication and may cause high postoperative morbidity and mortality rates. This chapter describes the correlation between nutrition and gastrectomy for gastric cancer and nutritional management of gastrectomized patients.

Malnutrition and Cancer

Malnutrition is defined as a nutritional status characterized by the deficiency of energy, proteins, or other specific nutrients, producing appreciable alterations of body physiology [1, 2]. Several studies showed that about 30-50% of inpatients suffer from malnutrition [3-6]. Prevalence of malnutrition in cancer patients ranges from 8% to 84% [6], depending on cancer population sample and methods of nutritional assessment [7].

Cancer patients can experience a weight loss of more than 10% of total body weight [8, 9], and about 20% of deaths are caused by malnutrition and its complications than by disease itself [10]. Patients affected by cancer of the esophagus, pancreas, head, neck, and stomach are more likely to suffer from malnutrition [11]. Malnutrition modifies prognosis by affecting both response to anticancer treatments and overall survival [10, 12, 13]. Increased morbidity [14] and prolonged hospital stay [15] cause high healthcare costs. Malnutrition is also associated to increased mortality, particularly in elderly patients [16] and those with poor QoL [17]. Cancer patients, therefore, need specific nutritional assessment, which can help to reduce complications of cancer-related nutritional depletion and to improve clinical outcomes. According to the guidelines of the European Society for Clinical Nutrition and Metabolism (ESPEN), severe nutritional risk is defined as the presence of at least one of the following criteria: weight loss < 10-15% over six months, body mass index < 18.5 kg/m2, Subjective Global Assessment (SGA) grade C, and serum level of albumin < 30 g/L [18].

Causes of Cancer-Related Malnutrition

Malnutrition occurs through different cancer-related mechanisms and through the effect of anticancer treatments on several physiological processes [19,20]. These mechanisms include loss of appetite, alterations in absorption and metabolism of nutrients and impaired organ functions [21]. Alterations in taste sensation, which are frequently reported by patients, are mainly due to anticancer therapies, and aversion to food is associated to cancer cachexia, which is a specific form of cancer-related malnutrition characterized by progressive, uncontrolled weight loss with depletion of lean-body mass and muscle wasting [20].

Psychological factors, such as fear, depression, or anxiety, influence also malnutrition in cancer patients. All these factors modify appetite and food intake thus affecting QOL [21, 22]. Analgesic therapy can alter food intake by decreasing appetite and cause erosions of the gastrointestinal mucosa and constipation [23]. An effective control on cancer-related symptoms could increase appetite [24].

Cancer-Related Malnutrition and Metabolic Alterations

Nutritional intake is decreased in cancer patients suffering from weight loss [25]. These patients may also experience anorexia, cachexia, nausea, vomiting, pain, fatigue, and alterations of sensations of taste and smell. Pathophysiological modifications occurring in specific areas of the central nervous system controlling food intake and sensation of taste/smell, are involved, indeed, in the development of anorexia, malnutrition, and cachexia, in cooperation with the production of multiple cytokines by monocytes and tumor cells [26, 27]. Tumor cells can excrete several agents, such as amino-acid-type substances, which can contribute to taste alterations [28].

Moreover, cancer symptoms such as odynophagia, dysphagia, early satiety, malabsorption, gastrointestinal obstruction, and pain could also affect food intake. Although reduced food intake may be the most important factor in nutritional decay in cancer patients, alterations in metabolism and changes in resting-energy consumption are also other relevant causes [29].

Bosaeus and colleagues [30] observed that weight loss was more closely related to increased resting-energy consumption than to decreased dietary intake. Barber and colleagues [9], however, suggested that reduction in physical activity may not modify total energy expenditure even though the resting-energy consumption is high. Other data suggest that competition for nutrients between cancer and the organism may result in an accelerated condition of starvation, which promotes further metabolic alterations, including increased metabolic rate and hence resting-energy consumption and energy inefficiency [29]. Hypermetabolism usually affects proteins, fat, and carbohydrates.

Abnormal levels and patterns of amino acids in plasma, increased gluconeogenesis or altered turnover of proteins in liver and muscles are, indeed, common alterations in cancer patients [31]. Decreased proteins catabolism and preservation of lean body mass by use of amino acids and visceral proteins as precursors of gluconeogenesis are adaptive mechanisms to energy consumption in healthy subjects but not in cancer patients, in which conversely, a significant proteins depletion and muscle atrophy occur through an increased proteins turnover, a reduced synthesis of muscle proteins, and an increased synthesis of hepatic proteins, [32].

Carbohydrate metabolism is also altered. Liver production of glucose is increased, but its use in peripheral tissues is poor due to insulin resistance and glucose intolerance [33]. Increased mobilization of peripheral fat and oxidation of fatty acids are the most relevant metabolic alterations occurring in cancer patients. Alterations of lipid metabolism can cause depletion of fat storage and weight loss [34].

Acute-phase protein reaction consisting in complex biomolecular processes in response to cancer's presence and for preventing tissue damage, also occurs in patients with advanced cancer. Acute-phase protein reaction induces increased production of specific blood proteins, such as acute-phase proteins, C-reactive protein and mannose-binding protein, which are synthesized in the liver in response to inflammation. Inflammatory cytokines such as interleukin-1 (IL-1), IL-6, and tumor necrosis factor (TNF) promote this reaction. Altered protein synthesis causes an acceleration of hypermetabolism and consequently weight loss [35] and poor survival in patients with advanced cancer [36].

Surgery-Related Malnutrition

Etiology of malnutrition is multifactorial and includes anorexia, iatrogenic starvation, postprandial symptoms, malabsorption, maldigestion, short bowel syndrome and bacterial colonization. Total gastrectomy may cause malnutrition by altering digestion and physiology of the gastro-esophageal junction [37, 38].

Loss of adipose and lean-tissue mass continues over several years after surgery. Patients may suffer from weight and muscle mass loss, impaired mobilization and increased morbidity. Although many specialists consider malnutrition an unavoidable consequence of total gastrectomy, few studies have focused on the nutritional alterations occurring after this procedure and nutritional method to perform after total gastrectomy has not been standardized. Total gastrectomy, indeed, reduces the size of the stomach and alters its innervation, causing the so-called small-stomach syndrome. Gastrectomized patients usually complain of satiety (48%), epigastric fullness (26%), gastroesophageal reflux (43%), diarrhea (22%), and nausea (17%). Moreover, anorexia, inappetence and postprandial abdominal pain can cause a significant reduction in caloric intake in most patients (about 85% of gastrectomized patients) [39].

Diarrhea occurs generally within one or two hours of a meal and induces nutrients loss. Major causes of diarrhea are: vagotomy, lack of gastric hormones, deficit of fat absorption caused by pancreatic deficiency, bacterial colonization, or short-bowel syndrome [40,41]. Absence of secretion of biliary and pancreatic induced by ingested food can support malabsorption.

Duodenum is surgically excluded from food transit causing a decreased absorption of iron, calcium, fat, and carotene. Moreover, stasis in the afferent loop can induce bacterial colonization and altered metabolism of bile salts. Malabsorption of dietary fat is proposed to be the primary cause of weight loss after total gastrectomy. A total of 50g/die of fat can be lost in stools, seven times greater than that in healthy patients [40,42]. Malabsorption of amino acids is also reported after gastrectomy, establishing a condition of persistent proteolysis of lean tissue mass for a long period after surgery [43]. Surgery can reduce food intake and increase nutritional demand in the early postoperative, but these effects may persist in case of gastrointestinal resection [44].

The rationale of "nihil per os" in the early postoperative is to prevent postoperative nausea and vomiting and to preserve anastomosis. Another mechanism of malnutrition is related to the temporary loss of taste and smell, which occurs in about half patients undergoing upper gastrointestinal surgery. Alterations in taste and smell sensation resolve generally within 6-12 months. Pathophysiological mechanisms at the base of these alterations are still unknown [45]. Since oral intake is not allowed before consolidation of the anastomosis (up to a week after surgery) patients, who are malnourished at diagnosis, may experience a further aggravation of nutritional status in the postoperative.

Impact of Malnutrition in Gastrectomized Patients

Prevalence and Role of Malnutrition in Postoperative Complications

In 1936, Studley [46] showed that postoperative complication rate after surgery for benign peptic ulcers in patients with a weight loss of more than 20% of total weight was 10 times higher than that in patients without weight loss. Moreover, several studies confirmed that patients affected by malignant gastrointestinal disease have a high incidence rate of weight loss before surgery and an additional weight loss of about 10% of total weight over the first postoperative months [47-50]. Several studies, in addition, showed that protein caloric malnutrition is a significant risk factor of postoperative complications in major abdominal surgery [1, 51, 52]. Protein caloric malnutrition also prolong postoperative recovery [53, 54]. Pacelli et al. [55] conducted a retrospective study on 196 patients affected by gastric cancer undergoing surgery in order to define the effects of malnutrition and weight loss on postoperative complications. They stratified patients according to the preoperative percentage of weight loss, serum levels of albumin, and body mass index. Authors concluded that weight loss and hypoalbuminemia do not increase the risk of mortality and morbidity in gastric cancer patients undergoing surgery. Anastomotic leakage rates, however, were higher in patients with a weight loss of more than 10% of total body weight, levels of serum albumin of less than 3.0 g/L or body mass index value of less than 18.5 kg/m^2, even though these results were not statistically significant. Conversely, over the last 30 years several studies demonstrated that malnutrition is actually a risk factor of postoperative complications in patients undergoing major surgery for abdominal or gastric cancer [56, 57]. Other Authors, however, do not agree with these studies [58].

Most studies consider malnutrition as an important risk factor of major postoperative complications after subtotal or total gastrectomy for gastric cancer [20, 59]. Evaluation of diagnostic parameters for nutritional depletion in all patients is mandatory. Ryu and Kim [53] evaluated 80 patients undergoing gastrectomy (9 total and 71 partial gastrectomies) for gastric cancer and found an overall malnutrition rate of 31% at first diagnosis. Analysis was performed by SGA tool.

Bae et al. [59] reported a preoperative mean body mass index (BMI) of 22.2 kg/m^2 and a postoperative mean BMI of 18.9 kg/m^2, 15% less than preoperative weight ($p=0.01$). They found no significant correlation between time from surgery and weight loss, but the latter increased even 4.2 years after total gastrectomy. In their study on 108 patients, Kiyama et al. [42] analyzed body compositional changes using bioelectrical impedance analysis and observed that loss of proteic mass or fat occurred at different times after surgery. Proteins loss occurred mainly in the first 14 days after surgery and continued over 6 months. From six months to one year after surgery, weight loss was caused by the loss of fat mass with no alterations of proteins. Mean weight loss in patients who underwent total gastrectomy was 8.9 ± 5 Kg over the first six months and 4 ± 3.4 Kg over the second six months after surgery. Same results are reported by Liedman et al [60] who showed an early weight loss (10% of pre-operative weight) after total gastrectomy and a decreased body fat rate of 40% over the first six months after surgery.

A prospective randomized trial by Kodera et al [61] showed that pancreatectomy and prolonged operative time were the most important risk factors of postoperative complications and body mass index of 25 kg/m2 or higher, pancreatectomy and age > 65 were significant predictors of major postoperative complications. Wu et al. [18] used multivariate analysis to show that splenectomy and nodal dissection were two independent risk factors affecting morbidity. Patients with severe malnutrition, (levels of serum albumin < 3.0 g/dl, weight loss < 10% or BMI < 18.5 kg/m^2) did not show higher incidence in postoperative complications. Ryan et al [39] reported a complication rate of 35% and a mortality rate of 4% after total gastrectomy for gastric cancer.

A weight loss of 10% of total body weight was associated to higher rates of complications and higher mortality rate than a weight loss of less than 10% of total body weight. Multivariate logistic regression analysis showed that a weight loss of 10% of body weight was the sole factor influencing postoperative complications (OR 3.1 95%, CI 1.0–9.6, p=0.04). Grossmann et al reported a postoperative complication rate of 38% and a 30-day mortality rate of 7.7% after 234 total gastrectomies for cancer [153]. Multivariate logistic regression analysis showed that a weight loss of more than 10% of body weight over six months before surgery was a predictive factor of the risk of 30-day mortality. Similar increasing of mortality rate was also observed by Sitges-Serra et al., showing that a weight loss higher than 20% of total weight caused higher mortality rate than a weight loss of less than 20% of total weight (23% versus 7%, $P < 0.05$) [155].

Other tests assessing nutritional status, such as the nutritional risk index (NRI) and the prognostic nutritional index (PNI) are also used for predicting postoperative complications. Rey-Ferro et al. found a significant correlation between severe malnutrition (NRI 83.5) and postoperative mortality and cellular immunosuppression by associating weight loss to albumin levels values in the NRI [154].

They reported an incidence of moderate malnutrition of 42.5% and an incidence of severe malnutrition of 15% in patients with gastric cancer. NRI-postoperative mortality rate was 33% in the severe-malnourished group and 6.5% in the moderate-malnourished group. These groups also showed cellular immunosuppression with poor CD4/CD8 ratios, which were related to postoperative mortality.

ESPEN guidelines suggest that NRI [NRI: 15.9 x serum albumin (g/dL) + 41.7 x (current weight/usual weight)] could also predict perioperative morbidity [62]. Sitges-Serra et al reported that a PNI of less than 50% is correlated to lower mortality rates than a PNI of 50%. This difference is attributed to the lower resistance to infections in patients who are severely malnourished. Death rate related to sepsis in this kind of patients is reported to be five times higher than rates in well-nourished patients [155].

Prognosis and Quality of Life in Malnourished Gastric Cancer Patients

Most studies have shown that malnutrition and weight loss are the major causes of morbidity and mortality in cancer patients [63]. Weight loss is also a significant survival-related factor after gastrectomy [64]. One study [65] has shown a prevalence of malnutrition of only 11% according to BMI alone; 76% of the patients were losing weight at first diagnosis, while 46% had severe weight loss. One third lose more than 10% of total weight, which is considered the cut-off. Progressive weight loss, indeed, is also a common sign in several types of cancer and is associated not only to a poor QoL but also to an increased risk of complications and to a shorter survival [66].

Progressive weight loss is also associated to a decreased response to chemotherapy and to an increased risk of chemotherapy-induced toxicity [67]. Moreover, a higher risk of postoperative complications is also reported: fatigue, poor wound healing, impaired immune competence or inflammatory response, impaired cytotoxic T cell activity are the most common complications which decrease survival [12].

Protein energy malnutrition affects QoL in terms of functional status and welfare [68, 69]. In patients with advanced gastrointestinal cancer, a weight loss of 2.5 kg or more over 2-6 weeks can induce significant alterations in performance status [70]. Amount and speed of weight loss are important key points.

A retrospective study by Andreyev et al [12] confirmed the influence of weight loss on clinical outcome in patients receiving chemotherapy for gastrointestinal cancer. More than 1500 patients were evaluated over six years. Weight loss at presentation was correlated with shorter failure-free and overall survival, decreased response, quality of life and performance status and the authors interpreted this poor outcome as the consequence of the lower dose of chemotherapy patients received. Patients complained of several side-effects caused in part by specific nutritional deficits such as vitamin B6 (pyridoxine) deficiency, palmar-plantar erythrodysesthesia, or association between mucositis and glutamine deficiency.

This study clearly supports the important role of early nutritional intervention in preventing weight loss and correlated poor outcomes. It is clear how malnutrition may cause increased duration of therapy, longer hospital stay and increased healthcare costs. Nutritional counseling and supplementation when needed are of great benefit to patients with low costs [71]. Malone et al [72] reported that malnutrition (defined as a weight loss of more than 10% of total weight over six consecutive months) is a significant preoperative risk factor of nosocomial infections (12.3% vs 7.1% infections of the surgical site, $P = 0.011$).

Malnutrition is also associated to poor prognosis as a cause of high morbidity and mortality rates. Nutritional assessment thus is an essential step in the management of cancer patients. Postoperative nutritional support, then, is mandatory in the early postoperative for all patients undergoing upper gastrointestinal surgery.

Delmore [73] showed a close correlation between low levels of plasma albumin and poor outcomes in cancer patients. Other studies demonstrated that low concentrations of serum albumin were correlated to longer hospital stay, higher medical complications and increased mortality [58, 74] especially in advanced stage disease [75, 76]. Levels of serum albumin are also considered as an independent prognostic factor of overall survival in several types of cancer [77], including gastric cancer [78].

Onate-Ocana et al [78] demonstrated that preoperative very low, low and medium levels of serum albumin were correlated with a median survival of 1.44, 1.96, and 2.62 years, respectively, while high levels of albumin were correlated with a mean survival of 10.68 years ($P < 0.001$).

A careful selection of food, avoiding hyperosmolar starchy food and large volumes, is mandatory in cancer patients [79].

Nutritional support must be offered in order to reverse malnutrition mechanisms, so initial assessment of patient nutritional status and continued evaluation before and after surgery play a key role in tailoring nutritional support. [80]

Diagnosing Malnutrition

Endpoints of nutritional assessment are: identification of those patients who are malnourished or at risk of malnutrition, gathering informations to establish an appropriate nutritional plan for each patient, preservation of adequacy of the plan [81], investigation on causes of malnutrition [82]. All nutritional parameters and indexes have to achieve acceptable sensitivity and specificity in order to best represent the course of malnutrition, from diagnosis to treatment. Evaluation of malnutrition should be combined with patient performance status and QoL in order to adjust nutritional support according to patient nutritional requirements [83]. A standardized tool, therefore, is mandatory as several studies have shown that any single tool used to assess nutritional status is insufficient for the scope. Investigators developed different nutritional indexes which could be used for identification of high-risk patients [84]. Nutritional status scoring systems are usually based on objective measurements such as body weight, oral energy intake, weight loss, levels of serum proteins, loss of subcutaneous fat and immune competence.

All these systems are easy to use, validated in several countries and institutions and accepted by physicians and nursing staff [85]. SGA is a screening tool for determining nutritional depletion, thus identifying patients at risk for malnutrition. It was developed by Detsky et al. [74] in 1987 and adapted to cancer patients by Ottery [86]. SGA is recommended by North America and European guidelines for clinical nutrition as the primary method to assess nutritional status in end-stage renal failure [87]. SGA is based on objective parameters and accurately predicts clinical outcome after major surgery with a sensitivity of 82% and a specificity of 72% [88]. Nutritional risk screening (NRS) is another nutritional index developed by Reilly et al [86]. NRS has been validated for adults and children and it is composed of five items through which it is possible to measure body mass index, appetite, ability to eat spontaneously, weight loss, and concurrent diseases. NRS index allows dividing patients into three categories: minimally, moderately, and severely malnourished patients. Its advantage is easy reproducibility not only by specialized teams but also by different nutrition specialists, such as dietitians and nutritionists. An Icelandic team developed another questionnaire including nine items.

It showed good correlation with objective data when used to identify malnourished inpatients or those at risk of malnutrition [89]. These clinical nutritional assessments, however, need to be combined with different objective variables [90] such as measure of anthropometric data, levels of serum proteins, and impedancemetry data, to complete provided informations.

Recent weight loss is a good indicator of nutritional deficit and it is used to divide patients into different groups according to the severity of malnutrition. Thus, a weight loss of 10% or more of total weight over the previous six months or 5% or more in the previous month indicates an alarming situation and well correlates to clinical outcomes (Table 1). Evaluation of body fat and fat-free mass [91] through subcapsular and triceps skinfold and mid-arm muscle circumference, however, is difficult to assess due to the influence of hydration status on results since range of hydration status values varies by country. These indexes are not validated in cancer patients [92] and reproducibility is poor [93]. Levels of serum proteins such as albumin, transferrin, and transthyretin are usually used to evaluate nutritional status and to control efficacy of nutritional support [94], but these measures may vary in different clinical conditions or diseases such as nephrotic syndrome, liver deficiency, or hyperhydration.

Albumin is usually considered a good marker of nutritional status and visceral proteins amount. NRI (nutritional risk index) was developed by Veteran's Affairs Total Parenteral Nutrition Group in 1991 for evaluation of efficacy of perioperative total parenteral nutrition in patients undergoing thoracic or abdominal surgery. NRI is based on the following equation [95]:

1.519 X [serum albumin] (g/L) + 0.417 X
(current patient weight/usual patient weight x 100).

A range score between 97.5-100 and 83.5-97.5 and a score value of less than 83.5 indicate mild, moderate, and severe malnutrition, respectively. Ryu and Kim [53] showed that NRI and levels of serum albumin exactly evaluated nutritional status of gastric cancer patients. Moreover, reduced levels of albumin, a protein with a half-life of 20 days, indicated a long period of nutritional deficit in absence of clinical conditions which might alter its levels. Several studies showed that malnutrition is not always correlated with low levels of serum proteins, and viceversa.

Levels of transferrin and transthyretin are useless in the evaluation of nutritional status due mainly to a short half-life [96]. These so-called nutritional proteins have been included into different indexes [91] but with limited value, because indexes are usually based on immunological parameters (i.e. lymphocyte count) which can vary regardless of patient nutritional status. New biological measurements, such as levels of IGF-1 (insulin growth factor), are better correlated to nutritional status and nitrogen balance [97]. Alterations in muscle physiological mechanisms occur before changes in levels of serum proteins, so the hand-grip strength test has been proposed as a good indicator of nutritional status [98].

Impedancemetry has been validated for intensive-care patients and has acceptable feasibility even in case of edema or other causes [99, 100]. Impedancemetry can also be used in oncological practice to evaluate nutritional status and assess efficacy of nutritional support. Data on the identification of patients at risk and nutritional assessment in cancer and hematologic patients can be used to build a decisional pathway, in which a specialized nutritional team should be considered, according to Ottery [88].

Screening of malnutrition allows physicians to divide patients into two groups: malnourished and not-malnourished patients. American Society for Parenteral and Enteral Nutrition (ASPEN) guidelines define malnutrition as an involuntary loss or gain of ≥10% of usual body weight in six months or ≥5% of usual body weight in one month [82].

European Society for Parenteral and Enteral Nutrition (ESPEN) guidelines for surgical patients suggest a systematic screening of malnourished patients based on additional criteria: severe nutritional risk defined by a weight loss greater than 10–15% of total weight over six months, BMI less than 18.5 kg/m2, SGA grade C, or serum-albumin concentration less than 30 g/L [62].

Difficulty in obtaining valid conclusions is generally related to the lack of a standardized method to evaluate malnutrition. Wu and colleagues [102] showed exactly this variability. They evaluated the nutritional status of more than four thoUSnd patients using different methods of nutritional assessment. Results varied according to method they used: 21.3% based on BMI and 50.6% based on triceps skinfold thickness assessment. Moreover, SGA or levels of serum prealbumin, showed a range between 35.4 and 38.8% while BMI was 24.2% according to levels of serum albumin. This variability was also experienced in Europe. Norman and colleagues [103] evaluated 287 patients and found that almost 30% of them presented with malnutrition according to SGA but only 3.8% according to BMI. The threshold for malnutrition was 18.5% if SGA was used alone. Method of nutritional assessment, then, influences early diagnosis and treatment of malnutrition.

Table 1. Classification of nutritional status according to weight loss and loss time interval. (Weight loss is calculated on the percentage of usual weight) [53]

Time	Mild malnutrition (Weight loss)	Severe malnutrition (Weight loss)
1 week	1-2 %	>2 %
1 month	5 %	>5 %
3 months	7.5 %	7.5 %
6 months	10 %	>10 %

Four parameters are usually used to assess patient nutritional status: loss of body weight, levels of plasma proteins, anthropometric measurements and prognostic nutritional indexes (PNI). All these tools provide useful informations when used singularly, but have some drawbacks, so none of them may be considered as the gold standard. Several methods assess nutritional status in cancer patients, but have both advantages and disadvantages [105]. The most frequently used are subjective global assessment (SGA) [106, 107], bioelectrical impedance analysis (BIA), and laboratory measurements of different parameters such as levels of serum albumin [108, 109], prealbumin, and transferrin [74, 110]. Other methods include anthropometric data [111, 112], such as weight loss, arm-muscle circumference, skin-fold thickness [113] and presence of edema and ascites [114].

SGA is an inexpensive and non-invasive, easy method to use, but it is operator-dependent. BIA is also easy to use, non-invasive, and reproducible. Measure of levels of serum albumin is a simple method to gather informations on visceral-protein functions. Normal range of this protein is 3.5-5.0 g/dl, in adults. Hypoalbuminaemia is a condition when serum albumin levels are less than 3.5 g/dl [115, 116]. Malnutrition and inflammation suppress synthesis of albumin [117]. Systemic inflammatory response to cancer causes, in addition, release of proinflammatory cytokines and growth factors with a consequential catabolic effect on patient metabolism [118, 119]. IL-6, indeed, induces liver to produce acute-phase reaction proteins (such as C-reactive protein and fibrinogen) which increase the request for specific amino acids. If those amino acids are not supplied in diet, they can be recycled from skeletal muscles with consequent fibers disruption. IL-6 also modulates production of albumin by hepatocytes, thus reducing concentration of serum albumin [120]. Tumor necrosis factor may increase permeability of the microvasculature allowing an increased transcapillary transfer of albumin. Liver micrometastases may induce kupffer cells to produce a variety of cytokines (IL-Ib, IL-6, or TNF), which may also modulate synthesis of albumin by liver cells. Levels of serum albumin decrease with disease progression [75, 76].

Level of serum albumin is, therefore, used to assess nutritional status, severity of disease, disease progression, and prognosis. Several studies correlated serum levels of albumin with hospital mortality [76, 121, 122], length of stay [123, 124] and nosocomial infections [125]. Levels of serum albumin are, therefore, considered not only as an indicator of patient nutritional status, but also as a predictor of outcome [126, 127]. Evaluation of levels of serum albumin is an inexpensive, reproducible, and powerful method [128] for establishing the need of aggressive nutritional approach [129]. It has also several biases, such as the difficulty of interpretation due to non-nutritional factors (i.e. hydration or disease process) which may alter the effects of nutritional depletion [130]. More studies are necessary to define the exact role of each method, to identify the gold standard, and make easier and reproducible evaluations in order to obtain valid conclusions.

Nutritional Support

Perioperative nutritional support can reduce postoperative complications in malnourished patients. There are, however, some risks, such as infections, etc. The use of nutrition support — total parenteral nutrition (TPN) or enteral feedings (EF) — before and after surgery depends on grade of malnutrition and type of surgical procedure (type of procedure and/or elective/emergency set). Several studies showed that specific subsets of patients have worse outcomes after administration of TPN than those submitted to standard care plan [73, 131-133]. A careful selection of patients who should receive nutritional support and a correct nutritional plan is mandatory.

Preoperative TPN

Several studies examined effects of preoperative TPN on patients outcome showing, however, heterogeneous results. Veterans Affairs Total Parenteral Nutrition Cooperative Study [73] provided important informations. Three hundred ninety-five malnourished patients, who required elective laparotomies or thoracotomies without vascular or cardiac procedures, were enrolled in this study. Fifty-one percent of these patients had gastrointestinal cancer. Patients were randomly assigned either to receive perioperative TPN (7-15 days preoperatively and three days postoperatively) or no TPN (control group). Analysis of results 90 days after treatment showed a prevalence of infectious complications, such as pneumonia or bacteremia, in TPN group (14.1% vs 6.4%; $P = 0.01$) while prevalence of noninfectious complications (cardiovascular and respiratory failure) was higher in the control group (22.2% vs 16.7%; $P = 0.2$). Authors justify the prevalence of infections in TPN group asserting that these patients received a high-caloric regimen (nearly 45 kcal/kg/day), which could cause hyperglycemia, a well-known risk factor for infections. Moreover, they found an excess of infections in all subgroups who received TPN with either borderline or mild malnutrition. Conversely, severely malnourished patients (NRI < 83.5) receiving TPN had fewer noninfectious complications than control group (5% vs 43%; $P = 0.03$) and no increase in infectious complications. This group had also fewer major complications with TPN (21% vs 47%; $P = 0.12$).

Bozzetti and colleagues [134] randomly assigned 90 patients diagnosed with gastric or colorectal cancer to perioperative parenteral nutrition or to control group (no TPN). Postoperative morbidity reduced by 20% ($P = 0.03$) in patients receiving TPN. A meta-analysis [135] of 27 randomized studies on perioperative TPN, however, concluded that TPN had no effect on mortality but was associated to fewer major complications. Authors found also a trend to fewer deaths and complications in TPN patients in studies published before 1988 but curiously not in later studies. The reason is still unknown, but they suggested that applied methods in later studies were superior in quality than previous methods.

Another study [136] showed that malnourished patients receiving preoperative TPN over 7-10 days had a reduction of postoperative complications by 10%. A meta-analysis of the American Gastroenterological Association Position Paper on TPN, however, found that preoperative TPN had no effect on perioperative complications [137]. This study included trials on patients with stomach and esophageal carcinoma and found a reduction of major complications with an estimated risk difference of 18%. Pooled data, however, failed to confirm that perioperative nutrition improves postoperative mortality rate, but this meta-analysis had some important biases such as significant heterogeneity of patients, small sample, treatment and method between studies, short duration of preoperative nutrition and unsuitability of caloric intake in several studies. More well-designed studies will be necessary to achieve valid conclusions. Despite these findings, patients with gastric cancer who undergo total gastrectomy usually receive TPN over 7–10 days after surgery because of the concern on the integrity of the esophago-jejunal anastomosis [35, 36].

Some authors argued against a role of artificial feeding after total gastrectomy because it fails to impact on postoperative complications. Ryan and colleagues [39] found that total gastrectomy is associated to high weight loss with a mean loss of 15.5 kg after three-month of follow up. This study showed that TPN reduces postoperatively in-hospital weight loss and further post-discharge weight loss. TPN patients seemed to benefit from nutritional support at long-term. Further randomized controlled trials on nutritional support in gastrectomized patients are needed.

Preoperative Enteral Nutrition

Few reports analyzed early enteral feeding after total gastrectomy either by nasojejunal tube feeding or percutaneous catheter jejunostomy. Lim et al. [138] found lower rates of morbidity and mortality in patients receiving TPN compared to enteral nutrition, but difference was not statistically significant. Sako et al. [139] found no difference in postoperative complications and mortality rates in patients who received preoperative TPN compared to those who received enteral nutrition.

Postoperative TPN

Several studies examined the effects of postoperative TPN on patients outcome. Yamada et al. [140] reported that cancer patients receiving postoperative TPN had fewer postoperative complications, higher survival rate, body weight, serum levels of albumin and total lymphocyte counts compared to those receiving oral intake. Authors argued that the reason of this better outcome would be a higher tolerance to chemotherapy. A meta-analysis by Klein et al. [136] showed an incidence of complications of more than 10% in patients receiving routine postoperative TPN. These results are also confirmed by Torosian et al. [141]. Conversely, Collins et al. [142] reported that TPN may help to increase wound-healing rates and showed a lower incidence of postoperative sepsis compared to amino-acid solution or oral intake regimen. Other studies [143, 144] found no reduction in colonic fistula rates after colonic anastomosis in patients submitted to a regimen of postoperative TPN for six days compared to oral intake alone and no difference in morbidity and mortality rates after major thoracoabdominal procedures in patients treated with postoperative TPN for seven days compared to a control group who received a standard regimen of common postoperative fluids.

Postoperative Enteral Nutrition

Few studies analyzed the use of enteral nutrition in the postoperative. Some studies showed that EN (enteral nutrition) may improve wound healing, may reduce septic complications, length of stay and hyper metabolic response. [145, 146]. A review of five studies which prospectively compared postoperative enteral vs parenteral nutrition, however, reported similar morbidity and mortality rates [147].

Heyland et al [135] asserted that enteral nutrition significantly reduces complication rate than TPN. In their meta-analysis, Braunschweig et al presented the effects of enteral or parenteral nutrition on adults suffering from gastrointestinal cancer and undergoing surgery. Pooled analysis showed that tube feeding was associated to lower risk of infection than TPN (relative risk 0.66, 95% CI 0.56–0.79). Mortality and infectious complications were higher in patients with severe protein caloric malnutrition [156].

Candidates to Receive Nutritional Support

Nutritional support is generally indicated in patients who are unable or unwilling to consume, digest, and assimilate adequate nutrients "per os". Not all patients who cannot eat for a few days, however, are candidates, but only those who may benefit from nutritional support with less risk. Preoperative support should be administered in case of severe malnutrition or if required by surgical procedure (i.e. major abdominal or thoracic surgery) or in case of elective surgery in which it is possible to submit patient to nutritional regimen for 7 to 10 days before surgery. This is the time needed for a correct preoperative nutritional support [148].

Nutritional support should be given enterally if the access to the gastrointestinal tract is available and formula tolerance is demonstrated. TPN is the preferred method of feeding if enteral nutrition is not applicable.

Postoperative nutritional support should be generally administered to mildly malnourished patients who cannot tolerate an oral diet for 7-10 days after surgery or to severely malnourished patients for 5-7 days after surgery [141]. Postoperative nutritional support may depend on preoperative surgical assessment which indicates patient not to suitable to resume oral intake within 7-10 days from surgery.

In conclusion, enteral nutrition is preferred to TPN, whenever possible, because it is safer, more cost-effective and associated to similar or better outcomes.

Immunonutrition: A Special Type of Nutritional Support

Immune-enhancing formulas are intended to strengthen immune system functions in stressed patients. These enteral formulas usually contain supplements of arginine, RNA, and omega-3 fatty acids. This area of research is relatively new, and several studies evaluated the use of these formulas in perioperative patients. Daly et al. [149] analyzed the effects of such a formula in patients undergoing elective surgery for gastrointestinal malignancies and found significant fewer infections and wound complications (11% vs 37%).

Other studies showed reduced length of hospital stay and postoperative complications [150, 151]. Summit on Immune-Enhancing Enteral Therapy [152] recommended the use of these formulas in specific groups of patients, including malnourished patients undergoing elective gastrointestinal surgery. Recommendations, however, were not officially endorsed by American Society for Parenteral and Enteral Nutrition. Better knowledge of content of this type of formulas and its indications are needed.

Conclusion

Malnutrition is common in gastrointestinal cancer patients, especially in gastrectomized patients and causes are often complex and multifactorial. Although several parameters are related to postoperative complications in patients who underwent gastrectomy for gastric cancer, preoperative weight loss seems to be the most important factor associated to higher risk of postoperative complications and higher mortality. Malnutrition affects, indeed, postoperative outcomes and, therefore, the prognosis, and, however, a key-role of perioperative nutritional support in reducing surgical risk or complications in malnourished cancer patients is equivocal. Nutritional support should be considered in postoperative patients who cannot eat for 7-10 days after surgery. Enteral nutrition is preferred to TPN, whenever possible, because it is safer and more cost-effective.

References

[1] Allison S. P. Malnutrition, disease, and outcome. *Nutrition*, 2000;16:590-593.

[2] Elia M. Guidelines for detection and management of malnutrition. Malnutrition Advisory Group (MAG), standing committee of BAPEN. 2000, Maidenhead.

[3] Walesby R. K., Goode A. W., Spinks T. J., Herring A., Ranicar A. S., Bentall H. H. Nutritional status of patients requiring cardiac surgery. *J Thorac. Cardiovasc. Surg.*, 1979;77:570-576.

[4] Bistrian B. R., Blackburn G. L., Vitale J., Cochran D., Naylor J. Prevalence of malnutrition in general medical patients. *JAMA*, 1976;235:1567-1570.

[5] Agradi E., Messina V., Campanella G., Venturini M., Caruso M., Moresco A., Giacchero A., Ferrari N., Ravera E. Hospital malnutrition: incidence and prospective evaluation of general medical patients during hospitalization. *Acta Vitaminol Enzymol*, 1984;6:235-242.

[6] Mullen J. L., Gertner M. H., Buzby G. P., Goodhart G. L., Rosato E. F. Implications of malnutrition in the surgical patient. *Arch. Surg.*, 1979;114:121-125.

[7] Doerr T. D., Marks S. C., Shamsa F. H., Mathog R. H., Prasad A. S. Effects of zinc and nutritional status on clinical outcomes in head and neck cancer. *Nutrition*, 1998;14: 489-495.

[8] Pablo A. M., Izaga M. A., Alday L. A. Assessment of nutritional status on hospital admission: nutritional scores. *Eur. J. Clin. Nutr.*, 2003;57:824-831.

[9] Bosaeus I., Daneryd P., Svanberg E., Lundholm K. Dietary intake and resting energy expenditure in relation to weight loss in unselected cancer patients. *Int. J. Cancer*, 2001;93:380-383.

[10] Bozzetti F. Nutrition support in patients with cancer. In Payne-James J, Grimble G, Silk DBA (Eds), *Artificial Nutrition Support in Clinical Practice*, 2nd Edition, 2001, Greenwich Medical Media, London, pp. 639-680.

[11] Ottery F. D. Cancer cachexia: prevention, early diagnosis, and management. *Cancer Pract.*, 1994;2:123-131.

[12] Andreyev H. J., Norman A. R., Oates J., Cunningham D. Why do patients with weight loss have a worse outcome when undergoing chemotherapy for gastrointestinal malignancies? *Eur. J. Cancer.*, 1998;34:503-509.

[13] Tian J., Chen J. S. Nutritional status and quality of life of the gastric cancer patients in Changle County of China. *World J. Gastroenterol.*, 2005;11:1582-1586.

[14] van Bokhorst-de van der S., van Leeuwen P. A., Kuik D. J., Klop W. M., Sauerwein H. P., Snow G. B., Quak J. J. The impact of nutritional status on the prognoses of patients with advanced head and neck cancer. *Cancer*, 1999;86:519-527.

[15] Lacquaniti A., Bolignano D., Campo S., Perrone C., Donato V., Fazio M. R., Buemi A., Sturiale A., Buemi M.. Malnutrition in the elderly patient on dialysis. *Ren. Fail.*, 2009;31:239-245.

[16] Kyle U. G., Pirlich M., Schuetz T., Lochs H., Pichard C. Is nutritional depletion by Nutritional Risk Index associated with increased length of hospital stay? A population-based study. *JPEN J. Parenter. Enteral. Nutr.*, 2004;28:99-104.

[17] Pirlich M., Lochs H. Nutrition in the elderly. *Best Pract. Res. Clin. Gastroenterol*, 2001;15:869-884.

[18] Wu C. W., Chang I. S., Lo S. S., Hsieh M. C., Chen J. H., Lui W. Y., Whang-Peng J. Complications following D3 gastrectomy: post hoc analysis of a randomized trial. *World. J. Surg.*, 2006;30:12-16.

[19] Gupta D., Lis C. G., Granick J., Grutsch J. F., Vashi P. G., Lammersfeld C. A. Malnutrition was associated with poor quality of life in colorectal cancer: a retrospective analysis. *J. Clin. Epidemiol.*, 2006;59:704-709.

[20] Rivadeneira D. E., Evoy D., Fahey T. J., 3rd, Lieberman M. D., Daly J. M. Nutritional support of the cancer patient. *C. A Cancer J. Clin.*, 1998;48:69-80.

[21] Mutlu E. A., Mobarhan S. Nutrition in the care of the cancer patient. *Nutrition in clinical care*, 2000;3:3-23.

[22] Lesko L. M. Psychosocial issues in the diagnosis and management of cancer cachexia and anorexia. *Nutrition*, 1989;5:114-116.

[23] Padilla G. V. Psychological aspects of nutrition and cancer. *Surgical Clinics of North America*, 1986;66:1121-1135.

[24] Beer T. M., Eilers K. M., Garzotto M., Hsieh Y. C., Mori M. Quality of life and pain relief during treatment with calcitriol and docetaxel in symptomatic metastatic androgen-independent prostate carcinoma. *Cancer*, 2004;100:758-763.

[25] Holmes S. Cancer Chemotherapy: A guide to practice. 1997, Asset Books, Leatherhead.

[26] Barber M. D., Ross J. A., Fearon K. C. Cancer cachexia. *Surgical Oncology*, 1999;8:133-141.

[27] Davis M. P., Dreicer R., Walsh D., Lagman R., LeGrand S. B. Appetite and cancer-associated anorexia: a review. *Journal of Clinical Oncology*, 2004;22:1510-1517.

[28] Tisdale M. J. Cancer anorexia and cachexia. *Nutrition*, 2001;17:438-442.

[29] Grant M., Kravits K. Symptoms and their impact on nutrition. Semin *Oncol. Nurs.*, 2000;16:113-121.

[30] Ravasco P., Monteiro-Grillo I., Vidal P. M., Camilo M. E. Cancer: disease and nutrition are key determinants of patients' quality of life. *Support Care Cancer*, 2004;12: 246-252.

[31] Langer C. J., Hoffman J. P., Ottery F. D. Clinical significance of weight loss in cancer patients: rationale for the use of anabolic agents in the treatment of cancer-related cachexia. *Nutrition*, 2001;17:S1-20.

[32] Heber D., Byerley L. O., Tchekmedyian N. S. Hormonal and metabolic abnormalities in the malnourished cancer patient: effects on host-tumor interaction. *JPEN J. Parenter. Enteral. Nutr.*, 1992;16:60S-64S.

[33] Smith K. L., Tisdale M. J. Increased protein degradation and decreased protein synthesis in skeletal muscle during cancer cachexia. *Br. J. Cancer*, 1993;67:680-685.

[34] Rofe A. M., Bourgeois C. S., Coyle P., Taylor A., Abdi E. A. Altered insulin response to glucose in weight-losing cancer patients. *Anticancer. Res.*, 1994;14:647-650.

[35] McAndrew P. F. Fat metabolism and cancer. *Surg. Clin. North Am.,* 1986;66: 1003-1012.

[36] Falconer J. S., Fearon K. C., Plester C. E., Ross J. A., Carter D. C. Cytokines, the acute-phase response, and resting energy expenditure in cachectic patients with pancreatic cancer. *Ann. Surg.*, 1994;219:325-331.

[37] Braga M., Vignali A., Gianotti L., Cestari A., Profili M., Carlo V. D. Immune and nutritional effects of early enteral nutrition after major abdominal operations. *Eur. J. Surg.*, 1996;162:105-112.

[38] Liedman B. Symptoms after total gastrectomy on food intake, body composition, bone metabolism, and quality of life in gastric cancer patients--is reconstruction with a reservoir worthwhile? *Nutrition*, 1999;15:677-682.

[39] Ryan A. M., Healy L. A., Power D. G., Rowley S. P., Reynolds J. V. Short-term nutritional implications of total gastrectomy for malignancy, and the impact of parenteral nutritional support. *Clin. Nutr.*, 2007;26:718-727.

[40] Bragelmann R., Armbrecht U., Rosemeyer D., Schneider B., Zilly W., Stockbrugger R. W. Nutrient malassimilation following total gastrectomy. *Scand. J. Gastroenterol Suppl.*, 1996;218:26-33.

[41] Armbrecht U., Lundell L., Lindstedt G., Stockbruegger R. W. Causes of malabsorption after total gastrectomy with Roux-en-Y reconstruction. *Acta. Chir. Scand.*, 1988;154:37-41.

[42] Bae J. M., Park J. W., Yang H. K., Kim J. P. Nutritional status of gastric cancer patients after total gastrectomy. *World J. Surg.*, 1998;22:254-260.

[43] Cristallo M., Braga M., Agape D., Primignani M., Zuliani W., Vecchi M., Murone M., Sironi M., Di Carlo V., De Franchis R. Nutritional status, function of the small intestine and jejunal morphology after total gastrectomy for carcinoma of the stomach. *Surg. Gynecol. Obstet.*, 1986;163:225-230.

[44] Bozzetti F., Gianotti L., Braga M., Di Carlo V., Mariani L. Postoperative complications in gastrointestinal cancer patients: the joint role of the nutritional status and the nutritional support. *Clin. Nutr.*, 2007;26: 698-709.

[45] Blackburn G. L., Bistrian B. R., Maini B. S., Schlamm H. T., Smith M. F. Nutritional and metabolic assessment of the hospitalized patient. *JPEN J. Parenter Enteral. Nutr.*, 1977;1:11-22.

[46] Falconer J. S., Fearon K. C., Ross J. A., Elton R., Wigmore S. J., Garden O. J., Carter D. C. Acute-phase protein response and survival duration of patients with pancreatic cancer. *Cancer*, 1995;75:2077-2082.

[47] Pham N. V., Cox-Reijven P. L., Wodzig W. K., Greve J. W., Soeters P. B. SGA and measures for muscle mass and strength in surgical Vietnamese patients. *Nutrition*, 2007;23:283-291.

[48] Copland L., Liedman B., Rothenberg E., Bosaeus I. Effects of nutritional support long time after total gastrectomy. *Clin. Nutr.*, 2007;26:605-613.

[49] Braga M., Molinari M., Zuliani W., Foppa L., Gianotti L., Radaelli G., Cristallo M., Di Carlo V. Surgical treatment of gastric adenocarcinoma: impact on survival and quality of life. A prospective ten year study. *Hepatogastroenterology*, 1996;43:187-193.

[50] Liedman B., Andersson H., Berglund B., Bosaeus I., Hugosson I., Olbe L., Lundell L. Food intake after gastrectomy for gastric carcinoma: the role of a gastric reservoir. *Br. J. Surg.*, 1996;83:1138-1143.

[51] Studley H. O. Percentage of weight loss: a basic indicator of surgical risk in patients with chronic peptic ulcer. *JAMA*, 1936;1936:4-459.

[52] Windsor J. A., Hill G. L. Risk factors for postoperative pneumonia. The importance of protein depletion. *Ann. Surg.*, 1988;208:209-214.

[53] Ryu S. W., Kim I. H. Comparison of different nutritional assessments in detecting malnutrition among gastric cancer patients. *World J. Gastroenterol*, 2010;16: 3310-3317.

[54] Giner M., Laviano A., Meguid M. M., Gleason J. R. In 1995 a correlation between malnutrition and poor outcome in critically ill patients still exists. *Nutrition*, 1996;12:23-29.

[55] Sungurtekin H., Sungurtekin U., Balci C., Zencir M., Erdem E. The influence of nutritional status on complications after major intraabdominal surgery. *J. Am. Coll. Nutr.*, 2004;23:227-232.

[56] Pacelli F., Bossola M., Rosa F., Tortorelli A. P., Papa V., Doglietto G. B. Is malnutrition still a risk factor of postoperative complications in gastric cancer surgery? *Clin. Nutr.*, 2008;27:398-407.

[57] Gil-Rendo A., Hernandez-Lizoain J. L., Martinez-Regueira F., Sierra Martinez A., Rotellar Sastre F., Cervera Delgado M., Valenti Azcarate V., Pastor Idoate C., Alvarez-Cienfuegos J. Risk factors related to operative morbidity in patients undergoing gastrectomy for gastric cancer. *Clin. Transl. Oncol.*, 2006;8:354-361.

[58] Gibbs J., Cull W., Henderson W., Daley J., Hur K., Khuri S. F. Preoperative serum albumin level as a predictor of operative mortality and morbidity: results from the National VA Surgical Risk Study. *Arch. Surg.,* 1999;134:36-42.

[59] Saito A., Noguchi Y., Yoshikawa T., Doi C., Fukuzawa K., Matsumoto A., Ito T., Tsuburaya A., Nagahara N. Gastrectomized patients are in a state of chronic protein malnutrition analyses of 23 amino acids. *Hepatogastroenterology*, 2001;48:585-589.

[60] Kiyama T., Mizutani T., Okuda T., Fujita I., Tokunaga A., Tajiri T., Barbul A. Postoperative changes in body composition after gastrectomy. *J. Gastrointest. Surg.*, 2005;9:313-319.

[61] Kodera Y., Sasako M., Yamamoto S., Sano T., Nashimoto A., Kurita A. Identification of risk factors for the development of complications following extended and superextended lymphadenectomies for gastric cancer. *Br. J. Surg.*, 2005;92:1103-1109.

[62] Weimann A., Braga M., Harsanyi L., Laviano A., Ljungqvist O., Soeters P., Jauch K. W., Kemen M., Hiesmayr J. M., Horbach T., Kuse E. R., Vestweber K. H.. ESPEN Guidelines on Enteral Nutrition: Surgery including organ transplantation. *Clin. Nutr.*, 2006;25:224-244.

[63] Harris A. M., Griffin S. M. Postoperative taste and smell deficit after upper gastrointestinal cancer surgery--an unreported complication. *J. Surg. Oncol.*, 2003;82:147-150.

[64] O'Gorman P., McMillan D. C., McArdle C. S. Prognostic factors in advanced gastrointestinal cancer patients with weight loss. *Nutr. Cancer*, 2000;37:36-40.

[65] Sanchez-Bueno F., Garcia-Marcilla J. A., Perez-Flores D., Perez-Abad J. M., Vicente R., Aranda F., Ramirez P., Parrilla P. Prognostic factors in a series of 297 patients with gastric adenocarcinoma undergoing surgical resection. *Br. J. Surg.*, 1998;85:255-260.

[66] Laviano A., Meguid M. M. Nutritional issues in cancer management. *Nutrition*, 1996;12:358-371.

[67] Tisdale M. J. Wasting in cancer. *J. Nutr.*, 1999;129:243S-246S.

[68] Liedman B., Andersson H., Bosaeus I., Hugosson I., Lundell L. Changes in body composition after gastrectomy: results of a controlled, prospective clinical trial. *World. J. Surg.*, 1997;21:416-420.

[69] Crogan N. L., Pasvogel A. The influence of protein-calorie malnutrition on quality of life in nursing homes. *J. Gerontol. A Biol. Sci. Med. Sci.*, 2003;58:159-164.

[70] Peltz G. Nutrition support in cancer patients: a brief review and suggestion for standard indications criteria. *Nutr. J.*, 2002;1:1.

[71] Edington J., Boorman J., Durrant E. R., Perkins A., Giffin C. V., James R., Thomson J. M., Oldroyd J. C., Smith J. C., Torrance A. D., Blackshaw V., Green S., Hill C. J., Berry C., McKenzie C., Vicca N., Ward J. E., Coles S. J. Prevalence of malnutrition on admission to four hospitals in England. The Malnutrition Prevalence Group. *Clin. Nutr.*, 2000;19:191-195.

[72] Malone D. L., Genuit T., Tracy J. K., Gannon C., Napolitano L. M. Surgical site infections: reanalysis of risk factors. *J. Surg. Res.*, 2002;103:89-95.

[73] The Veterans Affairs Total Parenteral Nutrition Cooperative Study Group. Perioperative total parenteral nutrition in surgical patients. *N. Engl. J. Med.*, 1991;325:525-532.

[74] Delmore G. Assessment of nutritional status in cancer patients: widely neglected? *Support Care Cancer*, 1997;5:376-380.

[75] McMillan D. C., Watson W. S., O'Gorman P., Preston T., Scott H. R., McArdle C. S. Albumin concentrations are primarily determined by the body cell mass and the systemic inflammatory response in cancer patients with weight loss. *Nutr. Cancer*, 2001;39:210-213.

[76] Sacks G. S., Dearman K., Replogle W. H., Cora V. L., Meeks M., Canada T. Use of subjective global assessment to identify nutrition-associated complications and death in geriatric long-term care facility residents. *J. Am. Coll. Nutr.*, 2000;19:570-577.

[77] Maltoni M., Amadori D. Prognosis in advanced cancer. *Hematol. Oncol. Clin. North Am.*, 2002;16:715-729.

[78] Onate-Ocana L. F., Aiello-Crocifoglio V., Gallardo-Rincon D., Herrera-Goepfert R., Brom-Valladares R., Carrillo J. F., Cervera E., Mohar-Betancourt A. Serum albumin as a significant prognostic factor for patients with gastric carcinoma. *Ann. Surg. Oncol.*, 2007;14:381-389.

[79] Friess H., Bohm J., Muller M. W., Glasbrenner B., Riepl R. L., Malfertheiner P., Buchler M. W. Maldigestion after total gastrectomy is associated with pancreatic insufficiency. *Am. J. Gastroenterol.*, 1996;91:341-347.

[80] Hill G. L., Blackett R. L., Pickford I., Burkinshaw L., Young G. A., Warren J. V., Schorah C. J., Morgan D. B. Malnutrition in surgical patients. An unrecognised problem. *Lancet*, 1977;1:689-692.

[81] Wong P. W., Enriquez A., Barrera R. Nutritional support in critically ill patients with cancer. *Crit. Care Clin.*, 2001;17:743-767.

[82] ASPEN Board of Directors and the Clinical Guidelines Task Force. Guidelines for the use of parenteral and enteral nutrition in adult and pediatric patients. *JPEN J. Parenter Enteral. Nutr.*, 2002;26:1SA-138SA.

[83] Grindel C. G., Whitmer K., Barsevick A. Quality of life and nutritional support in patients with cancer. *Cancer Pract.*, 1996;4:81-87.

[84] Ottery F. D. Supportive nutrition to prevent cachexia and improve quality of life. *Semin. Oncol.*, 1995;22:98-111.

[85] Jones H. J., de Cossart L. Risk scoring in surgical patients. *Br. J. Surg.*, 1999;86: 149-157.

[86] Detsky A. S., McLaughlin J. R., Baker J. P., Johnston N., Whittaker S., Mendelson R. A., Jeejeebhoy K. N. What is subjective global assessment of nutritional status? *JPEN J. Parenter Enteral. Nutr.*, 1987;11:8-13.

[87] Jones C. H., Wolfenden R. C., Wells L. M. Is subjective global assessment a reliable measure of nutritional status in hemodialysis? *J. Ren. Nutr.,* 2004;14:26-30.

[88] Ottery F. D. Definition of standardized nutritional assessment and interventional pathways in oncology. *Nutrition*, 1996;12:S15-19.

[89] Reilly J. J., Wilson J., Durnin J. V. Determination of body composition from skinfold thickness: a validation study. *Arch. Dis. Child*, 1995;73:305-310.

[90] Thorsdottir I., Eriksen B., Eysteinsdottir S. Nutritional status at submission for dietetic services and screening for malnutrition at admission to hospital. *Clin. Nutr.*, 1999;18:15-21.

[91] Nitenberg G., Raynard B. Nutritional support of the cancer patient: issues and dilemmas. *Crit. Rev. Oncol. Hematol.*, 2000;34:137-168.

[92] Durnin J. V., Womersley J. Body fat assessed from total body density and its estimation from skinfold thickness: measurements on 481 men and women aged from 16 to 72 years. *Br. J. Nutr.*, 1974;32:77-97.

[93] Constans T., Bacq Y., Bertrand P., Beaugerie A., Babault C., Delarue J., Lamisse F. The American anthropometric norms are not suitable to assess the nutritional status of a French population. *Clin. Nutr.*, 1990;9:168-171.

[94] Hall J. C., O'Quigley J., Giles G. R., Appleton N., Stocks H. Upper limb anthropometry: the value of measurement variance studies. *Am. J. Clin. Nutr.*, 1980;33:1846-1851.

[95] Inoue Y., Nezu R., Matsuda H., Takagi Y., Okada A. Rapid turnover proteins as a prognostic indicator in cancer patients. *Surg. Today*, 1995;25:498-506.

[96] Delgado-Rodriguez M., Medina-Cuadros M., Gomez-Ortega A., Martinez-Gallego G., Mariscal-Ortiz M., Martinez-Gonzalez M. A., Sillero-Arenas M. Cholesterol and serum albumin levels as predictors of cross infection, death, and length of hospital stay. *Arch. Surg.*, 2002;137:805-812.

[97] Ingenbleek Y., Carpentier Y. A. A. prognostic inflammatory and nutritional index scoring critically ill patients. *Int. J. Vitam. Nutr. Res.*, 1985;55:91-101.

[98] Donahue S. P., Phillips L. S. Response of IGF-1 to nutritional support in malnourished hospital patients: a possible indicator of short-term changes in nutritional status. *Am. J. Clin. Nutr.*, 1989;50:962-969.

[99] Kalfarentzos F., Spiliotis J., Velimezis G., Dougenis D., Androulakis J. Comparison of forearm muscle dynamometry with nutritional prognostic index, as a preoperative indicator in cancer patients. *JPEN. J. Parenter Enteral. Nutr.*, 1989;13:34-36.

[100] Fredrix E. W., Saris W. H., Soeters P. B., Wouters E. F., Kester A. D., von Meyenfeldt M. F., Westerterp K. R. Estimation of body composition by bioelectrical impedance in cancer patients. *Eur. J. Clin. Nutr.*, 1990;44:749-752.

[101] Desport J. C., Courat L., Preux P. M., Pillegand B., Sautereau D. Étude des malnutritions de l'adulte avec et sans œdèmes dépistées lors de la consultation de nutrition d'un hôpital universitaire. *Nutrition Clinique et Métabolisme*, 1999;13:25-34.

[102] Tchekmedyian N. S. Pharmacoeconomics of nutritional support in cancer. *Semin. Oncol.*, 1998;25:62-69.

[103] Wu G. H., Liu Z. H., Zheng L. W., Quan Y. J., Wu Z. H. [Prevalence of malnutrition in general surgical patients: evaluation of nutritional status and prognosis]. *Zhonghua Wai Ke Za Zhi*, 2005;43:693-696.

[104] Norman K., Schutz T., Kemps M., Josef Lubke H., Lochs H., Pirlich M. The Subjective Global Assessment reliably identifies malnutrition-related muscle dysfunction. *Clin. Nutr.*, 2005;24:143-150.

[105] Sarhill N., Mahmoud F. A., Christie R., Tahir A. Assessment of nutritional status and fluid deficits in advanced cancer. *Am. J. Hosp. Palliat. Care*, 2003;20:465-473.

[106] Bauer J., Capra S., Ferguson M. Use of the scored Patient-Generated Subjective Global Assessment (PG-SGA) as a nutrition assessment tool in patients with cancer. *Eur. J. Clin. Nutr.*, 2002;56:779-785.

[107] Gupta D., Lammersfeld C. A., Vashi P. G., Burrows J., Lis C. G., Grutsch J. F. Prognostic significance of Subjective Global Assessment (SGA) in advanced colorectal cancer. *Eur. J. Clin. Nutr.*, 2005;59:35-40.

[108] Gupta D., Lammersfeld C. A., Burrows J. L., Dahlk S. L., Vashi P. G., Grutsch J. F., Hoffman S., Lis C. G. Bioelectrical impedance phase angle in clinical practice: implications for prognosis in advanced colorectal cancer. *Am. J. Clin. Nutr.*, 2004;80:1634-1638.

[109] McIntosh E. N., Laurent L. L. Nutritional assessment of the hospitalized patient. *Am. Fam. Physician*, 1983;27:169-175.

[110] Boles J. M., Garre M. A., Youinou P. Y. Simple assessment of the nutritional status in the critically ill patient. *Resuscitation*, 1984;11: 233-241.

[111] Curtas S., Chapman G., Meguid M. M. Evaluation of nutritional status. *Nurs. Clin. North Am.*, 1989;24:301-313.

[112] Slaviero K. A., Read J. A., Clarke S. J., Rivory L. P. Baseline nutritional assessment in advanced cancer patients receiving palliative chemotherapy. *Nutr. Cancer*, 2003;46:148-157.

[113] Davies M. Nutritional screening and assessment in cancer-associated malnutrition. *Eur. J. Oncol. Nurs.*, 2005;9 Suppl. 2:S64-73.

[114] Duguet A., Bachmann P., Lallemand Y., Blanc-Vincent M. P. [Good clinical practice in nutritional management in cancer patients: malnutrition and nutritional assessment]. *Bull Cancer*, 1999;86: 997-1016.

[115] Di Fiore F., Lecleire S., Pop D., Rigal O., Hamidou H., Paillot B., Ducrotte P., Lerebours E., Michel P. Baseline nutritional status is predictive of response to treatment and survival in patients treated by definitive chemoradiotherapy for a locally advanced esophageal cancer. *Am. J. Gastroenterol.*, 2007;102:2557-2563.

[116] Ishizuka M., Nagata H., Takagi K., Horie T., Kubota K. Inflammation-based prognostic score is a novel predictor of postoperative outcome in patients with colorectal cancer. *Ann. Surg.*, 2007;246:1047-1051.

[117] Yeun J. Y., Kaysen G. A. Factors influencing serum albumin in dialysis patients. *Am. J. Kidney Dis.*, 1998;32:S118-125.

[118] Simons J. P., Schols A. M., Buurman W. A., Wouters E. F. Weight loss and low body cell mass in males with lung cancer: relationship with systemic inflammation, acute-phase response, resting energy expenditure, and catabolic and anabolic hormones. *Clin. Sci.* (Lond), 1999;97:215-223.

[119] O'Gorman P., McMillan D. C., McArdle C. S. Impact of weight loss, appetite, and the inflammatory response on quality of life in gastrointestinal cancer patients. *Nutr. Cancer*, 1998;32:76-80.

[120] Barber M. D., Ross J. A., Fearon K. C. Changes in nutritional, functional, and inflammatory markers in advanced pancreatic cancer. *Nutr. Cancer*, 1999;35:106-110.

[121] Longo W. E., Virgo K. S., Johnson F. E., Oprian C. A., Vernava A. M., Wade T. P., Phelan M. A., Henderson W. G., Daley J., Khuri S. F. Risk factors for morbidity and mortality after colectomy for colon cancer. *Dis. Colon. Rectum.*, 2000;43:83-91.

[122] Obialo C. I., Okonofua E. C., Nzerue M. C., Tayade A. S., Riley L. J. Role of hypoalbuminemia and hypocholesterolemia as copredictors of mortality in acute renal failure. *Kidney Int.*, 1999;56:1058-1063.

[123] Ryan T. A., Rady M. Y., Bashour C. A., Leventhal M., Lytle B., Starr N. J. Predictors of outcome in cardiac surgical patients with prolonged intensive care stay. *Chest*, 1997;112:1035-1042.

[124] Chima C. S., Barco K. , Dewitt M. L., Maeda M., Teran J. C., Mullen K. D. Relationship of nutritional status to length of stay, hospital costs, and discharge status of patients hospitalized in the medicine service. *J. Am. Diet. Assoc.*, 1997;97:975-978.

[125] Farinas-Alvarez C., Farinas M. C., Fernandez-Mazarrasa C., Llorca J., Casanova D., Delgado-Rodriguez M. Analysis of risk factors for nosocomial sepsis in surgical patients. *Br. J. Surg.*, 2000;87:1076-1081.

[126] Lien Y. C., Hsieh C. C., Wu Y. C., Hsu H. S., Hsu W. H., Wang L. S., Huang M. H., Huang B. S. Preoperative serum albumin level is a prognostic indicator for adenocarcinoma of the gastric cardia. *J. Gastrointest Surg.*, 2004;8:1041-1048.

[127] Gupta D., Lis C. G. Pretreatment serum albumin as a predictor of cancer survival: a systematic review of the epidemiological literature. *Nutr. J.*, 2010;9:69.

[128] Sun L. C., Chu K. S., Cheng S. C., Lu C. Y., Kuo C. H., Hsieh J. S., Shih Y. L., Chang S. J., Wang J. Y. Preoperative serum carcinoembryonic antigen, albumin and age are supplementary to UICC staging systems in predicting survival for colorectal cancer patients undergoing surgical treatment. *B. M. C. Cancer*, 2009;9:288.

[129] Lis C. G., Grutsch J. F., Vashi P. G., Lammersfeld C. A. Is serum albumin an independent predictor of survival in patients with breast cancer? *JPEN. J. Parenter Enteral. Nutr.*, 2003;27:10-15.

[130] Detsky A. S., Baker J. P., Mendelson R. A., Wolman S. L., Wesson D. E., Jeejeebhoy K. N. Evaluating the accuracy of nutritional assessment techniques applied to hospitalized patients: methodology and comparisons. *JPEN. J. Parenter Enteral. Nutr.*, 1984;8:153-159.

[131] Bellantone R., Doglietto G. B., Bossola M., Pacelli F., Negro F., Sofo L., Crucitti F. Preoperative parenteral nutrition in the high risk surgical patient. *JPEN. J. Parenter Enteral. Nutr.*, 1988;12:195-197.

[132] Fan S. T., Lo C. M., Lai E. C., Chu K. M., Liu C. L., Wong J. Perioperative nutritional support in patients undergoing hepatectomy for hepatocellular carcinoma. *N. Engl. J. Med.*, 1994;331:1547-1552.

[133] Brennan M. F., Pisters P. W., Posner M., Quesada O., Shike M. A prospective randomized trial of total parenteral nutrition after major pancreatic resection for malignancy. *Ann. Surg.*, 1994;220:436-441.

[134] Bozzetti F., Gavazzi C., Miceli R., Rossi N., Mariani L., Cozzaglio L., Bonfanti G., Piacenza S. Perioperative total parenteral nutrition in malnourished, gastrointestinal cancer patients: a randomized, clinical trial. *JPEN J. Parenter Enteral. Nutr.*, 2000;24:7-14.

[135] Heyland D. K., Montalvo M., MacDonald S., Keefe L., Su X. Y., Drover J. W. Total parenteral nutrition in the surgical patient: a meta-analysis. *Can. J. Surg.*, 2001;44: 102-111.

[136] Klein S., Kinney J., Jeejeebhoy K., Alpers D., Hellerstein M., Murray M., Twomey P. Nutrition support in clinical practice: review of published data and recommendations for future research directions. National Institutes of Health, American Society for Parenteral and Enteral Nutrition, and American Society for Clinical Nutrition. *JPEN J. Parenter Enteral. Nutr.*, 1997;21:133-156.

[137] Koretz R. L., Lipman T. O., Klein S. AGA technical review on parenteral nutrition. *Gastroenterology*, 2001;121:970-1001.

[138] Lim S. T., Choa R. G., Lam K. H., Wong J., Ong G. B. Total parenteral nutrition versus gastrostomy in the preoperative preparation of patients with carcinoma of the oesophagus. *Br. J. Surg.*, 1981;68:69-72.

[139] Sako K., Lore J. M., Kaufman S., Razack M. S., Bakamjian V., Reese P. Parenteral hyperalimentation in surgical patients with head and neck cancer: a randomized study. *J. Surg. Oncol.*, 1981;16:391-402.

[140] Yamada N., Koyama H., Hioki K., Yamada T., Yamamoto M. Effect of postoperative total parenteral nutrition (TPN) as an adjunct to gastrectomy for advanced gastric carcinoma. *Br. J. Surg.*, 1983;70: 267-274.

[141] Torosian M. H. Perioperative nutrition support for patients undergoing gastrointestinal surgery: critical analysis and recommendations. *World J. Surg.*, 1999;23:565-569.

[142] Collins J. P., Oxby C. B., Hill G. L. Intravenous aminoacids and intravenous hyperalimentation as protein-sparing therapy after major surgery. A controlled clinical trial. *Lancet*, 1978;1:788-791.

[143] Woolfson A. M., Smith J. A. Elective nutritional support after major surgery: a prospective randomised trial. *Clin. Nutr.*, 1989;8:15-21.

[144] Preshaw R. M., Attisha R. P., Hollingsworth W. J. Randomized sequential trial of parenteral nutrition in healing of colonic anastomoses in man. *Can. J. Surg.*, 1979;22:437-439.

[145] Kudsk K. A., Croce M. A., Fabian T. C., Minard G., Tolley E. A., Poret H. A., Kuhl M. R., Brown R. O. Enteral versus parenteral feeding. Effects on septic morbidity after blunt and penetrating abdominal trauma. *Ann. Surg.*, 1992;215:503-511.

[146] Moore E. E., Jones T. N. Benefits of immediate jejunostomy feeding after major abdominal trauma--a prospective, randomized study. *J. Trauma.*, 1986;26:874-881.

[147] Campos A. C., Meguid M. M. A critical appraisal of the usefulness of perioperative nutritional support. *Am. J. Clin. Nutr.*, 1992;55:117-130.

[148] Maxfield D., Geehan D., Van Way C. W. Perioperative nutritional support. *Nutrition in Clinical Practice*, 2001;16:69-73.

[149] Daly J. M., Lieberman M. D., Goldfine J., Shou J., Weintraub F., Rosato E. F., Lavin P. Enteral nutrition with supplemental arginine, RNA, and omega-3 fatty acids in patients after operation: immunologic, metabolic, and clinical outcome. *Surgery*, 1992;112: 56-67.

[150] Braga M., Gianotti L., Vignali A., Cestari A., Bisagni P., Di Carlo V. Artificial nutrition after major abdominal surgery: impact of route of administration and composition of the diet. *Crit. Care Med.*, 1998;26: 24-30.

[151] Heyland D. K., Novak F., Drover J. W., Jain M., Su X., Suchner U. Should immunonutrition become routine in critically ill patients? A systematic review of the evidence. *JAMA*, 2001;286:944-953.

[152] Anonymous. Proceedings from Summit on Immune-Enhancing Enteral Therapy. May 25-26, 2000, San Diego, California, *US JPEN J. Parenter Enteral. Nutr.*, 2001;25: S1-63.

[153] Grossmann E. M., Longo W. E., Virgo K. S., Johson F. E., Oprian C. A., Henderson W., Daley J., Khuri S. F. Morbidity and mortality of gastrectomy for cancer in Department of Veterans Affairs Medical Centers. *Surgery*, 2002;131(5):484-490.

[154] Rey-Ferro M., Castaño R., Oruzco O., Serna A., Moreno A. Nutritional and immunologic evaluation of patients with gastric cancer before and after surgery. Nutrition, 1997;13(10):878-881.

[155] Sitges-Serra A., Rafecas A., Jaurrieta E. Malnutrition, resectability and postoperative outcome in gastric cancer patients. *Br. J. Clin. Pract. Suppl.*, 1998;63:15-19.

[156] Braunschweig C. L., Levy P., Sheean P. M., Wang X. Enteral compared with parenteral nutrition: a meta-analysis. *Am. J. Clin. Nutr.* 2001;74(4):534-42.

Index

C

G

H

I

N

O

N

O

X

Y

Z